THE ETHICS OF ORGAN TRANSPLANTATION

ADVANCES IN BIOETHICS

Series Editors: Rem Edwards and Edward Bittar

Volume 1: Violence, Neglect and the Elderly
edited by L. Cebik, G. C. Graver, F. H. Marsh

Volume 2: New Essays on Abortion and Bioethics
edited by R. B. Edwards

Volume 3: Values, Ethics and Alcoholism
edited by W. N. Shelton and R. B. Edwards

Volume 4: Critical Reflections Medical Ethics
edited by M. Evans

Volume 5: Bioethics of Medical Education
edited by R. B. Edwards

Volume 6: Postmodern Malpractice
Edited by Colleen Clements

ADVANCES IN BIOETHICS VOLUME 7

THE ETHICS OF ORGAN TRANSPLANTATION

EDITED BY

WAYNE SHELTON

Albany Medical College, New York, USA

JOHN BALINT

Albany Medical College, New York, USA

2001

JAI

An Imprint of Elsevier Science

Amsterdam – London – New York – Oxford – Paris – Shannon – Tokyo

ELSEVIER SCIENCE Ltd
The Boulevard, Langford Lane
Kidlington, Oxford OX5 1GB, UK

First edition 2001

Library of Congress Cataloging in Publication Data
A catalog record from the Library of Congress has been applied for.

British Library Cataloguing in Publication Data
A catalogue record from the British Library has been applied for.

ISBN: 0-7623-0764-1

♾ The paper used in this publication meets the requirements of ANSI/NISO Z39.48-1992 (Permanence of Paper).
Printed in The Netherlands.

CONTENTS

LIST OF CONTRIBUTORS *vii*

DEDICATION *ix*

PREFACE *xi*

1. ORGAN DONATION AND TRANSPLANTATION: A BRIEF HISTORY OF TECHNOLOGICAL AND ETHICAL DEVELOPMENTS
   Robert P. Baker and Victoria Hargreaves *1*

2. DO WE ALL HAVE A RESPONSIBILITY TO DONATE OUR ORGANS?
   James Lindermann Nelson *43*

3. SHOULD WE ADOPT A MARKET STRATEGY TO ORGAN DONATION?
   Julia D. Mahoney *65*

4. ETHICAL ISSUES IN LIVING RELATED DONORS
   Aaron Spital *89*

5. WHO SHOULD RECEIVE DONOR ORGANS?
   Erich H. Loewy *125*

6. THE ETHICS OF ORGAN RETRIEVAL
   David C. Thomasma *149*

7. ETHICAL ISSUES IN NON-HEARTBEATING CADAVER DONORS
   Shelly Ozark and Michael A. DeVita *167*

8. THE ETHICS OF XENOTRANSPLANTATION
   Richard A. Demme *195*

9. PUBLIC POLICY MAKING IN ORGAN TRANSPLANTATION
Martin A. Strosberg and Ronald W. Gimbel 231

10. AN INTERNATIONAL PERSPECTIVE TOWARD HUMAN ORGAN DONATION AND TRANSPLANTATION
Mario C. Deng and Hans H. Scheld 255

11. THE RELIGIOUS AND SPIRITUAL PERSPECTIVE TOWARD HUMAN ORGAN DONATION AND TRANSPLANTATION
Laurence J. O'Connell 277

12. THE ROLE AND RESPONSIBILITY OF THE MEDIA IN RELATION TO ORGAN DONATION AND TRANSPLANTATION
Elisa J. Gordon 293

13. WOMEN, MINORITIES AND ORGAN DONATION IN TRANSPLANTATION
Etienne Juarez Phipps and Gala True 317

14. ORGAN TRANSPLANTATION ISSUES IN MINORS
Marilyn A. Fisher 339

LIST OF CONTRIBUTORS

Robert Baker	Union College, New York, USA
Michael DeVita	Associate Professor, University of Pittsburgh Medical Center, Pittsburgh, USA
Richard Demme	Assistant Professor, University of Rochester School of Medicine and Dentistry, New York, USA
Mario C. Deng	Director of Cardiac Transplantation Research, Colombia University College of Physicians and Surgeons, New York, USA
Marilyn Fisher	Albany Medical Center, New York, USA
Ronald Gimbel	Union College, Schenectady, USA
Elisa Gorden	Loyola University of Chicago, Illinois, USA
Victoria Hargreaves	Cornell University, New York, USA
Erich Loewy	Professor and Chair, University of California, California, USA
Julia Mahoney	Associate Professor of Law, University of Virginia School of Law, Virginia, USA
James L. Nelson	Michigan State University, Michigan, USA
Laurence J. O'Connell	President and CEO, Park Ridge Center, Chicago USA
Shelley Ozark	Center for Bioethics and Law, Pittsburgh, USA

Etienne Phipps	Associate Professor, Jefferson University, Philadelphia, USA
Hans H. Scheld	Chair of the Department of Cardiothoracic Surgery, Muenster, Germany
Aaron Spital	Associate Professor, University of Rochester School of Medicine, New York, USA
Martin Strosberg	Professor, Union College, Schenectady, USA
David E. Thomasma	Professor and Director, Loyola University Chicago Medical Center, Illinois, USA
Gala True	Assistant Professor, Thomas Jefferson University, Philadelphia, USA

DEDICATION

This book is dedicated to the "MOD Squad" – Mothers of Organ Donors – of the Center for Donation and Transplant in Albany, New York. These mothers selflessly offer their support in the hospital to families facing the loss of a loved one. Their extraordinary work, which was started over three years ago, serves as a model for replication at other sites in the state.

PREFACE

Organ transplantation has achieved much success in saving lives. It is now an accepted and expected part of the standard of care for qualified patients with end stage organ failure. This success has been based on scientific and technological accomplishments in the understanding of immunologic responses to foreign tissues, the technology of organ preservation, immune suppression, and surgical procedures. These milestones earned Nobel Prizes in medicine for Sir Peter Medawar and Dr. Macfarlane Burnet. Given the growth and significance of this whole undertaking during the past 30 years, we have planned this volume to provide readers of all levels, both expert and lay, with an overview of the major ethical, policy and even spiritual questions in organ donation and transplantation. We have brought together some of the leaders in their respective areas of specialization to address these questions.

In Chapter One Professor Robert Baker traces the evolution of this exciting medical technology, as well as the social and ethical adaptations needed to allow it to flourish; he sets the framework for some of the extremely hard questions to follow.

The great technical success of organ transplantation with long term graft and recipient survival rates now in excess of 10 years in more than 70% of solid organ transplants, has presented patients, transplant teams and society with a major challenge: there are now worldwide two to three times as many patients in need of a transplant as there are suitable donor organs available. This challenge or dilemma has prompted many responses aimed at increasing organ donation rates, which raise significant ethical issues. These issues are addressed in Chapters 2 through 5. Professor James Nelson in Chapter 2 discusses the question of whether all of us as members of the community, and indeed of the human race, have a duty to donate our organs when we can no longer use them. Such a "duty" conflicts with our societal ethic of individualism that might make enforcement of such a societal norm difficult. He asks the question: Should those who do not volunteer to be donors lose priority if they should ever need an organ transplant? Professor Julia Mahoney in Chapter 3 considers the option of adopting a market strategy to enhance organ availability. Such a policy would go against a strong societal sense that human organs must not be treated as a commodity. In Chapter 4 Professor Aaron Spital reviews the current status of organ donations by living related and unrelated donors. Questions are raised about the meaning of "related": should "related" apply only to those genetically related or include those emotionally related to the recipient? The issue of donation by altruistic strangers is also discussed. Should there be allowable differences in the level of acceptable risk to which living donors may be exposed depending upon the relationship to the recipient? Finally, in this group of essays, Professor Erich Lowey examines who should be acceptable recipients of organs in Chapter 5. He returns to the question asked by Professor James Nelson, whether those who do not volunteer to be potential donors or their families should be treated differently from those who do, should they themselves become patients in need of an organ. Professor Erich Lowey also explores concerns about whether those who develop end stage organ failure due to bad life style choices should be eligible to receive donated organs.

The next group of three chapters challenges us to consider the ethical issues involved in the definition of death, which leads us to ask, who can be and/or asked to be a donor? Professor David Thomasma in Chapter 6 explores concerns about who should ask for organ donations, when such a request is appropriate, as well as what is the definition of death? In Chapter 7, Ms. Shelly Ozark and Professor Michael DeVita examine the difficult ethical and social problems encountered in organ retrieval from patients who are not brain dead. The concept of brain death and the adoption of brain death as a criterion of death was itself a response to the need for organs with well preserved function for transplantation. This required that they be well perfused with oxygenated blood up to the time of removal from the dead donor's body. In an effort to increase organ retrieval the concept of non-heartbeating donation was proposed for potential donors who are kept alive on cardio-pulmonary life support, but who have no hope for recovery and whose families wish to donate their organs. Finally, in this group Professor Richard Demme in Chapter 8 examines ethical issues arising in the use of organs from other species such as chimpanzees, baboons and pigs: the emerging field of xenotransplantation. These issues include the risks of transmitting non-human pathogens to humans, with potentially devastating effects. Other concerns involve anthropocentrism and genetic engineering of non-human species by gene transfer to render their organs less immunogenic in humans.

In Chapter 9, Professor Martin Strosberg and Mr. Ronald Gimble reviews the policy and political issues surrounding the management of organ distribution in the U.S.A. Should organ allocation be left to a non-governmental non-profit agency of experts such as UNOS or should it be controlled by governmental or legislatively mandated regulations? Should organs be used primarily in the region where they were donated or distributed nationally? In Chapter 10, Professors Mario Deng and Hans Scheld contrast the policies developed in

Europe in answer to the questions discussed by Professor Strosberg and Mr. Gimble. The European response to these difficult policy issues reflects their more communitarian social philosophies.

The last group of essays examines some broader issues related to organ donation and transplantation: discrimination and its effects on women and minorities, the role of the news media in formation of societal attitudes and the ethical issues raised at the beginning of life. Dr. Lawrence O'Connell in Chapter 11 describes and examines the various faith traditions, moral and religious perspectives toward the use of donor organs for transplantation. In Chapter 12 Professor Elisa Gordon examines some of the pivotal instances in which public attitudes and opinions have been greatly affected by how the news media reported particular stories. In Chapter 13 Drs. Etienne Phipps and Gala True provide us insight into the often overlooked area of the treatment of women and minorities in organ donation and transplantation, which raise serious problems of fairness. Finally, Professor Marilyn Fisher in Chapter 14 examines some the perplexing ethical problems in organ donation that occur at the beginning of life; specifically, whether or not organs should be used from anencephalic infants, and tissue be used from aborted fetuses?

Many of the ethical concerns regardiing organ transplantation in our society revolve around the issue of organ shortages and how they can be overcome. At the same time it is easy to forget some simple facts. For example, about 50% of all liver transplants are for end stage liver failure from the ravages of hepatitis C and past alcohol abuse. Both these conditions could be preventable with better precautions for hepatitis C and better treatment of alcohol abuse. Similar considerations apply to end stage heart and kidney failure caused by poorly controlled hypertension and diabetes, urinary tract infections and hyperlipidemia. Thus a central question: should we use our resources for improved preventive and curative health care, or for the provision of more organs for transplantation by genetic manipulation of other species or in vitro creation of organs for transplantation from embryonic stem cells? These questions need careful and detailed public debate. We hope this volume will stimulate the readers to think on these issues.

We would like to thank all of the authors who made this volume possible; their dedication and patience are greatly appreciated. We would also like to give a special thanks to Line Callahan who provided invaluable secretarial and editorial support.

Wayne Shelton, Ph.D. and John Balint, M.D.
Albany Medical College, Albany, NY
October, 2000

1. ORGAN DONATION AND TRANSPLANTATION: A BRIEF HISTORY OF TECHNOLOGICAL AND ETHICAL DEVELOPMENTS

Robert P. Baker and Victoria Hargreaves

> It was on a dreary night in November that I beheld the accomplishment of my toils. With an anxiety that almost amounted to agony, I collected the instruments of life around me that I might infuse a spark of being into the lifeless thing that lay at my feet . . . by the glimmer of the half-extinguished light I saw the dull yellow eye of the creature open; it breathed hard, and convulsive motion agitated its limbs (Shelley, 1969).[1]

So begins the tale of the first total organ transplant.[2] Written by Mary Wollenstonecraft Godwin Shelley to while away some rainy days, the tale unfolds as a series of first person narratives. The section quoted above is narrated by Dr. Victor Frankenstein. "The creature" to whom he refers, and from whom he fled in horror, is an organ recipient. "Learn from me," Dr. Frankenstein warned, " how dangerous is the acquirement of knowledge, and how much happier that man is who believes his native town to be the world, than he who aspires to become greater than his nature will allow (Shelley, 1969)." Many have heeded Dr. Frankenstein's warning that any alteration of nature may provoke fearsome retribution. Shelley's sympathies, however, lay with "the creature," the organ recipient. Intending her tale, subtitled "the Modern Prometheus," as a parable about the complex relationship between

The Ethics of Organ Transplantation, Volume 7, pages 1–42.
2001 by Elsevier Science Ltd.
ISBN: 0-7623-0764-1

creators and their creations,[3] Shelley's message was that biomedical innovations become monstrous only if we fail to take responsibility for them. Her bioethical parable was thus meant to champion biomedical progress and the new forms of life it would create – including organ transplantation and organ recipients.

Shelley's parable is almost universally misread. Today, the term 'Frankenstein' is not used to designate those who, like Dr. Frankenstein, irresponsibly turn their backs on innovation, it is used to demonize biomedical innovations, much in the way that Frankenstein himself demonized his innocent creature. 'Frankenstein foods' is thus an epithet used for the blanket condemnation of genetically modified food organisms; although, had her audience understood her tale, 'Frankenstein' would have more appropriately served as a way of condemning those who irresponsibly turn against the idea of innovation, including genetically modifying food organisms. Yet, even as popular culture has inverted the moral of Shelley's bioethical parable, it has preserved one of her deepest insights: biomedical innovations are socially meaningful because they tend to provoke profound questions about who and what we are ourselves.

Shelley bespeaks the social prejudices of her day when she has Dr. Frankenstein remark:

> I kept my workshop of filthy creation . . . The dissecting room and the slaughter-house furnished many of my materials; and often did my human nature turn with loathing from my occupation, whilst, still urged on by an eagerness which perpetually increased, I brought my work near to a conclusion (Shelley, 1969).

The sources of Dr. Frankenstein's loathsome materials, organs, were the "dissecting room and the slaughter-house," that is, human cadavers and butchered animals. What filled Dr. Frankenstein with "loathing," was that his materials were "dead"; he was thus attempting "transcendence." He was trespassing on a foundational social taboo by violating the boundary between death and life. Thus, as Shelley quite presciently saw, transplantation could only become a normal social practice if transcendence came to be accepted as a life-giving, rather than death-dealing, process. Indeed, there is a historical conception of transplantation as a "gift of life" that dates back to the Renaissance: the miracle of Saints Cosmas and Damian. These saints are said to have transplanted the leg of a (black) Moor onto the body of a (white) Christian, whose leg had to be removed because of a cancer (Carmichael & Ratzan, 1991).[4] Shelley, who was probably familiar with this tale and thus with concept of transplants as life-giving, asked the provocative question: how would such a creature, an organ recipient, be received in society? She evidently decided that the greater the extent of the transplant, the more likely it was that society would reject the recipient as a freak or a monster. Social acceptance of transplant recipients would thus require that recipients be transformed, so that they were no longer viewed as "creatures," or monsters, but simply as humans with new organs.

Some societies, most notably Japan's, have been reluctant to accept either transcendence of the organ source or transformation of recipients. Not unnaturally, therefore, in these societies, organ transplantation is not standard medical practice. What intrigues, in the light of the horror surrounding Frankenstein's "loathsome" activities, and the perpetuation of Dr. Frankenstein's views in the mass media, is not that Japan is one of the very few technologically sophisticated countries to resist organ transplantation, but why other societies came so readily to accept it. How did we learn to see Frankenstein's "loathsome" acts in terms of the miracle of Cosmas and Damian? How did we learn to see organ recipients not as "creatures" or "monsters" but as "recipients," or more simply, as "people with transplanted organs?"

TRANSCENDING GHOULISHNESS

Dissection and Gallows Corpses

Several watershed events were crucial to what might be called "transcendence," that is, transcending the social taboo prohibiting the desecration or mutilation of dead bodies. Dissection was universally deemed desecration in all cultures, including those of the West. Society creates rituals of closure and passage to cope with death. The corpse, itself, tends to play a central role to these rituals. Intrusions upon the body of the corpse become symbolically significant, and thus states have often asserted their power over individuals through the desecration of their corpses. The *ancien régimes* of Europe, for example, desecrated the corpses of those considered guilty of high crimes; to move deeper into the past, recall that Antigone died to protest state desecration of her brother's corpse (Foucault, 1979).

By the Renaissance, states began to use criminal corpses for utilitarian as well as punitive purposes. They enacted gallows corpse dissection laws, giving anatomists legal access to the corpses of criminals, thereby increasing the fearsomeness of punishment, even as they assisted in the training of surgeons. As early as 1540, an Act of Parliament under Henry VIII gave the Guild of Barbers and Surgeons access to four "gallows corpses" for public dissection (Richardson, 1989). The law was renewed as late as 1752 in the British Murder Act, which forthrightly declared dissection a "further terror and peculiar mark of infamy . . . added to the punishment" of criminals (Harrison, 1983). Public dissection of gallows corpses also provided a spectacle for the amusement of the public (De Moulin, 1988).

Medical Progress, Resurrectionism and Riots

Some jurisdictions, however, prohibited any desecration of corpses and thus forbade public dissection. In so totally protecting the dead body, these jurisdictions made no legal provision for access to corpses for purposes of surgical education. Surgical educators were thus forced to choose between their duty to obey the law and their commitment to educate competent surgeons. Many medical educators, including those at New York Hospital, placed professional integrity above the law.

> Things came to a head on 13th April, 1788 when a mob gathered round the New York Hospital, broke into the dissection rooms and found a number of cadavers in the process of being dissected. The mob then attacked the doctors who were suspected of being involved in grave-robbing and 'anatomizing'. The doctors wisely took refuge in the city jail. Governor Clinton, Secretary John Jay and Baron Steuben tried to stop the mob – the latter two were injured by the rioters. Finally the militia had to fire on the mob to disperse them. . . . The immediate effect of this 'Doctors' Mob' was to have the legislature pass a law prohibiting grave-robbing. Subsequently the legislature permitted the legal dissection of the bodies of executed criminals – thus making the teaching of anatomy easier (Chakravorty, 1998; Linden, 1951; Blake, 1980; Numbers, 1980; Wilf, 1989; Sappol, 1997; Sappol, 2000).

New Yorkers were behind the times in first enacting gallows corpse laws at the end of the eighteenth century. Such laws offered an elegant compromise between the needs of medicine and the values of society – although, by restricting dissection to criminals, they also reinforced the primal identification of dissection with desecration. By the end of the eighteenth century, however, the gallows-corpse compromise was being overtaken by a series of revolutionary changes in the nature of medicine itself.

Dissection had always been considered an essential tool of surgical pedagogy, since apprentice surgeons needed to master human anatomy; but it was not considered integral to the education of apothecaries (general practitioners) or of physicians. The educational needs of physicians changed, however, after the Italian, Giovanni Battista Morgagni (1682–1771), called attention to clinico-pathological correlations – the tracks that diseases left in organ systems. Physicians now had reason to take an interest in their patients' corpses. More specifically, physicians had reason to perform autopsies, that is, post-mortem examinations of diseased organs and parts of the body.[5]

Autopsies, moreover, were thought to be more consonant with the physician-patient relationship than dissections. Where dissections were usually public events that exposed their subject to the eyes of indifferent spectators, autopsies could be discrete. They could be conducted privately, in a physician's office or in a patient's home; they could focus on specific diseased organs; and they could be regarded as a final gesture of care for the patient. Perhaps of greater symbolic importance: whereas dissection tended to destroy the appearance of a body, autopsy could remove corruptible organs and thus help to preserve a corpse's appearance, facilitating, rather than disrupting, grieving and closure (Harely, 1994).

Medical education reformers – from the French surgeon Marie François Xavier Bichat (1771–1802), to such influential American physicians as Benjamin Rush (1745–1813) – urged the integration of autopsy into the normal medical education and into the routine practice of physicians. In *The Birth of the Clinic: An Archaeology of Medical Perception*, Michel Foucault has argued that the integration of autopsies into medical education radically altered physicians' perception of their patients, teaching them to regard their patients through the prism of the autopsy – to perceive living patients in terms of their pathological anatomy (Foucault, 1975). Whether or not one accepts Foucault's thesis, by the early nineteenth century autopsy was considered as integral to the initial and continuing education of physicians as it was to the education of surgeons.

Burke and Hare

Custom and law lagged behind these changes in medical theory – except in Revolutionary France, where physicians were permitted to appropriate the corpses of the hospitalized poor for both autopsy and dissection (Outram, 1989). In other jurisdictions, demand for cadavers soon exceeded the supply of gallows corpses. Consequently, a black market in bodies and body parts arose. Grave robbers, or "resurrectionists," as they were sometimes called, began to supply this market. Some were medical students willing to appropriate the bodies of others, typically of the lower classes, in the name of science; most were simply entrepreneurs with strong stomachs and weak scruples. The constraints limiting the supply of bodies to persons already deceased inhibited profit margins, and so a few entrepreneurial souls began to look upon the living as a potential source of cadavers. The most notorious instance of this involved two Willams–Burke (1792–1829) and Hare (1792–1890) – who suffocated people to sell their corpses and body parts. Burke and Hare were tried in 1829. On the evidence of Hare (who entered into a plea-bargain), Burke was convicted, hung, publicly anatomized and flayed; his skin was tanned and sold to the public by the strip – reinforcing the association between dissection and desecration (Porter, 1997).

Medicine and society had reached an impasse. As long as autopsy and dissection were associated with desecration, society would restrict them to those whose bodies were appropriately desecrated – and the supply of legal cadavers would be limited to gallows corpses. Medical practitioners thus found themselves on the horns of a dilemma. As they saw it, they could permit custom and law to stifle medical education and medical progress, or they could allow themselves to become complicit in criminal activities.

The Utilitarian Critique of the Gallows Corpse Laws

A few nineteenth-century physicians tried to dissolve this dilemma by challenging the social equation of dissection with desecration. Anticipating the bioethics movement of the late twentieth century, they aligned themselves with those trained to analyze and critique the received culture, i.e. philosophers, and they began to develop a philosophical critique of the taboo against dissection. Leading this movement was T. Southwood Smith (1788–1861), a physician who served as a Unitarian minister on Sundays. Adumbrating twentieth-century bioethicists, Smith combined his knowledge of theology and medicine with philosophical analysis. He crafted his arguments using a framework developed by his friend and mentor, Jeremy Bentham (1748–1832), founder of modern Utilitarianism. In a forceful, widely reproduced and instantly classic essay, "Use of the Dead to the Living," published in the Utilitarian journal, *Westminster Review,* in 1824, Smith urged expanding the supply of cadavers by appropriating the unclaimed bodies of the poor. The issue, Smith argued, was: "whether the surgeon shall be allowed to gain knowledge by operating on the bodies of the dead, or driven to obtain it by practising on the bodies of the living." Noting that surgeons learn their trade in charity hospitals (the equivalent of today's academic or teaching hospitals), Smith remarked that "if the dead bodies of the poor are not appropriated to this use, their living bodies will and must be." "It is time," Smith concluded, "that the physicians and surgeons of England should exert themselves to change a system which has so long retarded the progress of their science, and been productive of so much evil to the community."

Yet, it was neither a physician nor a surgeon who provided the catalyst for reforming the gallows corpse laws; it was a philosopher. On June 9, 1832, three days after his death, following the dictates of a will drafted in 1769 and reaffirmed in his declining days, the body of Jeremy Bentham was publicly dissected at the Webb Street Anatomy Theatre by his friend and disciple, Southwood Smith. As Bentham's biographer, Ross Harrison observes:

> Bentham's last act is just another example of the kind of [reformist utilitarian] political activity in which [Bentham and] his disciples [were] engaged. However, it illustrates, particularly well, the kind of thinking behind [their] proposed reform[s]. Instead of natural feelings, instead of irrational fears or superstitions, such as the horror of dissection, is to be substituted rational thought and calculation, such as the demonstration that dissection increased utility [by promoting the greatest good for the greatest number] (Harrison, 1983).

Legal Reform: Anatomy Acts Permit the Use of the Dead for the Living

Later in 1832, inspired by Bentham's dramatic act, and mindful of the outrages perpetrated by Burke and Hare, the British Parliament passed the Anatomy Act. The act rescinded all laws requiring dissection as punishment. It also created two legal sources of cadavers: voluntary donations (following the precedent set by Bentham) and unclaimed corpses. It stipulated further that bodies used in dissection must be given decent burial.

Within a few decades, almost every jurisdiction in Western Europe and North America had similar laws. Thus, by the end of the nineteenth century, the countries of Western Europe and North America had considerable experience with the demands of medical science for bodies and organs. A sophisticated system had been invented to accommodate these demands to the values of the greater society. Bentham had set a memorable precedent: voluntarism was the ideal. Indeed, in certain circles, donating one's body to medical science was even considered a hallmark of enlightenment. On the other side of the debate, resurrectionism and the anti-resurrectionist riots had hardened Western attitudes against the involuntary exploitation of corpses. The excesses of Burke and Hare had also left their imprint, setting a precedent that effectively precluded the commodification of corpses, body parts, or organs. (In 1984, the National Organ Transplant Act would prohibit the buying and selling of organs, calling them a "national resource.") In this framework, there was one decidedly gray area: non-voluntarism, the appropriation of unclaimed corpses. The practice was deemed permissible because it served a public purpose, and because it seemed to violate no one's proclaimed wishes, but non-voluntary appropriation could easily shade into the prohibited area of involuntary exploitation of the dead – desecrating their memories through their bodies.

When, in the mid-twentieth century, medical researchers began to experiment with organ transplantation, they worked in an environment in which Victor Frankenstein's "loathing" of organs had been transcended, except in a few religious traditions (Rosner, 1986).[6] A normative-legal framework was in place that supported autopsy/dissection, provided it was voluntary, or, at least, not obviously involuntary. Only commodification and the appropriation of corpses against the express wishes of the deceased or their families were prohibited (Caplan, 1995).[7] The policies that later evolved for organ donation in America and Europe followed the basic outlines of those developed for cadavers, with one significant difference. So-called "opt-out" schemes tried to capture the tradition of appropriating unclaimed corpses for medical purposes. In these schemes, organs would be automatically "donated," unless "donors," or their families, formally declared their objections. Opt-out schemes had greatest appeal in Continental Europe where historical roots are deepest. France enacted an opt-out policy in 1976; Austria and Belgium have similar policies (Caplan, 1995). These schemes, however, have proved contentious. Unlike schemes for the medical appropriation of unclaimed bodies, opt-out organ donation schemes affect everyone insufficiently diligent in filling out official forms. They thus affect not merely the poor and the homeless, but the more influential upper and middle classes – articulate groups who can effectively protest the prospect of having their corpses appropriated for post-mortem use against their will (Caplan & Coelho, 1998).[8]

The Legacy of Normative Reform

Normative frameworks are less tangible than physical objects. The edifices of the past impose themselves upon us; by contrast, past normative accomplishments appear elusive. Perhaps the best way to bring into focus the importance of the gallows corpse debate and the significance of the Utilitarian critique is to turn to a culture that did not engage in this debate. Japan, for example, was isolated from the Enlightenment – and hence from the critiques of Bentham and his disciples. So, just as most Japanese cities lack Enlightenment street plans, with their squared blocks and orderly numbered houses, Japanese culture never engaged in a Utilitarian dialogue about the "Use of the Dead to the Living." Lacking the West's earlier experience with gallows corpse laws, resurrectionism, and anatomy acts, Japan had to face the questions raised by organ transplantation *without* the sort of normative structures that had evolved in the West. Not surprisingly, the initial Japanese reaction to organ transplantation was to prohibit it. Recently, the Japanese have become less rejecting of transplantation; nonetheless, their original rejection highlights the role that the normative frameworks that evolved to deal with gallows corpse shortage played in setting a precedent for organ transplantation (Locke, 1999; Youngner et al., 1999; Miller & Hagihara, 1997; Wise, 1997).

TRANSFORMING SURGERY: TECHNICAL ADVANCES AND THEIR SOCIAL ACCEPTANCE

Surgery in Mary Shelley's Era

Organ transplants could not have become routine medical practice without a normative framework that transcended the horror of desecration and that permitted medicine access to the bodies and organs of others, living and dead. Access to organs, however, presupposes the techniques of modern surgery. As historian, Martin Pernick, reminds us, modern surgical procedures were simply "inconceivable" in the pre-anesthesia era in which Mary Shelley wrote *Frankenstein*. Dr. Valentine Mott (1785–1865), often called the father of American vascular surgery, described with horror,

> how often have I dreaded that some unfortunate struggle of the patient would deviate the knife a little from its normal course, and that I, who fain would be the deliverer, should involuntarily become the executioner, seeing my patient perish in my hands by one of the most appalling forms of death (Boland, 1950).

Pre-anesthesia, patients dreaded surgery even more than physicians did. Here is a short but vivid excerpt from the novelist Fanny Burney's account of her mastectomy – a procedure which she credits with saving her life. The operation was performed by the most famous French surgeon of the day, Napoleon's Surgeon General, Baron Dominique Jean Larrey (1766–1842), inventor of the ambulance and of the concept of triage (Baker & Strosberg, 1991).

> M. Dubois placed me upon the Mattress, & spread a cambric handkerchief upon my face. It was transparent, however, & I saw through it that the Bed stead was instantly surrounded by the 7 men and my nurse, I refused to be held; but when, bright through the cambric, I saw the glitter of polished steel – I closed my eyes . . .
>
> Yet – when the dreadful steel was plunged into the breast—cutting through veins – arteries – flesh – nerves – I needed no injunctions not to restrain my cries. I began a scream that lasted unintermittingly during the whole time of the incision – & I almost marvel that it rings not in my Ears still! so excruciating was the agony. When the wound was made, & the instrument was withdrawn, the pain seemed undiminished, for the air that suddenly rushed into those delicate parts felt like a mass of minute but sharp & forked poniards, that were tearing the edges of the wound – but when again I felt the instrument – describing a curve – cutting against the grain, if I may so say, while the flesh resisted in a manner so forcible as to oppose & tire the hand of the operator, who was forced to change from the right to the left – then, indeed, I thought I must have expired, I attempted no more to open my eyes. . . . The instrument this second time withdrawn, I concluded the operation over – Oh no! presently the terrible cutting was renewed – & worse than ever, to separate the bottom, the foundation of this dreadful gland from the parts to which it adhered . . . yet again all was not over (Porter, 1997).

Such was the state of surgery in the summer of 1816, when Shelley wrote her tale of transplantation (as part of a competition with her husband, Percy Shelley, their friend, Lord Byron and Byron's physician, Dr. John Polidori). Surgery was so brutal, that it was easier even for Shelley's lively imagination to contemplate the creation of life from death, than to imagine a living recipient surviving the brutality of a transplant. Transplants into living organ recipients were literally inconceivable in the pre-anesthesia era.

Anesthesia, Asepsis and the Development of Modern Surgery

Laughing gas, nitrous oxide, was the first of the modern anesthetics. It was discovered in 1795 by the English scientist, Sir Humphry Davy (1778–1829) (Porter, 1997), who speculated that it " may probably be used with advantage during surgical operations (Porter, 1997)." An American dentist, Horace Wells (1815–1848) became intrigued with the gas, and, in an act of autoexperimentation, had a fellow dentist remove one of his decayed teeth, using the gas to deaden the pain. Unfortunately, when Wells tried to repeat the demonstration on a volunteer, the volunteer screamed. The medical community thus dismissed nitrous oxide as unreliable. William Thomas Morton (1819–1868) was captivated by Wells' unsuccessful demonstration, and, on the advice of chemist Charles T. Jackson (1805–1880), experimented with applying ether to dull the pain of tooth removal. It worked. On October 16, 1846, Morton successfully demonstrated the use of ether in surgery at the Massachusetts General Hospital.

The era of modern anesthesia might have been stillborn, however, had the Drs. Frankenstein of the day triumphed. Anesthesia was denounced as unnatural, "artificial death" (Pernick, 1985). Fortunately, the newly formed American Medical Association lent its imprimatur to the new technique in 1848, as did British and European medical and surgical societies shortly thereafter. The emphatic embrace of organized medicine prevented would-be Drs. Frankenstein from suppressing anesthesia, opening the way for the development of modern surgery.

Technical problems still prevented complex surgery, however. Foremost among these was sepsis, or infection. "It is like a plague," wrote one British surgeon, "no operation dare be performed, every cure stands still, every wound becomes a sore, and every sore is apt to run into gangrene." Influenced by the work of the French chemist and microbiologist, Louis Pasteur (1822–1895), the Glasgow surgeon Joseph Lister (1827–1912) argued that infection was a disruption of the healing process, caused by ubiquitous infection-causing elements. To prove his point, he used phenol-soaked lint to disinfect surgeon's hands and surgical instruments, as well as surgical incisions (a technique discovered by François Jules Lemaire (1814–1886)). Sepsis, decreased markedly. Pasteur contributed to the development of aseptic technique in 1874, when he recommended that surgical instruments be boiled to kill germs. In 1890, the American surgeon (and inventor of the radical mastectomy) William S. Halsted (1852–1922) introduced rubber gloves. His intent was to alleviate one nurse's allergic reaction to the disinfectant (she was, incidentally, his fiancée). Facemasks were first used by Johannes von Mikulicz-Radecki (1850–1905), a Polish surgeon in 1897, to act as a barrier to disease transmission from physician to patient.

By the beginning of the twentieth century, the operating theatre had acquired its modern garb: anesthesia, asepsis, gowns, masks and rubber gloves. One surgeon described the transformation from the pre-aseptic/antiseptic days to post- as follows:

> Operating theatres, which resembled a shambles in 1860, are replaced by rooms of spotless purity containing scintillating metal furniture and ingenious electric lights. All concerned in the operation are clothed from nose-tip to toe-tip in sterilized linen gowns, and their hands are covered with sterilized rubber gloves (Bynum & Porter, 1993).

Alexis Carrel and the Development of Transplant Surgery

These apparent advances were still not enough to address the technical problems that had to be resolved to perform the sort of transplantation that Mary Shelley had envisioned. One small but crucial problem was that surgical stitches, or sutures, leaked. Removing an organ from a body was thus easier than reattaching it to another, since severed blood vessels would need to be reattached in a leak-proof manner.

The problem of leaking sutures was solved by Noble prize-winning French-American surgeon, Alexis Carrel (1873–1948). After observing the work of a lace maker, Carrel developed a new suturing procedure in which the everted ends of the blood vessels were sewn together on their outsides. This method created tight leak-proof connections with no thread in the interior of the vessel (reducing the possibility of clot formation).

The technical means of transplantation now appeared possible. Of the three possible sources of organs – animals (xenografts), cadavers, or living donors – animals seemed to pose the fewest moral problems. In 1905, Carrel and Charles Claude Guthrie (1880–?) used the new suturing technique to transplant a heart from a small dog into the neck of a larger dog. Despite their initial success, these experiments revealed yet another barrier to successful transplants. Carrel noticed that when kidneys were transplanted within one-and-the-same animal (an autograft), both the kidney and the animal had a better chance of survival than when a kidney was transplanted into another animal (an allograft). Carrel had rediscovered a phenomenon reported in tissue grafts by the Italian surgeon Giuseppe Baronio (1758–1811) in 1800, the atrophy of the transplanted organ, more commonly referred to as "rejection."

Sir Peter Medawar and the Problem of Rejection

It was not until 1943 that immunologist Sir Peter Brian Medawar (1915–1987) identified organ rejection as an immune system response. Medawar suggested that a recipient's immune system produced antigens in an attempt to "fight off" the new organ, treating it as if it were an invader, sending in defensive "troops" in the form of lymphocytes and antibodies. Lymphocytes circulate through the blood, infiltrating the organ, and wreaking havoc. The antibodies serve as a second line of offense, targeting the blood vessels. Medawar hypothesized that, if the invasion metaphor was apt, drugs that forestalled or overpowered the immune system could prevent or delay rejection. In 1951, he experimented with cortisone, an immunosuppressive drug. In 1959, Roy Calne and J. E. Murray drew on Medawar's experiments to create azathioprin, a more potent immunosuppressor. In 1960, Medawar was awarded a Nobel Prize.

HUMAN EXPERIMENTATION IN THE ERA OF HIGH MINDED PATERNALISM

Experimentation vs. Therapy

Medawar's initiatives lay the foundations for what might be called the era of "false hope," an era in which faith in surgery, and the hope stimulated by the development of immunosuppressive drugs, encouraged widespread experimentation with transplantation. Although it is unclear where and when experiments were initiated, in the 1950s some institutions engaged in experimental transplants of cadaver kidneys into terminal patients with end stage renal disease. These experiments failed (although one organ recipient at Peter Brent Brigham Hospital, in Boston, survived for 175 days (Jonsen, 1998)); nonetheless, they laid the foundation for later successful forays into transplantation.

These early experiments appear, in retrospect, to have been purely investigative, but the bright line that we tend to draw between investigation and therapy was rather dim in the pre-bioethical era. It was not clear, either to the investigator or to the patient, whether an experiment was being conducted primarily as an investigation to benefit medical science, or as therapy to benefit the particular patient who was the subject of the experiment. The ethic informing experimentation in the pre-bioethical era was "high-minded paternalism." Researchers believed, to quote the Moseley Professor of Surgery at Harvard Medical School, and Surgeon-in-Chief of Peter Brent Brigham Hospital, Francis D. Moore, in the "essentially ethical nature of the scientific process" itself (Moore, 1969). This meant that, although the subjects of research were "given a clear picture of the hazards involved and allowed to join in the discussion," nonetheless, "the final decision [would] not be left in the hands of the patient [who] has not the education, the background nor dispassionate view necessary to make the decision in his own best self-interest (Jonsen, 1998)." In the end, Moore believed that only the virtuous character of researchers could act as guarantor of the integrity of the research process. Thus, like most researchers in his day, Moore resisted the National Institutes of Health's proposal to submit their research efforts to scrutiny by institutional review committees (IRCs). "The ethical acceptability of therapeutic innovation documented in a research application," Moore contended, "is far better attested by the nature of the scientific consultants working on the project, than by the nature of the hospital panel that is to review each case (Moore, 1969)."[9]

Using Living Donors: Kidney Donation and The Herrick Twins

It was Moore's own surgical service, however, that first raised issues transcending questions about the integrity and character of researchers. On December 23, 1954, Drs. Joseph Murray and John Merrill of Peter Brent Brigham Hospital removed a healthy kidney from a twenty-four-year-old, Ronald Herrick, transplanting it to his twin brother Richard. Richard survived the operation, living for another eight years. The controversy that emerged turned, not on questions about the integrity of Drs. Murray and Merrill, not on their treatment of their subject/patient, Richard, the organ recipient, but rather on the appropriateness of the removal of Ronald's healthy organ.

Hitherto, cadavers had been the standard source for organs used for transplants. Since the norms governing cadaver organ usage had been worked out over one hundred years earlier, the source of organs was not morally problematic. Indeed, cadaver organ donation would soon become legally acceptable as well, at least throughout the U.S. and Europe. In 1968, for example, the U.S. National Conference of Commissioners on Uniform State Laws drafted a model law, the Uniform Anatomical Gift Act (UAGA), extending the conventions in place for cadaver body donation to cadaver organ donation. The UAGA also recognized the right of specific family members to donate organs on behalf of the deceased, provided that the deceased had never specifically expressed opposition to serving as a donor. By 1971, all 50 states had adopted this act, and many allowed potential organ donors to indicate their willingness to donate on their driver's licenses.

However, no moral consensus existed for living donors. Drs. Murray and Merrill's actions were unprecedented and precipitated a controversy that, to reiterate, had nothing to do with the integrity of surgeons or of their science. The controversy was engaged on two levels. On one level, experimenters needed to ask whether it was permissible for them, as *medical* professionals, to remove a healthy organ from a healthy person, even with that person's consent. On another level, *society* needed to face the question of whether consent could legitimate the donation, or sale of a person's own organs – even for noble purposes.

Both questions raised profound issues. Perhaps the deepest tenets of Western medicine – tenets first articulated in the Hippocratic Oath and routinely reiterated in the canonical texts of the tradition—are that medicine's goal is to help patients (the principle of beneficence), and not to injure or to harm them (the principle of non-maleficence). The Herrick transplantation required the violation of the principle of non-maleficence with respect to Ronald, in order to apply the principle of beneficence to Richard. Nevertheless, if it was not permissible to rob Peter of his organs to benefit Paul, did Ronald's consent suffice to render it permissible to take his organs to benefit Richard? Researchers replied that kidneys were redundant organs (everyone, in effect, had one to spare) and insofar as kidney donation was voluntary and would pose only limited risks to donors, it should be considered permissible. (For this reason, in the 1950s and early 1960s 'transplant' became almost synonymous with 'kidney transplant' – although other "redundant" tissues, such as skin and eye were also transplanted (Murray, 1992).) Nonetheless, the surgeons were harming Ronald to help Richard. Were such acts of beneficent harm permissible for *a doctor*, provided only that the donor consented?[10]

The correlative question turned, not on the actions of the surgeons, but on the actions of Ronald, the organ donor. Society needed to resolve the issue of whether it was permissible to donate a kidney to help one's brother, or one's sister, or one's cousin, or one's neighbor, or even a stranger in need. The Burke and Hare debacle had imprinted the dangers of commodification on societal memory; thus, little serious consideration was given to offering organs for sale (although the issue is seriously debated today) (Caplan & Coelho, 1998).[11] On the contrary, Bentham's precedent, and, perhaps more importantly, the universal experience with Red Cross blood drives, created a strong normative preference for permitting altruistic voluntary contributions – provided that these contributions did not significantly endanger the donor's life or health.

Religious Objections to Live Donors: The Principle of Totality

The religious traditions dominant in the background culture, moreover, raised significant obstacles. Catholicism distinguished between mutilation and surgery by relying on the Principle of Totality (*Summa Theologica* II-II, q. 65 a. 1). In general, it is impermissible for Catholics to destroy or to mutilate their own bodies, with one exception: if the removal of a bodily part saves the totality of the rest of the body. Removing Ronald's kidney did not save the totality of Ronald's body, so the act seemed to violate the principle of totality. Yet, Ronald's sacrifice seems to reflect less a rejection of the sanctity of life than reverence and respect for the life of his brother, Richard. Ultimately, the idea that triumphed was that organ donation represented a "gift of life." As such, it was an affirmation of life's value, entirely consonant with the religious tenet that life is sacred. In the mid-1960s, a normative consensus began to solidify supporting organ donation as an affirmation and gift of life (Wolstenhome & O'Connor, 1966).[12]

Moral problems were exacerbated, however, as experimenters began to move from twins to related but non-twin donors. Mortality rates due to organ rejection rose correlatively. In 1963, there were 103 non-twin transplants and a 90% three-month mortality rate (Fox & Swazey, 1978). Death rates at this level raise questions about the rationality of the living donor's gift. These questions were not addressed in the context of kidney donation, however, society faced them in the context of a different transplant procedure, involving an organ more deeply freighted with symbolic significance than the kidney.

Heart Transplants

On December 3, 1967, Dr. Christiaan Barnard of Groote Schuur Hospital in Cape Town, South Africa, performed an operation that other transplant surgeons had feared to initiate. Using a heart-lung machine (a device that had been developed by John Gibbon (1903–1973)) that had been shipped from the U.S. by his mentor from the University of Minnesota, Dr. Owen Wagenansteen, Barnard performed the world's first heart transplant. He excised the heart from the chest of twenty-two year-old Protestant, Denise Daarvall, who had been terminally injured in an automobile accident, and transplanted it into the chest of a fifty-five year-old Jew, Louis Washkansky. Barnard claimed that he waited a full three minutes after Daarvall's heart had stopped beating before harvesting it. After the transplant, Barnard shocked the heart into beating.

Predictably, Washkansky's body rejected the new heart. He died eighteen days later. Nonetheless, the operation attracted the media. *Time* called it "the ultimate operation."

Co-starring with Barnard as darling of a media spectacular was the second Capetown transplant recipient, white dentist, Philip Blaiberg. On January 3, 1968, Blaiberg received the heart of a twenty-four year old "cape colored" (i.e. black) man, Clive Haupt. Blaiberg survived for 594 days, celebrating the first anniversary of his operation with his family, basking in the limelight of worldwide media attention. Tales of Christian hearts in Jewish bodies, and black hearts in white bodies made great headlines, recalling miracle of Saints Cosmas and Damien (Jonsen, 1998).

The media reception of the "miracle of Capetown," soon overwhelmed the moral and medical scruples of other transplant surgeons. On January 6, 1968, Norman Shumway and his Stanford University team performed their first heart transplant; transplant teams around the world followed suit. The media christened 1968, "Year of the Transplant (Jonsen, 1998; Fox & Swazey, 1978)."

The Moratorium on Heart Transplants

The sun set swiftly on the era of false hope. Just a year later, on January 21, 1969, the Montreal Heart Institute announced a moratorium on heart transplants. Other transplant teams, the media, and the lay public reacted to the moratorium announcement much as one reacts to any psychological trauma: denial, anger, negotiation, acceptance. At first, everyone denied the overwhelming mortality rates accompanying non-twin transplants. Later, there were angry statements from figures like Dr. Denton Cooley, Professor of Surgery at the Baylor College of Medicine, who proclaimed that "one should not surrender to the enemy just because one has lost a few battles (Fox & Swazey, 1978)." Others tried to negotiate expectations, explaining, as did Dr. John Najarian, a pediatric surgeon from the University of Minnesota, in testimony before the U.S. Senate, that a 16% survival rate was acceptable for an experimental procedure (Jonsen, 1998). In fact, Najarian was putting an optimistic spin on dreary statistics. In 1971, the National Heart Institute's "Summary of heart transplants as of survival, September 1, 1970," documented 165 transplants, 103 in the U.S., 62 elsewhere. There were, as Najarian's figure suggests, 22 survivors and 140 deaths; however, only two people had survived for over 24 months, and only fourteen for over 15 months (Fox & Swazey, 1978). The media accepted this data as conclusive, pronouncing heart transplantation a failure. Dr. Francis Moore, who was now at another Harvard teaching hospital, Massachusetts General Hospital, announced a moratorium on heart transplants on his service; by the end of 1970, this moratorium was nearly universal (Fox & Swazey, 1978).

What had gone wrong? The moratorium on heart transplant demonstrated the weakness of Moore's ethic of researcher virtue. Moore, who had acted with integrity, characterized the period as "the only example . . . in the history of transplant medicine where everyone went nuts (Pence, 2000)." Virtue alone was clearly insufficient to constrain the forces of egoism and chauvinism. Further constraints were needed. Yet, perhaps because they themselves were such paragons of integrity, partisans of researcher virtue ethic, like Moore, and his Harvard colleague, Henry Beecher (1904–1976), still resisted formal codes regulating researcher conduct, like the 1947 Nuremberg Code (Beecher, 1970). Their position was dominant in the 1960s, and was expressed in the 1964 World Medical Association's Helsinki (I) Declaration on research on human subjects (Beecher, 1970).

Helsinki and Animal Experimentation

The Nuremberg Code had required demonstrable success in animal experiments, as a prerequisite to experiments on humans. Helsinki I, however, skirted this requirement. It recognized a category of "therapeutic experiments." Conscientious physicians were permitted to engage in therapeutic experiments, provided the experiments held out a prospect of directly aiding the patient. Therapeutic experiments were thus considered permissible, even in the absence of prior successful animal or human research (and even in the absence of informed consent (Pence, 1990)[13]). Transplants fell squarely in the category of "therapeutic experiments."

It is important to appreciate that animal experiments predicted high mortality for heart transplants through rejection or infection. Experiments conducted on dogs by Shumway and his associates at Stanford demonstrated "early survival," from four to 21 days, but no significant long-term survival (Fox & Swazey, 1978). These data were consistent with the experience of non-twin kidney transplants. Cumulative experience with both animals and humans thus indicated that, until medical researchers could control rejection, almost all heart transplants from non-related donors would culminate in rejection and death. This data was known to everyone in the transplant field, but they were not understood by the media or the public.

Rules Rather Than Virtues Regulate Research

Following the ethics of researcher virtue lauded by Beecher and Moore, Norman Shumway and other leading transplant surgeons had demonstrated moral restraint, declining to experiment with human heart transplants. Barnard, a recently trained transplant surgeon working in the backwaters of the research community, was not so constrained. What followed was a memorable illustration that Gresham's Law (that bad money drives out good) applies in the realm of conscience and character. Once the world press lauded Barnard's success, leading transplant surgeons in the field no longer restrained their scalpels. The consequent fiasco and the subsequent moratorium were predictable. The debacle demonstrated not only the foolishness of researchers rushing in when accumulated animal and human data predicted failure but also the fragility of a research ethic dependant entirely on the conscience and character of researchers. One bad actor, like one bad apple, could contaminate the entire barrel – especially since the media limelight seemed capable of corrupting all but the strongest sense of conscience. Partially as a consequence, in the 1970s, the current system of formal regulation and review of human subjects research was developed to supplement the older system of researcher virtue.

Heart transplants also raised important questions about moral agency. Barnard had acted as physician to *both* Daarvall and Washkansky. When he asked Denise Daarvall's father for permission to use Denise's heart, was he acting in Denise's interest? in Washkansky's interest? or, in his own interest? The conflict was most dramatic at the point where Barnard had to pronounce Daarvall dead. Daarvall's interests required certitude, caution, and thus delay; but Washkansky's interests as a patient – and Barnard's as a researcher – required haste, to prevent deterioration of Daarvall's heart. We have only Barnard's word that he chose to be cautious. In the aftermath of the Barnard case, conventions developed to disambiguate these roles. Separate teams care for the patient-donor and for the recipient. Today, the team that cares for the donor acts independently of the transplant team, especially at the point when the death of the donor is pronounced.

CYCLOSPORIN: THE ERA OF TRUE HOPE

Dausset's Hypothesis

Although 1968 did not live up to its official title, "Year of the Transplant," it did see two important breakthroughs, one technical, the other normative. Jean

Dausset proposed that the white blood cells known as "leuckocytes" could be "tissue typed," much as, in 1900, red blood cells had been typed into the familiar A, B, AB, O system by the Austrian, Karl Landsteiner (1868–1943). Dausset theorized that one cause of rejection was the mismatching of white cell types. Mindful of this hypothesis, transplant surgeon Thomas Starzl proposed a six-month moratorium on transplants at the University of Colorado, so that past operations could be reanalyzed to see whether rejection could be attributed to tissue mismatching. The reanalysis of past transplants, supplemented by prospective trials combining new tests of histocompatibility with serological methods to match donor and recipients, seemed to confirm Dausset's hypothesis. In 1980, Dausset was awarded a Nobel Prize for his research (even though, actual consequences of a policy of systematic tissue typing for histocompatibility proved more equivocal than Dausset's hypothesis suggested).

The National Organ Transplantation Act and UNOS

Tissue typing required a radical reorganization of the institutional basis of transplantation. Up to this point, transplantation had been both experimental and entrepreneurial: each transplant team acted independently, pairing donors with waiting recipients. Compatibility requirements complicated this simple and straightforward pairing procedure, requiring a more complex organizational structure to match histocompatible donors with waiting recipients. Consequently, informal organ-sharing arrangements arose to share compatible organs. As arrangements were made, not only to distribute organs, but also, to preserve and transport them, organ-sharing systems became increasingly complex. In 1984, Congress passed the National Organ Transplantation Act, that, in addition to prohibiting the commodification of organs, tried to rationalize the hodgepodge of organ sharing arrangements that had evolved. The Act envisioned a national organ-sharing system that would be fair and rational. In 1987, this vision was implemented in the form of a quasi-non-governmental organization, or a quango, the United Organ Sharing Network (UNOS). Dausset's hypothesis thus served as the catalyst for a national system for sharing organs.

The Invention of Brain Death

The year 1968 was pivotal for development of transplantation in another respect. An Ad Hoc Harvard Committee, led by Henry Beecher, developed a new concept of death. Cardiopulmonary criteria (absence of pulse or heartbeat, no spontaneous breathing, and so forth) had been used by Western physicians to determine death, ever since the Hippocratic period. The Ad Hoc Committee proposed replacing these criteria, and thus the traditional concept of death of the body, with new criteria and, correlatively, a new concept of death: "brain death," or death of a person. "Brain death" was to be determined by neurological criteria (absence of reflex responses, flat-line electroencephalograph reading, and so forth). The Ad Hoc Committee was forthright in stating its reasons for advancing these new criteria. A new class of irreversibly comatose intensive care (ICU) patients had been created by the advent of the artificial ventilator. Sometimes their "heart continues to beat but [their] brain is irreversibly damaged." The Ad Hoc Committee proposed pronouncing these irreversibly comatose patients "dead" because they placed "a burden on families, on hospitals, and on those in need of hospital beds already occupied by these comatose patients." The Committee also remarked that "obsolete criteria for the definition of death can [also] lead to controversy in obtaining organs for transplantation (Beecher, 1968)." A new definition of death would thus not only clarify the status of irreversibly comatose ICU patients, it would also open the door to using brain dead patients as organ donors.

The Ad Hoc Committee was remarkably successful. Jurisdiction after jurisdiction in the U.S. and elsewhere accepted the concept of brain death. In 1980, the President's Commission for the Study of Ethical Problems in Medicine and Biomedical and Behavioral Research drafted the Uniform Determination of Death Act (President's Commission, 1981), which set the legal standard for death in most U.S. jurisdictions. Moreover, as the Ad Hoc Committee had hoped, the brain dead bodies became a major source of donor organs.

Cyclosporin

In the 1980s, organ transplantation crossed a threshold, leaving its status as an experimental therapy to enter the realm of standard medical practice. A fungus opened the door. The Sandoz Pharmaceutical Corporation had a long-standing policy of asking workers to bring fungi and other promising drug sources back with them from vacation. After examining a fungus brought from Norway in the Sandoz laboratory, J. F. Borel discovered that it had immunosuppressive properties. He led the development of the new drug, "cyclopsporin," through careful testing, first in animals, and then, in 1978, in small groups of human subjects. In 1981, an editorial in the prestigious *New England Journal of Medicine* hailed "the advent of cyclosporin A [a drug that] offers hope that the legendary success of two third-century saints of the healing profession

[Cosmas and Damian] will become a fait accompli of modern medical practice." Two years later (1983), the Food and Drug Administration (FDA) approved cyclosporin as an immunosuppressive for organ recipients.

The age of transplantation had finally arrived. The moratorium on heart transplants was lifted and all forms of transplantation increased radically. Cyclosporin also broadened the sources available for organ donation by making cadaver organs tolerable to recipients. In 1983, the first year of the era of effective immunosuppressive therapy, the 12 U.S. programs approved to perform heart transplants by the federal government's Medicare program performed 172 transplants. By 1989, in contrast, 131 approved programs performed 1,673 heart transplants. In that same year, Medicare-approved programs performed 8,886 kidney transplants, 2,160 liver transplants, 412 pancreas transplants, 89 lung transplants, and 79 heart-lung transplants (Fox & Swazey, 1992). Medicare does not reimburse experimental therapies. Between the years 1983 and 1989, therefore, transplantation exited the experimental stage; it was now considered standard medical practice.

COPING WITH SCARCITY: BRIDGING, INCREASING SUPPLY, RATIONING

SCARCITY

Success created scarcity. After the formation of UNOS in 1987, scarcity became manifest in formal waiting lists. As early as 1991, more than 1,500 people were on waiting lists for cadaver livers, and more than 2,000 were on the list for hearts. Some would be removed from the list after receiving transplants; but 9.9 % of those awaiting livers and 16.7% of those awaiting hearts would be removed by death (Evan et al., 1992). Since transplantation was now considered standard practice, these deaths came to be perceived as avoidable.

By the 1990s, three complementary sets of strategies evolved for eliminating avoidable deaths. One strategy focuses on developing bridge technologies to prolong the lives of people on the waiting lists. A second strategy focuses on increasing the supply of organs. A third strategy focuses on controlling demand by developing and refining formal principles of allocation.

BRIDGE TECHNOLOGIES

Perhaps the most direct way of dealing with waiting lists involves bridge technologies – bioartificial livers, Left Ventricular Assist Devices (LVADs), insulin pumps, renal dialysis, and so forth. These technologies prolong and protect the lives of those wait listed by preserving their vital functions until suitable donor organs are available.

Renal Dialysis

Renal dialysis, the grandfather of all bridge technologies, was derived from the artificial kidney invented by Dutch physician Willem Kolff. He developed the prototype of the artificial kidney in Nazi-occupied Netherlands, in the waning years of the Second World War, using old washing machine parts. The artificial kidney was effective in relieving acute renal failure but proved problematic for treating chronic kidney failure. The cannula, or the tube, which linked the dialysis machine to arteries or veins, tended to destroy the patient's blood vessels, until, eventually, patients ran out of blood vessels.

A solution to this problem came to Dr. Belding Scribner of the University of Washington, in a dream he had, after the death of one of his renal patients. He wrote:

> Then one morning about 4:00 a.m. I woke up and groped for a piece of paper and a pencil to jot down the basic idea of the shunted cannulas which would make it possible to treat people . . . again and again with the artificial kidney without destroying two blood vessels each time. And, indeed, basically it was such a simple idea – just connect the tube (cannula) in the artery to the cannula in the vein by means of a connecting tube or *shunt*, and the blood would rush without clotting and maintain the cannulas in functional condition indefinitely. Then when an artificial kidney treatment was needed, we could simply replace the shunt with the blood circuit of the artificial kidney.
>
> The most amazing thing about this was that unlike most such ideas it worked from the start (Fox & Swazey, 1978).

In the 1960s, Scribner's shunt made renal dialysis a way of life for many patients, and a practical bridge therapy for some. Ironically, although such therapies were designed to circumvent the problems of waiting lists, demand for dialysis machines rapidly outstripped supply, replicating the very problem of access that the bridge therapy was designed to circumvent – as we shall see later.

The Artificial Heart

Another bridge technology that developed in tandem with the artificial kidney was the artificial heart. In 1965, the NIH committed forty million dollars to developing an artificial heart. In 1969, Dr. Denton Cooley, of the Baylor

College of Medicine, implanted an artificial heart into a patient Haskell Karp, who died within 36 hours. Like Barnard, Cooley avoided review by the institutional research committee (IRC), on the grounds that this was a "therapeutic experiment." The U.S., however, is a more litigious society than South Africa, and Karp's family sued Cooley for breach of "therapeutic privilege." They lost the suit, and so, two years later, when Cooley again implanted an artificial heart, he again circumvented review by the IRC.

In 1982, working with the permission of the Food and Drug Administration (FDA) and the blessing of an Institutional Review Board (IRB) – bioethically empowered successors to IRC's, that approached researchers with principles, powers, and "an attitude" – Willem DeVries of the University of Utah took an entirely different approach. He had been working with Willem Kolff's protégé, Robert Jarvik, to develop an artificial heart. The seventh version of this heart (Jarvick–7) had undergone extensive testing in sheep. Some of the sheep had lived for 268 days, and the University of Utah IRB thought these results promising enough to approve experimental testing on humans. Unlike previous heart transplant subjects, the IRB demanded that the subject of DeVries' experiment, Barney Clark, be given full disclosure of the animal results and sign an eleven-page informed consent document as a prerequisite to the experiment.

The sixty-one year-old Clark, a lifelong one- or two-pack a day smoker who was dying of heart failure (idiopathic cardiomyopathy), chronic obstructive lung disease, and emphysema, was desperate. He volunteered to be a subject despite the daunting consent process. On the night of December 1, 1982, the implant operation commenced. Clark died 112 days later, on March 23, 1983. The University of Utah had invited the media to cover the story, which the distinguished *New York Times* medical correspondent, Dr. Lawrence Altman called "one of the most dramatic moments in medical history (Jonsen, 1998; Pence, 1990)."

Yet, questions concerning cost were to doom the artificial heart project. Clark's transplant had cost a quarter of a million dollars. As George Lundberg, editor of the *Journal of the American Medical Association* observed, no health care system could afford to make such an expensive technology available to everyone suffering coronary failure (Pence, 1990). In 1982, the U.S. Government's Office of Technology Assessment estimated that if 60,000 Medicare recipients used artificial hearts, the cost would be 5.5 billion dollars annually. In 1988, the NIH called for a moratorium on artificial heart research. In the 1990s, artificial hearts were commonly used only as bridge technologies for patients awaiting heart transplants.

INCREASING SUPPLY

Bridge technologies provide a technological fix for the normative problem of allocating scarce resources. Another way of addressing the problem is to increase supply. By the mid-1980s there were approximately 50,000 people waiting for organs, and approximately 200,000 people being declared brain dead in the U.S. annually (Schwartz, 1985). Yet, fewer than 20% of Americans signed the donor cards on their driver's licenses, and organs were being obtained from only about 2,000 brain dead corpses annually.

Presumed Consent and Required Request Laws

The profound mismatch between the potential and the actual supply led some bioethicists to propose the concept of "presumed consent." This is an "opt out" scheme in which persons are presumed to consent to organ donation, unless they or their families had declared their objections to donating. Arthur Caplan, who is now Director of the Center for Bioethics of the University of Pennsylvania, but who was then a Fellow at the Hastings Center, was the leading proponent of this plan. In 1981 Virginia attempted to pass presumed consent legislation. Religious objections quashed the initiative. Caplan subsequently modified his position, championing "required request" laws, requiring hospital personnel to seek permission for donation from all families of brain dead patients (Jonsen 1998). Although such laws have been enacted in many jurisdictions, they have not significantly increased the supply of donor organs.

Xenotransplants: Animals as Suppliers of Transplantable Organs

Other mechanisms have also been explored to increase the supply of organs for transplant. On October 26, 1984, Dr. Leonard Bailey of Loma Linda Hospital, near Riverside, California, transplanted a baboon heart from a ten-month-old baby baboon, Goobers, into a fifteen-day-old baby, known (for reasons of confidentiality) as Baby Fae. Baby Fae had been born prematurely with hypoplastic left heart syndrome (HLHS), a condition that is estimated to affect approximately 500 infants annually. The IRB had approved an experimental xenograft, but as in the Barnard and Jarvick-7 experiments, animal models predicted precipitous failure. To quote from an editorial in the November 1984 *Journal of Heart Transplantation*:

> From the experimental data, and past clinical attempts, there is nothing to indicate that primate hearts will be tolerated by a human infant for months or years, using today's means to induce and control tolerance. The Loma Linda surgical team had not informed the

medical community, as yet, of any new evidence that might suggest the contrary (Losman, 1984).

Predictably, Baby Fae died in eleven days. Yet, a decade-and-a-half post-Barnard, the community of transplant surgeons recognized the folly of proceeding without successful prior animal experimentation.

A further problem with this particular xenograft is the nature of the animal whose heart was transplanted. Human societies are, for the most part, omnivores, who carnivorously exploit and consume other animals, such as the sheep that served as "guinea pigs" for the Jarvick hearts. While there are arguments for animal rights, given the omnipresence of steak houses and burger restaurants in our society, there is no moral reason for singling out xenografts as particularly objectionable. Apes are another matter. These biological cousins seem to be self-aware creatures, capable of language recognition and learning. If they are not clearly "persons," they are uncomfortably close. Apes seem to demand our moral respect. PETA (People for the Ethical Treatment of Animals) strongly criticized using Goobers as a donor for Baby Fae's transplant. Many bioethicists, who have little sympathy for the animal rights movement generally, tended to agree that apes like Goobers should not serve as guinea pigs.

Any form of xenograft, moreover, raises the specter of the trans-species spread of viruses and other disease agents. Such fears are not groundless. Bovine Spongiform Encephalitis, more popularly known as "Mad Cow Disease," jumped species from cattle to humans. The HIV virus also appears to have crossed the species barrier. The design of the Goobers-Baby Fae xenograft was flawed because it did not speak to these concerns. Currently, researchers are experimenting with cloning animals, and genetically modifying animal organs, in the hope of perfecting disease-free, reject-proof, xenotransplantable hearts and other organs. This line of research, however, may be shut down by the widespread protests against cloning and genetic engineering.

Anencephalic Infants as a Source of Organs for Transplant

Frustrated in his efforts to pursue xenografts, Dr. Bailey, sought another source of organs. Bailey's Loma Linda transplant program had successfully performed infant heart transplants 207 times in 277 attempts over the past decade and a half (Pence, 2000). Were more organs available, more infants could be saved. Desperate for new organ sources, Bailey considered the bodies of anencephalic infants as potential donors. 'Anencephalic' characterizes a range of gross congenital defects involving the non-formation of the brain (the cerebrum and cerebellum), beyond the brainstem. This relatively rare condition occurs in about 1 in 500 pregnancies. When it is detected in the uterus (by ultrasound and other means), most parents choose to abort; nonetheless, about 2,000 anencephalic infants are born in the U.S. each year. In 1987, a small group of bioethicists and surgeons, evoking the spirit of Jeremy Bentham and using impeccable utilitarian logic, proposed that instead of simply allowing these infants to die, they should be kept alive on respirators, so that their organs are properly harvested after they are pronounced dead (Pence, 2000; Harrington & Meilaender, 1986; Capron, 1987; Churchhill & Pinkus, 1980). The Ontario initiative also proposed that every six hours the infant's respirator be turned off to determine whether it could breathe without assistance. If the baby then was determined to be "dead," according to brain death criteria, its organs would be harvested.

The Ontario criteria tested the boundaries of acceptability. One parameter limiting the use of the dead had been set by Bentham's personal example, which established the permissibility of voluntary post-mortem donation. The Richard and Ronald Herrick case had expanded the zone of permissibility to permit voluntary organ donation from living donors. Yet donation was limited by another darker parameter: the Burke and Hare example, which established the impermissibility of killing anyone in order to obtain bodies or their parts (this boundary is sometimes misleadingly referred to as the "dead donor rule"). Permitting physicians to turn off ventilators, and then challenging a non-brain dead body in order to provoke brain death, seems remarkably Burke and Hareish. Nonetheless, in 1988 Dr. Bailey, tried to implement the Ontario protocol at Loma Linda hospital approximately a dozen times. He met with no success. By the end of the year, Bailey imposed an informal moratorium on anencephalic donors.

In 1992, Laura Campo and Justin Pearson, parents of an anencephalic infant brought their baby daughter, Theresa, to term. They hoped that her organs could help others and so they petitioned the courts to have their daughter declared dead. Their home state, Florida, accepted the Uniform Determination of Death guidelines, and hence the Harvard brain death criteria. As is typically the case with anencephalics, Theresa's brain stem was fully functional. She did not have a flat EEG and thus she was not brain dead according to Harvard criteria. The Florida Supreme Court refused to declare her dead (T.A.C.P., 1992).

Non-Heart-Beating-Cadavers (NHBD) as Organ Sources

A second, somewhat more successful attempt, to breach the Burke-Hare parameter was initiated by the University of Pittsburgh Presbyterian Medical

Center, one of the largest transplantation centers in the U.S. In 1993, Pittsburgh developed a protocol to obtain organs from patients declared dead using cardiopulmonary criteria. The protocol used the infelicitous and confusing name "non-heart-beating-cadavers" (NHBD) to distinguish donors declared dead, in this way, from brain dead donors, who are heart-beating-cadavers. Unlike traditional cardiopulmonary criteria, however, the Pittsburgh Presbyterian NHBD protocol, does not make irreversible loss of cardiopulmonary function a prerequisite to a declaration of death. The NHBD protocol permits the physician to declare a patient "dead," even though the patient's heart could be restarted by cardiopulmonary resuscitation – provided that the patient and/or an appropriate surrogate has requested a "Do Not Resuscitate" (DNR) order. Patients are thus declared "dead," in part, because they, or their surrogates, have requested that they are not to be resuscitated. The Pittsburgh protocol also permits physicians to administer anti-coagulants and vasodilators in order to perfuse, and thus to preserve, a patient's organs. The NHBD protocol thus seems to breach the Burke-Hare parameter. The justification offered is that: the intent to donate organs, when conjoined with consent to DNR, legitimates "managing" a terminal patient's death with the objective of preserving organs rather than prolonging the patient's life during the dying period.

Controversy over NHBD heated to the boiling point in 1997, when a Cleveland bioethicist Mary Ellen Waithe, revealed that the Cleveland Clinic had been using an NHBD protocol for two decades. The Cleveland Clinic protocol permitted the administration of an anti-coagulant, heparin, to donors in a manner that, in the opinion of some, could hasten a donor's death. NHBDs and the use of anti-coagulants remain controversial topics, as does the appropriateness of bioethicist publicizing such practices. What the NHBD controversy shares with debates dating back to the public dissection of Bentham's corpse, however, is a concern for beneficence and the consequent drive to make the dead and the dying useful to the living. These initiatives inevitably raise the question: when do our duties of beneficence toward the salvageable sick overstep their bounds to become disrespect for the rights of the dying or desecration of the dead?[14]

RATIONING: IMPLICIT AND EXPLICIT

There is yet another way to deal with the demands of the living: one can restrain them. Restraint in the face of scarcity means "rationing." Although, in political parlance, 'ration' tends to be a six-letter "four-letter word (Baker, 1994)," the term derives from 'ratio', or "reason." The core idea of rationing is to use reason to organize scarcity to ensure that its burdens are borne fairly. To organize scarcity, however, one must admit that it exists. Such admissions have been difficult in nations, such as Britain and Spain, that have government-sponsored national health *services* (in contrast to the mixed governmental and private national health *insurance* programs of France, Germany and the Netherlands). Once a government commits to providing health care in a more or less direct fashion for all of its citizens, any admission that care is not provided takes on an appearance of dereliction of duty.

Implicit Rationing of Kidney Dialysis and Transplants in Britain

The British National Health Service (NHS), in particular, has been loath to admit to patients that its resources are inadequate to their medical needs. Consider, for example, the waiting list for a surgical procedure invented by the British themselves, hip replacement prosthesis. Developed in 1972 by John Charnley (1911–1982), a surgeon at the Manchester Royal Infirmary, this technological miracle enables the halt, the lame and the wheelchair-bound to walk normally once again. Demand for Charnley's prosthesis was instantaneous. Yet, because the NHS budget had not expanded to meet the demand, waiting periods grew exponentially.

> In 1977 routine cases waited an average of thirteen to fourteen months and urgent cases an average of four months; barely concealed within these averages were extreme delays of up to five years, with even urgent cases waiting two or three years. Waiting lists grew 31% between 1977 and 1979 (Aaron & Schwartz, 1984).

Mention of waiting lists suggests a formal system. In fact, because the NHS was reluctant to acknowledge any scarcity of effective medicine, for decades it developed no rationing plan. Until relatively recently, rationing in the NHS was implicit in the way things were done, rather than in any formal explicit rationing scheme.

The NHS took a similarly implicit approach to kidney dialysis and transplantation in the post-cyclosporin era. Even as these procedures came to be internationally accepted as a standard medical practice, the NHS made only modest increases in its budget to accommodate them. Consequently, demand rapidly outstripped resources. Yet, in the absence of formal publicly accepted rationing criteria, doctors found it difficult to explain this situation to their patients. The results were documented in two studies: one conducted by economist Henry Aaron and physician William Schwartz, and published in 1984 by the Brookings Institution; and a second, conducted by political scientist Thomas Halper, and published by Cambridge University Press in 1989 (Halper, 1989). Both studies found informal age rationing hidden behind a façade of deception.

Here is how Aaron and Schwartz characterize the situation:

> Resource limitations put [NHS] doctors in a position that many of them find awkward. Trained to treat illness, they find they are unable to provide all the care from which their patients might derive benefit. . . . Doctors gradually redefine standards of care so that they can escape the constant recognition that financial limits compel them to do less than their best.
>
> By various means physicians . . . try to make the denial of care seem routine or optimal. . . . The British nephrologist tells the family of a patient . . . that dialysis would be painful and burdensome and that the patient would be better off without it; or he tells the resident alien from a poor country that he should return home, to be among family and friends who speak the same language – where, as it happens, the patient will die because dialysis is unavailable. . . .
>
> In each instance physicians are asserting that the treatment is *medically* optimal or very close to optimal, that the patients denied care or provided alternative forms of care because of budget limits lose essentially nothing of medical significance. For the undialyzed patient who dies . . . this view is unpersuasive. . . . But it enables doctors to avoid the painful realization that they are doing less than their best for the patient (Aaron & Schwartz, 1984).

Here, for example, is one nephrologist's description of how he would deal with a hypothetical case of a sixty-five year-old patient with end-stage renal disease (ESRD).

> Obviously the patient is sixty-five and therefore does not come within the regional dialysis [or transplantation] program. I would say [to the family] that mother's or aunt's kidneys have failed or are failing and that there is very little that anybody can do about it because of her age and general physical state, and that it would be my suggestion, or my advice that we spare her any further investigation, any further procedure and we do what we can to make her as comfortable as we can for what remains of her life (Aaron & Schwartz, 1984).

Notice that the nephrologist did not inform this woman, or her family, that she is being denied dialysis on the grounds of old age. Instead, she is told that "there is very little that anybody can do about it because of [your] age." This ambiguous characterization will be heard as one of medical fact – although dialysis could extend a sixty-five year-old woman's life for a decade or two. Nothing in the statement will suggest to the patient, or to her family that she is actually being denied dialysis and/or transplantation because the regional program does not accept anyone over the age of 55. A rationing decision is disguised as a medical judgment. This disguise denies the patient and her family more than access to dialysis and transplantation. They are denied the opportunity to seek alternative sources of dialysis or transplantation (by spending their own money, or by seeking funds from family, friends, neighbors, and private charities). They are also disenfranchised, denied the right to protest the regional dialysis center's policies, or to demand a change in the funding priorities that underlay this denial.

Age-Rationing in Britain

A second major finding of the two studies, evident in the above quotation, is that chronological age is a major criterion informally employed by the NHS to deny access to transplantation and dialysis. Although age rationing is often condemned as "ageism,"[15] i.e. as morally unjustifiable discrimination based on chronological age, several well-known philosophers believe that it can be morally justifiable. Among these philosophers are John Harris in Britain (Harris, 1985), and Daniel Callahan (Callahan, 1987) and Norman Daniels (Daniels, 1988) in the United States. Their arguments hinge on conceptions of the appropriate goals of medicine. Daniels believes that medicine's goal is to provide everyone with a fair opportunity to live a normal life. Consequently, in his view, medical resources are more properly expended on the young than the old, since the young have had the fewest opportunities to lead a normal life. Callahan and Harris argue that age rationing is permissible because medicine's aim is to assist people to live healthily through their natural life span. Thus it is no misfortune, Harris claims, to die at the end of one's natural life span, but it is a misfortune to die before the end of one's natural life span.

Robert Baker and other critics respond that medical resources are ideally allocated in response to medical need. Since medical need is typically greatest in the beginning decades and in the last few decades of life, medical resources are properly allocated to both the beginning and the end decades of persons' lives. Baker is also skeptical of the idea of a normal or natural life span, noting that, in the developed world, life spans have almost doubled between the first year of the twentieth century and the first year of the twenty-first. Moreover, by reanalyzing European Union data, Baker demonstrated that, since women outlive men by about a decade, and thus experience a later onset of organ failure, using chronological age to ration dialysis and transplantation inevitably discriminates against women. Age rationing in medicine is thus not only ageist, it is inevitably sexist. Finally, Baker challenges the legitimacy of any form of rationing, including that practised in the pre-Thatcher NHS (Robinson & Judge, 1988; Robinson et al., 1988),[16] that is not publicly visible and acceptable, in principle, to those affected by it (Baker, 1991; Baker, 1993; Strosberg et al., 1988).

Triage and the Explicit Rationing of Medical Resources

In the U.S., medical rationing has tended to be discussed more openly than in Britain. The tradition of public discussion of the allocation of scarce medical resources dates back to at least the Second World War, when there was public debate over the allocation of penicillin (Adams, 1989). For Western medicine, more generally, contemporary norms governing allocation for scarce resources date back to the patterns of "triage" that emerged with the invention of the modern hospital in the late eighteenth and early nineteenth centuries.

Initially, hospital admission and discharge policies were based on social criteria (such as, whether the sick person had lived a life that merited her or his admission to the hospital). These criteria were set by governing boards of lay persons, who represented the donors whose charitable contributions supported the hospital. Medical practitioners, however, sought to gain control over the process by developing rules based on technical criteria that aimed at minimizing morbidity and mortality (by, for example, separating maternity patients from fever patients, whose illnesses might be contagious).

In Britain, as such practitioners as John Aiken (1747–1822) and his protégé, Thomas Percival (1740–1804) gained control over the admissions process, they tended to draft admissions policies in a way that would efficiently optimize outcomes (Aiken, 1771, Percival, 1803). French medicine, on the other hand, began to assume its modern form in the context of the Revolution, when the practice of what we today call "triage" was invented by Napoleon's surgeon general, Baron Dominique Jean Larrey (1766–1842). Larrey was outraged by the unnecessary loss of life caused by the unsystematic treatment of battlefield casualties he found when he joined Napoleon's Grand Army. Prior to the revolution, the French army had been staffed by professional soldiers who supplied their own camp followers to act, not only as personal cooks and as valets, but as "corpsmen", administering first aid and fetching surgeons for their employers. The ordinary citizens who joined the ranks of the Grand Army lacked the resources to fund this traditional support system and so the wounded were treated haphazardly.

Larrey, applying the ideals of Enlightenment to the chaos he found on the battlefield, replaced happenstance with system. "Prompt and methodical succor received by the wounded on the field of battle," was to be delivered by "ambulance," a system of soldiers assigned to transport the wounded to mobile medical stations, positioned close to the field of battle. The "methodical" aspect of this system of "succor" required field surgeons to "sort," or, to use the French term, "triage" – the wounded by assigning treatment priorities. Here is Larrey's description of triage:

> Those who are dangerously wounded must be tended first, entirely without regard to rank or distinction. Those less severely injured must wait until the gravely wounded have been operated on and dressed. The slightly wounded may go to the hospital [behind the front] line; especially officers, since they have horses and therefore have transport – and regardless, most of these have but trivial wounds (Larrey, 1832).

Larrey does not mention the dying, but it is clear from a contemporary painting by Antoine-Jean Gros (1771–1835), that those who were hopelessly dying formed a third category, that was left untreated on the battlefield (Gros, 1807; Southgate, 1997).

As Surgeon General to an army that marched under the banner of "Liberty, Equality, Fraternity" (not efficiency, not the greatest good for the greatest number), Larrey emphasizes egalitarianism, giving each and every dangerously wounded but potentially salvageable patient a chance. His egalitarian triage contrasts strikingly with the British efficiency-oriented admissions and discharge tradition. Thus, where Larrey prioritizes in favor of treating the sickest salvageable patient first, the British prioritize in favor of treating those who can most effectively be made well, even if they are not the sickest. Oddly, both of these ways of *sorting* sick people came to be called 'triage' and both serve as the basis for modern admission/discharge and "triage" practices (Baker & Strosberg, 1991).

The conflation of these two seeming antithetical ideals – egalitarianism and efficiency – might seem bizarre, but they share one common overarching feature: they use technical criteria to wrest control of admission/discharge/allocation decisions from non-medical authorities. In a deep sense, moreover, both the British and French criteria assert the priority of medical need, and medical effectiveness over such non-medical considerations as military rank, social status, or moral desert. They thus reach back to a tradition of moral neutrality, deeply rooted in the canonical texts of the Western medical tradition, which urges medicine to treat all suffering humanity, irrespective of wealth, class, rank, or political allegiance. In urging technical, as opposed to social, criteria for admission/discharge decisions, Larrey and his British counterparts were thus envisioning a humanistic medicine that transcended the issues of class, politics, rank and social status.

Utilitarian Rationing Using Social Criteria: The Seattle Experience

Not surprisingly, it was a twentieth-century American, an unselfconscious heir to America's egalitarianism, who experimented with the reintroduction of social criteria into medical allocation. The experimenter was Belding Scribner, inventor of the Scribner shunt (which made long-term dialysis for chronic renal disease a practical reality). Scribner's success had created a problem of scarcity. The problem was inescapable and had to be dealt with, in some way or other, by each of the 87 medical centers experimenting with chronic kidney dialysis in the 1960s. All but eight of the centers used triage-based criteria to select a few dozen subjects from among hundreds of applicants. These criteria emphasize medical need, as well as therapeutic effectiveness and efficiency. Thus, when these dialysis centers were surveyed in 1969, all claimed to use medical suitability for dialysis as a primary determinant of admissibility. In addition, 86% also tried to assess a subject's "willingness to cooperate in the treatment regimen"; 79% tried to weigh-in the likelihood of long-term success; 69% considered the correlative criterion of absence of other disabling diseases. Less commonly, 34% of the centers considered the patient/families ability to understand and thus comply with the requirements of chronic dialysis; 32% considered the likelihood that the patient could return to work. A smaller 29% of centers considered the subject's chronological age, while 25% used psychiatric evaluations to consider suitability. Any indication that a patient/family could not, or would not, comply with the complex experimental dialysis regimen was automatically grounds for excluding a patient. Thus, 68% of all centers excluded patients with mental deficiencies. A smaller number, 29%, excluded patients with a family environment suggestive of difficulties; 25% excluded patients with criminal records; 21% excluded indigents; 20% excluded patients with poor employment records. Finally, 17% excluded patients who lacked transportation, or who were not residents of the state in which the center was located (Fox & Swazey, 1978).

While one might have suspicions that several of these criteria infuse social considerations into the selection process, those applying these criteria believed that they were using triage principles, predicated on notions of equality, effectiveness and efficiency. Eight of the 187 centers experimenting with dialysis, however, took a forthrightly different course. They experimented with breaching the triage tradition by reintroducing lay judgments about moral and social worth into the allocation process. The most famous of these eight centers was the center at Swedish Hospital in Seattle, which was headed by Belding Scribner himself. Access to dialysis at the Swedish Hospital was determined by a seven-member committee. Originally the members were: a banker, a housewife, a labor leader, a lawyer, a minister, a state government official, and a surgeon. There were also two physician advisors. In deciding which medically suitable candidate would receive dialysis, the committee factored in age (no one over forty-five received dialysis), marital status and number of dependents, income, net worth, educational achievements, occupation, and "past performance and future potential." Applicants submitted the names of people who could act as their references. In a case in which the committee considered four applicants for one open dialysis slot, it selected "a 33 year-old whose seven dependents almost certainly would become dependent upon state aid if he were unable to continue to work (Fox & Swazey, 1978)."

The committee might have served its function in quiet anonymity, had not Scribner called the public's attention to its existence. In a quest for additional funding, in 1962 Scribner and one of his dialysis patients attended a newspaper convention. The pathos of the patient proved newsworthy and Scribner's program attracted the media. *Life* magazine dispatched one of its reporters, Shana Alexander, to Seattle to cover the story. In the resulting article, "They Decide Who Lives, Who Dies: Medical Miracle Puts a Burden on a Small Committee (Alexander, 1962)," Alexander characterized the committee as a "God Committee." Alexander's articles attracted worldwide attention to the Seattle program but not in the way that Scribner anticipated.

> All of us who were involved felt that we had found a fairly reasonable and simple solution to an impossibly difficult problem by letting a committee of responsible members of the community choose which patients [would receive treatment] among several who were medically ideal. . . . In retrospect, of course, we were terribly naïve. . . . We simply could not understand why everyone was more interested in the existence and operation of the lay selection committee than in the fact that in two years we had taken a disease, end stage kidney disease, and converted it from a one hundred percent fatal prognosis to a ninety-five percent two year survival (Fox & Swazey, 1978).

Scribner was utterly oblivious to breaching the wall of moral neutrality that had permitted modern medicine to flourish, protected from social and political turmoil, for almost two centuries. He failed to appreciate that when the public read these accounts they feared that when next *they* needed treatment, they would be judged by physicians' perception of their social worth, rather than in terms of their medical need.

Scribner was unwittingly unraveling the carefully wrought framework of normative neutrality welded by Aiken, Larrey and Percival, that had successfully provided the foundation for modern medicine. Some of his colleagues, however, were quick to appreciate this point. Perhaps the most pointed and memorable critique of Scribner's experiment in abandoning moral neutrality was penned by the psychiatrist-lawyer team of David Sanders and Jesse Dukeminer.

> The ethical muddle of selection committee comparing human worth is well illustrated by the operations of the selection committee at the Seattle Artificial Kidney Center. The descriptions of how this committee makes its decisions . . . are numbing accounts of how close to the surface lie the prejudices and mindless clichés that pollute the committee's deliberations. . . . [They] paint a disturbing picture of the bourgeoisie sparing the bourgeoisie, of the Seattle committee measuring persons in accordance with its own middle-class value system: scouts, Sunday school, Red Cross. This rules out creative non-conformists who rub the bourgeoisie the wrong way but who historically have contributed so much to the making of America. The Pacific Northwest is no place for a Henry David Thoreau with bad kidneys (Sanders & Dukeminer, 1968).

Allocation in the Era of Physiological Criteria

After the Seattle debacle, when UNOS was established in 1987, it, and its sister agencies in Europe (U.K. Transplant and Eurotransplant) developed elaborate point systems based on physical and physiological criteria to allocate organs. These criteria involve such factors as: geographical location, tissue type, the match between the size of organ and the size of the recipient, blood type, degree of medical urgency, time spent on the waiting list, and so forth. Although such physical and physiological criteria provide a shield of moral neutrality insulating medical decision making from social and political pressures, questions about values still arise. They tend, however, to be parsed in technical language.

A Physiological Bias Against Minorities

Physiological criteria, for example, can be read as slanted against physiological minorities. A legacy of discrimination foments minority distrust of the majority culture, including the health care system. Minority members are thus naturally less inclined to donate organs than the majority counterparts. Consequently, when minority individuals experience organ failure, since there are fewer minority organs to be distributed, they are less likely to find a physiological match than members of the majority. A legacy of discrimination and a heritage of mistrust thus conspire to bias seemingly neutral physiological criteria against minority individuals (Gaston et al., 1993; Kjellstrand, 1988).[17]

Alcohol-Related End-Stage Liver Disease (ARESLD) Patients

Benthamite efficiency seems forever at odds with Larrey's egalitarian desire to give each and every desperately ill but salvageable patient a chance at life, even at the expense of efficiency. This age-old debate between efficiency and egalitarianism reappears in technical guise in the debate over the appropriateness of alcohol-related end-stage liver disease (ARESLD) patients as liver recipients. Any relapse to alcoholism will endanger newly transplanted livers, hence liver transplants are less likely to be successful in ARESLD patients, compared to non-ARESLD patients (whose liver failure has nothing to do with alcoholism). Benthamite efficiency thus demands that, since ARESLD patients tend to have worse outcomes than non-ARESLD patients do, we should maximize the number of successful transplants, by assigning ARESLD patients lower priority for transplants (Caplan & Coelho, 1998). Egalitarians, on the other hand, are likely to argue that ARESLD patients should have the same chance as everyone else, irrespective of whether alcoholics are considered ill, or merely weak-willed. If alcoholism is considered a moral failing, then discrimination against alcoholics is merely a revival of the discredited social worth criterion. If, on the other hand, alcoholism really is an illness, then, or so an egalitarian can claim, it should be treated no differently than diabetes or any other illnesses. Thus alcoholics, like diabetics, should be given a first chance, and even a retransplant, should the first transplant fail.

Retransplants

These issues come into focus more sharply if we consider the more general question of retransplantation. Approximately ten to twenty percent of available hearts and livers (including those given to ARESLD patients) are retransplants, allocated to patients whose first transplant has failed. Retransplant patients fare significantly worse than first transplant patients. From October 1, 1987 through December 31, 1991, 81.6% of the 4,830 first heart transplant patients survived for over one year; in contrast, only 56.7% of the 86 retransplant patients survived for over one year. Thomas Starzl and other transplant surgeons are aware of this difference, but reason, in the tradition of Larrey, that while it is unfortunate, physicians have an obligation *not to abandon* their desperately ill patients. Robert Arnold, Arthur Caplan, and Peter Ubel, on the other hand, evoke the spirit of Benthamite efficiency in arguing that UNOS criteria ought to be revised, so that first transplant patients have priority over retransplant patients (Balint and Shelton). The debate is conducted in the post-UNOS physiological jargon of twenty-first-century medicine, but the issue is as old as modern medicine itself: is medicine about efficiently saving the *most* lives, or is it about providing *each* salvageable patient an opportunity to survive, no matter how inefficient this process may be.

Eliminating Scarcity by Throwing Money at It

Discussions of rationing often evoke nostalgia for some mythical period before resources were scarce. It should be apparent, however, that, for the most part, medical scarcity is an artifact of medicine's success. Nonetheless, there is a reflexive desire to eliminate scarcity by increasing resources to the point that scarcity vanishes. In 1971, the U.S. Congress was persuaded to engage in one such experiment. The persuader was Shep Glazer, President of the American Association of Kidney Patients. Shep had himself dialyzed in front of the House Ways and Means Committee. In a dramatic gesture he disconnected a cannola tube and let the blood flow onto his hands. "If you don't fund more machines," he said, "you'll have this blood on your hands" (Ubel et al., 1993). Thirty minutes later, the Committee approved Public Law 92-603; on October 30, 1972, President Richard Nixon signed the law, thereby making dialysis and transplantation available, at government expense, to all patients with end stage renal disease (ESRD).

This generous, impulsive, and humane gesture solved the dialysis machine shortage, but it was a financial disaster. Treatment of ESRD rose exponentially, even in cases where dialysis was only marginally effective. In the 1990s, on average, over 50,000 patients were dialyzed annually, at a cost of over one billion dollars a year. Medical resources to support this program were cannibalized from others; Congress was so traumatized by the cost of this gesture that it has been skeptical of any further attempts to expand government commitments in healthcare. Throwing money at problems, it seems, does not always solve them in a satisfactory way.

CONCLUDING REMARKS

The brief summary of the parallel evolution of the medical techniques and ethical norms involved in transplants was designed to serve as more than a prologue. Bioethics tends to be thought of in "presentist" terms. Each problem is discussed as if it had no past, as if it were *sui generis*, as if the experience of prior generations were irrelevant. In bioethics, however, the past is more than prologue, it sets the parameters for the present. Our present policies governing organ donation and transplantation evolve from our experience with gallows corpse laws, resurrectionists, the Burke and Hare trials, and Bentham's donation of his own corpse for public dissection. Had Bentham never arranged for his own public dissection, it is possible that the Drs. Frankenstein of the world would have prevailed. One can easily imagine a Western world where, as in Japan, it would still be considered unconscionable to appropriate the dead for the use of the living. In such a world, there would be no organ transplants.

We are thus as much the beneficiaries of the moral examples and innovations of Bentham and Beecher, as we are of the Nobel Laureates Carrel, Dausset and Medawar. However, if we are the beneficiaries of the past, we are also its prisoners. Consider Belding Scribner's unwitting breach in the wall of moral neutrality surrounding medical decision making. By undoing the achievements of Aiken, Larrey and Percival, Scribner found, to his chagrin, that, instead of being lauded as a hero for saving previously unsalvageable patients, he was condemned for intruding social values into medical judgments. Ignorance of the past, and, in particular, failure to understand the evolution of the norms that evolved from past experience, can thus jeopardize scientific success.

The history of transplantation is also a tale of social and human experimentation. Experiments are by nature experimental. Some must fail. This is thus a story of moratoria: a moratorium on social evaluation (after Scribner's Seattle debacle); Moore's moratorium on heart transplants (on the basis of the 1968 mortality data), and Strazl's moratorium on liver transplants (to assess the significance of tissue typing). Scientists and society alike had to assess the results of these experiments in order to decide how best to proceed. Moreover, just as there are no a priori answers in science, there are no a priori solutions to ethical and social problems. We cannot know which norms appropriately govern new medical innovations, like transplants, without social experimentation. If the history of transplantation teaches any lesson at all, it instructs us in the error of those who, misreading Mary Shelley's message, follow Dr. Frankenstein in condemning, on a priori grounds, the latest biomedical innovation as "unnatural." It is human nature, and thus natural to humanity, to save the lives of their fellow humans. There is thus something quintessentially human and humane about the hundreds of thousands of people who live out their lives as organ recipients, but who would have died an earlier death, except for transplantation. This said, some very real problems face clinicians, researchers and bioethicists, who, unlike Dr. Frankenstein, do not flee from biomedical innovations, but who, instead, are wrestling with the very real moral quandaries surrounding organ donation and transplantation. The remainder of this volume addresses these quandaries.

NOTES

1. Although this passage now opens Chapter Five, it originally opened Mary Shelley's tale.
2. In 1990, Robert White performed a procedure he called a "total-body transplant" in which he transplanted the head of one monkey onto the body of another and vice versa (Porter, 1997).
3. For Shelley, Dr. Frankenstein's monster is "the new Prometheus," who holds his creator responsible for his creation. The concept is alluded to in Shelley's prefatory quote from John Milton's Paradise Lost: "Did I request thee, Maker, from my clay/ To mould Me man? Did I solicit thee/ From darkness to promote me?" (Paradise Lost, X.743–5).
4. A sixteenth-century picture of this remarkable operation is reproduced in this text by Carmichael and Ratzan (1991). No one comments on whether the Moor gave his informed voluntary consent for his donation of a leg. One thus suspects that this myth is as much about the exploitation of those considered to be "other," as it is about miracles or medicine.
5. The Royal Physician, William Harvey (1578–1657), was a pioneer in this respect.
6. Orthodox Judaism still rejects autopsy and dissection.

7. Non-Western countries, which have not gone through the gallows-corpse debate and which lack the Burke and Hare precedent, have been more tolerant of commodification. Brazil, China, Haiti, India, the Philippines, the countries of the former Soviet Union, and Turkey legally permit, or unofficially tolerate, financial compensation to living organ donors, and/or to the families of cadavers used for donation.

8. For the current state of the debate over "opt-out" appropriation schemes, see this volume Chapter Two.

9. Moore, here, argues for a virtue ethics, dependent upon the virtuous character of scientists, rather than a formal ethics of duties enforced via peer review.

10. See this volume, Chapter Four.

11. See this volume, Chapter Three.

12. The best indication of the state of ethical discussion in the mid-1960s, prior to the advent of heart transplantation, is the proceedings of a conference convened by the British transplant surgeon, Sir Michael Woodruff, with the support of the CIBA foundation (Wolstenhome & O'Connor, 1966).

13. Barnard kept Washkansky alive by performing a tracheotomy repair against Washkansky's express wishes. Today, this would be a clear violation of accepted standards of research ethics. At the time, however, the ethic of enlightened paternalism permitted such interventions.

14. See this volume, Chapter Nine, for further discussion.

15. There is some reason to suspect endemic ageism in British culture. Americans typically refer to anyone over sixty-five years old as a "senior citizen," emphasizing the notion of seniority, with its connotations of entitlement and citizenship, which also connotes a sense of entitlement. In contrast, the British refer to persons aged sixty and over as "old age pensioners," emphasizing age and dependency.

16. From 1987 to 1990 Prime Minister Baroness Thatcher reformed the NHS by introducing a plan for a "social market" or "internal market." These reforms radically altered the NHS, but it is not clear, at this point, how they have affected its proclivity for age rationing.

17. See this volume, Chapter Twelve.

REFERENCES

Aaron, H., & Schwartz, W. (1984). *The painful prescription: rationing hospital care* (pp. 37, 59, 101). Washington D.C.: The Brookings Institution.

Adams, D. P. (1989). Wartime bureaucracy and penicillin allocation: the committee of chemotherapeutic and other agents, 1942–1945. *The Journal of the History of Medicine and Allied Sciences*, *44*, 196–217.

Aiken, J. (1771). *Thoughts on hospitals*. London: J. Johnson.

Alexander, S. (1962). They decide who lives, who dies: medical miracle puts a burden on a small committee. *Life*, *53*, 102–125.

Baker, R. (1990). The inevitability of health care rationing: a case study of the British National Health Service. In: M. Strosberg et al. (Eds), *Rationing America's Health Care* (pp. 208–230). Washington, D.C.

Baker, R. (1993). Visibility and the just allocation of health care: a study of age-rationing in the British National Health Service. *Health Care Analysis*, *1*(2), 1–22.

Baker, R. (1993). Professional integrity and global budgeting, a study of physician gatekeeping in the British National Health Service. *Professional Ethics*, *2*, 1–34.

Baker, R. (1994). Rationing, rhetoric, and rationality: a review of the health care rationing debate in America and Europe. In: J. Humber & R. Almeder (Eds), *Allocating Health Care Resources* (pp. 53–84). Totowa, NJ: Humana Press.

Baker, R., & Strosberg, M. (1991). Triage and equality: a historical reassessment of utilitarian analyses of triage. *Kennedy Institute of Ethics Journal*, *2*, 103–124.

Beecher et al. (1968). A definition of irreversible coma. *Journal of the American Medical Association*, *205*, 337–339.

Beecher, H. J. (1970). *Research and the individual: human studies* (pp. 277–279). MA: Little Brown and Company.

Blake, J. B. (1980). *The education of American physicians* (pp. 34–38). Berkeley: UC Press.

Boland, F. (1950). *The first anesthetic* (pp. 18–19). Athens: University of Georgia Press.

Bynum, W., & Porter, R. (Eds) (1993). *Companion encyclopedia of the history of medicine* (p. 992). London: Routledge.

Callahan, D. (1987). *Setting limits: medical goals in an aging society*. New York: Simon and Shuster.

Caplan, A. L. (1995). Organ and tissue transplants: ethical and legal issues. In: W. Reich (Ed.), *Encyclopedia of Bioethics* (pp. 1892–1893). New York: Macmillan.

Caplan, A. L., & Coelho, D. (1998). The ethics of organ transplants: the current debate. Buffalo: Prometheus Books. Part II, 139–192. Part III, 193–246, 260–274. Part IV.

Capron, A. M. (1987). Anencephalic donors separate the dead from the dying. *Hastings Center Report*, *17*, 5–9.

Carmichael, A. G., & Ratzan, R. (1991). *Medicine: treasury of art and literature* (p. 65). New York: Macmillan.

Chakravorty, R. C. (1998). Medicine in early New York. *Veterans Health Systems Journal*. 61–65.

Churchill, L. R., & Pinkus, R. (1980). The use of anencephalic organs: historical and ethical dimensions. *The Milbank Quarterly*, *68*, 147–169.

Daniels, N. (1988). *Am I my parents' keeper: an essay on justice between the young and old*. Oxford: Oxford University Press.

De Moulin, D. (1988). *A history of surgery*. Dordrecht, NL: Kluwer Academic Publishers, 114–118.

Evans, R. W., Orians, C. E., & Ascher, N. L. (1992). The potential supply of organ donors: an assessment of the efficiency of organ procurement efforts in the United States. *Journal of the American Medical Association*, *267*, 239–246.

Fox, R., & Swazey, J. (1978). *The courage to fail: a social view of organ transplantation and dialysis* (pp. 71, 77, 111–115, 202–203, 227, 231, 233). Chicago: University of Chicago Press.

Fox, R., & Swazey, J. (1992). *Spare parts: organ replacement in American society* (p. 7). New York: Oxford University Press.

Foucault, M. (1975). *The birth of the clinic: an archaeology of medical perception*. New York: Vintage Books.

Foucault, M. (1979). *Discipline and punish: the birth of the prison* (p. 5). New York: Vintage Books.

Gaston et al. (1993). Racial equality in renal transplantation: the disparate impact of HLA-based allocation. *Journal of the American Medical Association*, *270*, 1352–1356.

Gros, A. J. (1807). *Napoleon on the Battlefield of Eylau*. Toledo Museim of Art. Toledo, Ohio.

Halper, T. (1989). *The misfortunes of others: end-stage renal disease in the United Kingdom*. Cambridge, U.K.: Cambridge University Press.

Harley, D. (1994). Political post-mortems and morbid anatomy in seventeenth-century England. *Journal of the Social History of Medicine*, *10*, 1–28.

Harrington, M. R., & Meilaender, G. (1986). The anencephalic newborn as organ donor. *Hastings Center Report*, *16*, 21–23.

Harris, J. (1985). *The value of life*. London: Routledge & Kegan Paul.

Harrison, R. (1983). *Bentham* (pp. 6–7). London: Routledge & Kegan Paul.

Humber, J., & Almeder, R. (Eds) (1994). Allocating health care resources. *Biomedical Ethics Reviews*, 55–84.

Jonsen, A. R. (1998). *The birth of bioethics* (pp. 197, 199, 200–202, 205–206, 208–211, 225). New York: Oxford University Press.

Kahane, B. D. (1981). Cosmas and Damian in the 20th century. *New England Journal of Medicine*, *305*, 280.

Katz, A. H., & Proctor, D. M. (1969). Social-psychological characteristics of patients receiving hemodialysis treatment for chronic renal failure. Washington D.C.: Public Health Service, Kidney Disease Control Program. In: Fox & Swazey, 230–231.

Kjellstrand, C. M. (1988). Age, sex, and race inequality in renal transplantation. *Archives of Internal Medicine*, *148*, 1305–1309.

Larrey, D. J. (1832). *Surgical memoirs of the campaign in Russia* (p. 109). Philadelphia: Cowey & Lee.

Linden, F. E. (1951). Resurrection riots during the heroic age of anatomy in America. *Bull. Hist. Med.*, *25*, 178–184.

Lock, M. (1999). The problem of brain death: Japanese disputes about bodies and modernity. In: Yougnen et al. (pp. 239–250).

Losman, J. (1984). *Journal of Heart Transplantation*, *4*, 10–11, quoted at Pence (2000), 346.

Miller, A. S., & Hagihara, A. (1997). Organ transplanting in Japan: the debate begins. *Public Health*, *111*(6), 367–372.

Moore, F. D. (1969). Therapeutic innovation: ethical boundaries in the initial clinical trials of new drugs and surgical procedures. *Daedalus: Journal of the American Academy of Arts and Sciences*, Spring, 513–514, 519.

Murray, J. E. (1992). Human organ transplantation: background and consequences. *Science*, *256*, 1411–1415.

Outram, D. (1989). *The body and the French Revolution*. New Haven, CT: Yale University Press.

Pernick, M. (1985). *The calculus of suffering*. New York: Columbia University Press.

Pence, G. E. (1990) *Classic Cases in Medical Ethics*. New York: McGraw Hill, 215.

Pence, G. E. (2000). *Classic cases in medical ethics: accounts of cases that have shaped medical ethics with philosophical, legal, and historical backgrounds* (pp. 215, 225–250, 293, 338, 360). New York: McGraw Hill.

Percival, T. (1803). *Medical ethics*. London: J. Johnson.

Porter, R. (1997). *The greatest benefit to mankind* (pp. 317, 365–366, 622). New York: W. W. Norton.

President's commission for the study of ethical problems in medicine and biomedical and behavioral research. (1981). *Defining death: medical, ethical, and legal issues in the definition of death*. Washington D.C.: U.S. Government Printing Office.

Richardson, R. (1989). *Death, dissection, and the destitute*. Middlesex: Penguin Books.

Rhodes, R. (1999). Minorities in medicine. *Mount Sinai Journal of Medicine*, 66.

Robinson, R., & Judge, K. (1988). *Efficiency and the NHS: a case for internal markets. Health Unit Paper.* No. 2.

Robinson et al. (1988). *Health finance: assessing the options.* London: Kings Fund Institute.

Rosner, F. (1986). *Modern medicine and Jewish ethics.* New York: Katav Publishing House and Yeshiva University Press, Chapter Three.

Sappol, M. (1997). *The cultural politics of anatomy in 19th-century America* (Doctoral Dissertation, Columbia University).

Sappol, M. (2000). *A traffic of dead bodies.* NJ: Princeton University Press.

Schartz, H. S. (1958). Bioethical and legal considerations in increasing the supply of transplantable organs. *American Journal of Law and Medicine, 10*, 397–438.

Southgate, M. T. (1997). The Cover. *JAMA, 278*, 349.

Shelley, M. (1969). *Frankenstein: or the modern Prometheus* (1818). (pp. 53, 55). Oxford: Oxford University Press.

Strosberg et al. *Rationing America's health care: the Oregon plan and beyond.* Brookings Institution, 208–230.

T.A.C.P. (1992). *Southern Law Reporter.* 2nd Series, Supreme Court of Florida, 588–595.

Ubel et al. (1993). Rationing failure: the ethical lessons of the retransplantation of scarce organ resources. *Journal of the American Medical Association, 270*, 2469–2474.

Wilf, S. R. (1989). Anatomy and punishment in late eighteenth-century New York. *Journal of Social History, 22*, 507–30.

Wise, J. (1997). Japan to allow organ transplants. *British Medical Journal, 314* (7090), 1298.

Wolstenhome, G. E. W., & O'Connor, M. (Eds) (1966). *Ethics in medical progress: with special reference to transplantation.* London, J & A Churchill Ltd.

Youngner et al. (Eds). *The definition of death: contemporary controversies* (pp. 239–256). MD: Johns Hopkins University Press.

2. DO WE ALL HAVE A RESPONSIBILITY TO DONATE OUR ORGANS?

James Lindermann Nelson

INTRODUCTION

Organ Transplantation and What We Owe Each Other

In the latter part of the 20th century, human bodies acquired what is widely seen as an unsettling new ability – their vital organs now have the power to sustain the lives of other human bodies. This new ability has extended the lives of tens of thousands of people around the world, providing the recipients of these organs and those with whom they live with the potential for active, fulfilling years and continued rich relationships that otherwise would be denied them.

It has also spawned enormous difficulties. Some patients have found transplantation, or the associated burdens required to avoid rejecting their new organs, troublesome, unsatisfactory, or unsuccessful, so that little in the way of good quality extra time was provided at all, or was provided only at great cost. Social burdens have been considerable as well, although it is difficult to calculate them accurately, since it is not clear how great have been what might be called the opportunity costs of transplantation medicine. What might have been the outcome of devoting to primary care for inner city kids the resources earmarked for organ transplantation? Would medical, as opposed to surgical, responses to end-stage organ failure be considerably further advanced had less of our resources and attention been directed to developing and improving

The Ethics of Organ Transplantation, Volume 7, pages 43–64.

ISBN: 0-7623-0764-1

transplantation? At the end of the day, might our enthusiasm for transplantation have actually resulted in a net loss of years of life saved?

These are worrisome questions. But there are aspects of organ transplantation just as disturbing as either its demonstrable or its speculative inefficiency as a means of extending human lives. The medical and social decision to invest so heavily in transplantation as a way of dealing with end-stage organ disease has forced us to make what Guido Calabresi and Philip Bobbit called in their celebrated book, *Tragic Choices*, "exposed choices against life" (1978). Notoriously, the supply of transplantable organs persistently lags far behind the demand, requiring society to put together elaborate rationing frameworks. These schemes are, of course, fair game for criticism by bioethicists, philosophers and other scholars. More significantly perhaps, the fairness of prevailing allocation schemes has been challenged by public policy makers, patients, families and citizens generally. This is only to be expected, as notions of what justice demands of us in the allocation of scarce, precious resources are complex, varied, and highly contested. But the disagreements are not academic; insofar as potential donors, for example, find the allocation system unjust, they are the less likely to contribute to it, thus exacerbating the very problem the rationing system must try to solve.

To avoid, or at least relieve, the challenges of rationing, either demand must be reduced – scarcely likely in a time when transplant programs are increasingly willing and able to provide their services to people previously barred from consideration by reason of age or disease states – or supply increased. This essay is about certain neglected moral issues involved in what might be called "supply-side" strategies.

The morality of organ procurement is heavily trodden ground; the literature is full of discussions of the ethics of various plans aimed at increasing their availability. However, I hope to travel this terrain in some different directions. I will ask whether the persistent difficulties in meeting the need for transplantable organs point to something more than glitches in how we advertise and promote donation, or natural and acceptable limits in the degree of altruism we can expect from people, particularly in the tragic circumstances in which organs are so often solicited. I also hope to guide attention away from the growing interest in turning human body parts into marketable commodities as a response to organ shortages. The question that will concern me here can be put this way: might this enduring pattern of allowing organs that could save human lives, to molder away in dead bodies, hint at deep problems within our basic ideas about the social arrangement of contemporary American society?

My pursuit of this question requires re-imagining the new ability of parts of our bodies to sustain other people. I will propose that we see organ transplantation not merely as a technological tour de force, but as a pointed invitation to understand differently the character of our relationships to one another. Responses to the moral challenges occasioned by organ transplantation have taken entrenched moral and political understandings largely as given, and have attempted to fit various procurement and allocation schemes to prevailing normative notions. My aim here is to invert this approach. Specifically, I will be arguing that our collective reluctance to provide more organs to those who need them reflects in some part those features of our culture that encourage us to think of ourselves, and of human goods, in too individualistic a fashion. Liberalism as a political philosophy, or, perhaps more accurately, as a political ideology, may bear some of the blame here, as may certain beliefs and anxieties bound up with certain normative understandings of gender roles. I will argue further that organ transplantation can reasonably be portrayed in ways that may help erode this kind of atomism; indeed, that it invites such portrayal. The image of organ transplantation I hope to make attractive can align itself with less dominant, less aggressively individualistic moral understandings of social and political relationships in general, and in particular, lead to a better appreciation of what we owe each other as potential organ donors.

ORGANS, METAPHORS AND MODELS

I have referred to the potential of sustaining other lives with the use of one's one organs as a " new ability," but people for whom pregnancy has been an experience or is a prospect may not find it quite so novel – female bodies have, after all, always typically possessed a certain form of this ability. But the analogy with pregnancy – or, more accurately, "pregnability" – is not one that has been much invoked in discussions of human organ transplantation. We have not turned to characteristically female reproductive powers and the social meanings that accompany them, as a model for more clearly understanding how we ought to live in the light of the new powers and relationships made possible by organ transplant technology. In fact, the chief acknowledgment of possible analogues between organ provision and pregnancy has moved in quite the opposite direction: it has been argued that since fathers, for instance, cannot be legally forced to provide organs, or even renewable tissues such as bone marrow, for their children, mothers should not be legally forced to provide their body to maintain the lives of fetuses that might become their children.

In the United States we have, rather, turned to metaphors of gift, construing the decision to make organs available or to withhold them as fundamentally a private matter, an expression of charity, rather than an expression of social solidarity, of care for the vulnerable, that we have reasonable grounds to expect of each other. That "gift" rather than "gestation" has been the metaphor of choice may not, on reflection, seem odd: not only are there clearly disanologies between organ provision and pregnancy, but the meaning of pregnancy itself, and of the relationships between gravid women and the fetuses they harbor, is much contested. "Gift," in contrast, is an extremely commodious and not particularly contentious conceptual category. The psychic and social complexities of gifts are hidden by at least a surface agreement on what they are and what they mean. One might even say that it is not metaphoric at all to speak of organs made available for transplant as gifts; under the present dispensation, they are quite literally gifts, so concerns about disanologies are beside the point.

Yet, as I will try to show, thinking of organs as gifts occludes important moral considerations, despite its apparent transparency, while thinking of our ability to use our bodies to support the lives of others in ways influenced by ideas about pregnancy will bring these considerations to the fore, despite the limits of the pregnability metaphor. While the conceptual and moral issues involved with women's reproductive powers are complex, and women's right to control those abilities are of the first importance – indeed, this can scarcely be emphasized sufficiently – pregnancy and pregnability have discernable social and moral meanings that go beyond serving as a backdrop for disputes about whether and when women may choose to reject relationships. At the level of a cultural theme – not to be confused with the level of individual psychology – the kind of intimate nurturing that pregnancy symbolizes is plausibly construed as part of why the idea of the female has been associated with an image of rich and concrete human interconnectedness as the basic moral *mise en scene*, and with care and compassion as both natural tendencies and leading moral ideals. This contrasts with how maleness as a cultural theme has been associated with a more Hobbesian conceit: a sketch of a world within we must always keep our self-interest centrally in view as we try to create somewhat precarious moral relationships with others. Individualism, self-reliance, and contractual relations are the guiding leitmotifs; care beyond contract is seen as wholly or largely discretionary, at least outside of the private sphere.

Some scholars – famously, Gilligan – have argued that women and men do tend to employ different strategies of moral imagination and practical reasoning that reflect these patterns (1982). Yet it is important to stress that acknowledging the presence, power and gendered associations of these themes is not necessarily to enter a claim about how real women and men always or even typically think about their lives and their relationships; there are surely plenty of women who rate independence from others very highly in their own conceptions of the good, plenty of men who cherish relationships intensely, and it's a good thing, too.

The notion, rather, is that such ideas as "connectedness," "relationship," and "caring" tend to cluster both together, and with the idea of femaleness, or perhaps with the feminine, much as "independence," "individuality" and "contract" tend to cluster together and with the idea of maleness or masculinity. These connections make up part of the "ideologies of the moral life" that are prominent in our culture, to borrow a phrase of Cheshire Calhoun's (1988) – ideas that form the horizon of moral imaginations, that incline us to look in certain directions for problems, solutions, and justifications, and nudge us to accept certain moral intuitions, analogies, and metaphors, without themselves pretending to be sound arguments for, or even good reasons to accept, any of these ideas (which is not, of course, to say that there may not be good reasons for promoting a certain ideology of the moral life, as well as good reasons for resisting others). The ways in which moral and political notions, images, and narrative threads have been bundled and gendered have significant effects on how we live and think publicly and communally, even if they may have only tenuous relationships with how particular individuals might experience and make sense of their own lives.

That these ideas have been so bundled and so gendered in our common imagination is in some sense an empirical claim, but one I take to be at least relatively uncontroversial: evidence is available from psychology (e.g. Gilligan, 1982), intellectual and philosophical history (e.g. Lloyd, 1993), and from countless contacts with popular culture that are commonly experienced by people in contemporary America: when Garrison Keeler closes the "News from Lake Woebegone" with the tag line, "All the women are strong, all the men are good looking, and all the children are above average," part of the humor resides in an inversion of standard gender associations; it is Ally McBeal, and not some male sit-com counterpart, who is haunted by a ghost baby. And so forth.

It has also been well established that notions that enjoy an association with the idea of maleness, if not necessarily with the subjectivities of actual men, have had a persistent edge in the competition for effective influence over cultural and political practice. When one turns to important political theorists such as Rawls, what one finds are images of rational self-interested individuals hammering out the terms of their lives together from their ignorance about themselves, not of compassionate agents acting out of their knowledge of each other. When one looks at the pecking order within academic disciplines such as philosophy or economics, what tends to be most prized is the most formal, the most abstract, the least connected with living everyday life, particularly as life is lived in familiar and intimate settings. And, particularly crucial for my purposes here, reigning moral and political theories strongly tend to start with an assumption that it is our distinctness, our separateness that most faithfully signifies what is morally special about persons, and that it is those forms of human activity that broach the barriers between us that need special monitoring and justification.

But one needn't dismiss the importance of Rawls' views, the heuristic richness of formal methods, nor the moral significance of the separateness of selves in observing that there is nothing necessary about either their associations with certain ideas of gender, nor with the way we allow those associations to make gratuitous additions to the cultural authority such ideas deserve on their own merits. In principle, we can both unbundle and reassociate these ideas, and in practice, we have no need to start from scratch. Ways of thinking about culture, philosophy, politics, and policy that are both carefully motivated argumentatively and which draw less on notions identified with the masculine are available to us – feminist approaches, most conspicuously, as well as some understandings of communitarianism – and these approaches may lead to justifying, and even installing, forms of practice that are more effective in responding to real needs. They may also help us clarify, and resonate more deeply with, our best impulses. Insofar as they do, they themselves become more plausible as general pictures of what we should be most concerned with as we direct our own lives, and how we should live with one another. That they lack the imprimatur of a set of social practices that stubbornly continue to privilege what is associated with the masculine over what is associated with the feminine hardly counts as a reason to think otherwise.

Organs as Gifts

Yet before considering what might follow from looking at organ transplantation through the metaphor of pregnability, the claims of the current model need further consideration. The reigning attitude in the U.S. is that organs are not only items that we *may* regard as "gifts," but are, in fact, *essentially* gifts: we may freely withhold or freely give them, but we may not sell them, nor claim them from others as a matter of right, nor even regard the provision of organs as something that is a default assumption of how decent people living in a decent society will treat each other.

To think of human organs as gifts in this specially restricted way has the great merit of practically underscoring the notion that people are morally important in ways that go beyond how they may be resources for each other – the Kantian notion that persons have "dignity but not price" is reinforced here – as well as acknowledging the special relationship between persons and their bodies. The respect owed to persons is itself a scarce and precious resource: any kind of cavalier approach to that of which we are made might with some plausibility be seen as a threat to the coherence of moral attitudes that need protection and continuous renewal.

Yet, whatever its philosophical merits, the gift model has been disastrous for the growing number of people whose lives could be substantially extended via organ transplantation: according to the United Network for Organ Sharing, 4855 people died while on waiting list for organs in 1998 alone; the UNOS total for the years 1988–98 is 32,449 (UNOS OPTN Scientific Registry Data, current as of February 1999, available at www.unos.org). How many people might have lived longer had organs been available, but who never even made it to waiting lists, is unknown, as is the number of life-years that will be lost in the future, if current patterns prevail.

There has been a good deal of ingenuity and effort exerted within the gift model to try to close the lethal gap between generosity and need – U.S. states have "required request" laws, which mandate that family members be asked to donate organs from the bodies of relatives who have died in ways that make them organ procurement candidates, driver's licenses include check-off boxes with which one can identify oneself as a donor, and images of cultural heroes, such as Michael Jordan, are employed to nudge people into being conscious of, and friendly to, the prospect of providing organs to others. Yet the gap remains.

Alternatives: Artifacts, Animals, and the Market

With altruism seemingly stymied, there has been persistent interest in what is surely one of American society's strong suits, technological innovation. As enough transplant organs are not available as gifts, perhaps the solution is to build better artificial organs, or to unlock the intriguing potential of human stem cells to produce human organs, or to deepen our understanding of genetic engineering, so that human bodies can reliably employ retooled animal organs.

Thus far, however, these approaches have run into both technical disappointments and moral challenges of their own. The story of the so-far futile effort to create a totally implantable, permanently indwelling artificial heart, for example, is a cautionary tale of the labyrinthine complexities of both the biology of circulation and politics of technology; xenograft inspires increasing worries, not simply about the moral status of animals who might provide organs to humans, but about the potentially grave public health risks of crossing species barriers in this way (Purdy, 1999). Human embryonic stem cells, with their apparent ability to generate all types of human tissues, are intriguing, but at this point, little more. Further, the process of obtaining such cells, harvested as they are from the inner cell mass of human blastocysts, or from fetal gonadal tissue, is scarcely innocent of moral controversies (Nelson, 2000).

There seems no good reason, therefore, to think that human organs are going to be rendered technologically redundant any time soon. Consequentially, there has seemed to some to be growing reason to turn to America's other strong suit – the market. If conceptualizing organs as essentially gifts does not meet our needs, perhaps we should abandon that notion, and with it the idea that there is something morally objectionable about commodifying non-renewable human body parts. If the law of supply and demand, as understood in free markets, were allowed to operate, then, so experience tends to indicate, supply will rise.

It would be unfair to think that unsettling the gift model in favor of seeing organs as saleable goods recommends itself solely to those who believe that the market is the fundamental form of moral relationship between people. Commodifying organs does not necessarily entail the prospect of people being surgically mutilated for profit during their life-times; that sort of transaction might well still be legally blocked, if enthusiasm for the market does not go so far as to welcome the prospect of impoverished people lining up to sell kidneys and liver lobes. What has been seriously suggested is a more modest, more pragmatic sort of approach to enhancing organ availability through judicious application of mild economic incentives. We might, for example, test how supply is enhanced by providing families of recently deceased potential organ donors with various kinds of fiscal inducements, from defraying funeral or hospital expenses to straight cash payments. People might also be willing to sell "future interests" in their organs, receiving payments in return for a binding undertaking that their organs be used for transplantation, should they happen to die in circumstances that lend themselves to this activity.

There are signs, then, that the social consensus that organs should be regarded as gifts essentially is fraying. While the reluctance to turn objects so closely related to human beings as their non-renewable organs into objects that take on a market value remains fairly robust, it faces a problem: by reserving human body parts from the market we underscore the special significance of the idea of a human being, but in so doing, we may in effect be endorsing the premature deaths of quite concrete instances of that class. This is precisely the dilemma of the gift model: it underscores that special significance, but fails to produce sufficient organs to meet a need whose deep seriousness is a function of that very significance itself. The market model promises to mobilize more transplantable organs, but encroaches on one of the most meaningful ways we have of proclaiming the special moral status of human beings: even in an era of the triumph of markets, humans retain a value that markets cannot calculate. This seems to be just the kind of situation that calls out for new ways of thinking, different models for understanding what is at stake.

Pregnable Selves

Let's return, then, to the notion that organ transplantation creates a new way in which we can be responsible for each others' lives, a way that chips away at the picture of human beings as fundamentally discrete, separate selves, joining their lives intimately only rarely, and only with those they choose, or to whom they are related, as we say, "by blood." Organ transplant makes available a sense in which we are all potentially related to each other "by blood." We now all face the chance that we may be in a position to save another person's life in a way that crucially involves sharing our bodies with those we save.

Does this fact provide us with reason to think of sharing organs as a practice we should, in general, expect from each other? That failure to do so should not be regarded simply as a purely discretionary matter? That we have in fact a duty to provide organs useless to ourselves, but vital to others, unless we have special reason to withhold them?

Not independently of other premises, surely. However, such premises seem very much ready to hand. In fact, it might be maintained that there are arguments concerning our duties to provide needy others with organs not currently of any use to ourselves that are sufficiently strong as to render speculations about new ways of thinking about human selves and their relationships quite beside the point.

BENEFICENCE AND EASY RESCUES

The moral notion of beneficence is key to a simple, plausible argument for a presumptive duty to provide others with organs that may be vital to them but are useless to us. Beneficence is often characterized as the obligation to provide help to those in need, particularly in serious need, if the help can be rendered at little cost to the agent. Accepting such a duty seems to cohere closely, if not strictly follow from, the barest acknowledgment that people other than one's self (and those with whom one may have particular emotional ties) matter morally, and hence that their needs, interests and projects have at least a presumptive moral value too.

It's worth stressing how minimal this assumption is. Accepting beneficence as a moral principle does not require accepting any substantial notion of impartiality, as utilitarianism tends to advocate (Rachels, 1999, p. 115); you needn't think that everyone's interests should count alike in your practical deliberations. What *is* necessary is merely to believe that other people's interests count for something that is not altogether negligible. Someone who dissented from this very weak form of beneficence, and yet who wanted to maintain that she did not regard other people as altogether bereft of moral worth, would presumably have to see the freedom to direct one's own agency in whatever way she chose as having an extraordinary kind of super-value, one that comes within hailing distance of trumping all other moral reasons. Such a position is not without adherents, but it is, to put the matter gently, strongly counterintuitive.

Just how counterintuitive can be vividly appreciated by considering the "duty of easy rescue" most familiarly illustrated (and motivated) by stories about children tripping, hitting their heads, and falling insensate into shallow ponds. Confronted with such stories, most people will allow that not extracting from their predicament any such children as we might come across is gravely wrong, at least absent very strong reasons for acting otherwise. If personal freedom were a value strong enough to trump beneficence, then any contrary whim would be enough to exempt a non-rescuer from the charge of grave wrongdoing.

Easy rescue examples can be multiplied without strain, particularly if we are willing to settle for TV standards of fidelity to ordinary experience: one of those run-away trolley cars beloved of contemporary moral philosophers threatens to run over five people helplessly tied to the tracks, and, quite without inconvenience, you can push a switch diverting it to an unoccupied siding. Can individual liberty, worthy of reverence though it is, justify you in not pushing the switch?

But there's really no need to visit the philosophical trolley yard. There's nothing outlandish about imagining an encounter with someone absorbed in thought, who wanders into the path of an oncoming car. A sharp shout from you will effectively bring her to a more realistic grasp of her situation. Inaction in such cases may be in principle excusable, but as most will surely agree, you'd need to be supplied with unusually good reasons to avoid the conclusion that you had done something very wrong indeed if you kept your mouth shut. Freedom of the individual does not seem up to the job.

What can be learned from such examples? At least this, I think: there is a strong presumption that refusing to save another person's life, when doing so is virtually costless to the person in a position to act, is seriously wrong. And it might seem that the implications of this point for a duty to provide your organs to those in need, should it occur that you no longer have any need for them, are quite straightforward: absent some consideration that makes allowing one's organs to save the lives of other unusually burdensome, we all have a duty to take such steps as are readily available to bring it about that our organs are provided to others in need, should we happen to die in the appropriate ways.

Is this inference drawn too quickly? As I have already allowed, it is, for example, at least open to question whether organ transplantation is, all things considered, an appropriate way for societies to allocate their resources. Accordingly, so some might argue, any "duty to donate" might be defeated by considerations of justice. However, even if some system other than organ procurement and transplantation might be more efficient a method of extending life years, it is not clear how that circumstance frees us from the duty in question. Building fences might be a more reliable way of keeping children from drowning in tempting ponds than is relying on the adventitious proximity of someone willing to get her sleeves wet. But the superior efficiency of fences hardly gives anyone good grounds not to rescue the child they happen to come across.

What does require extended attention is the idea that a person's relationship to parts of her body is not the same as her relationship to the things that she possesses, or, perhaps, even to the deeds she does. On the plausible notion that we do not so much own, but rather are our bodies, granting others the use of our organs, even if those organs no longer form parts of a living whole, is a matter of letting others have some of us. And once we realize this, or so someone might suppose, we will be less likely to think that the dire need of others underpins a beneficence, "easy rescue" based duty such that the posthumous provision of organs is virtually costless, except to those with somewhat idiosyncratic values. For willingness to provide our organs to others after our own deaths is can reasonably be seen as agreeing to a kind of intimacy that cannot be expected as a matter of a duty.

So the "easy rescue" argument may not be able to show on its own that a willingness to provide organs upon your death is a reasonable moral default assumption. It is precisely in response to this concern that the reason organ transplantation provides to reorient how we think of ourselves among others may turn out to be useful.

ORGAN DONATION AND/AS INTIMATE RELATIONSHIP

The idea that serving as an organ source involves a kind of intimate sharing of one's self is powerfully illustrated in Richard Selzer's short story, "Follow Your Heart" (Selzer, 1990). The story revolves around a woman named Hannah, whose husband Samuel died three years before the story's start, on his thirty-third birthday, shot in the head while helping someone change a tire by the side of road. Hannah agreed that Samuel's organs should be harvested for transplant, and later receives a letter informing her that

> your husband's liver has gone to a lady in McAlpine: the right kidney is functioning in Dallas; the left kidney was placed in a teenage girl in Galveston; the heart was given to a man just your husband's age in a little town near the Arkansas border; the lungs are in Fort Worth, and the corneas were used on two people right here in Houston . . . (p. 52).

Hannah is not comforted by this letter. In fact, she starts to think of herself as suspended in limbo, not quite a wife, not quite a widow, her husband not alive, but not altogether dead. One night she dreams of her husband and another man, and watches as a surgeon extracts Samuel's heart and places it in the other man's chest, who then sits up, puts on his shirt, and goes on his way.

On awakening, Hannah is immediately clear about what she must do:

> What was instantly made clear to her – it was so simple – was that she must go to find that man who was carrying Samuel's heart. If she could find him and listen once more to the heart, she would be healed (p. 55).

And, of course, after overcoming many obstacles and much reluctance on the part of the recipient, Mr. Pope, that is just what she does.

> Then Hannah bent her head and slowly lowered her ear toward his left, his secret sharing, nipple . . . Oh, it was Samuel's heart, all right. She knew it the minute she heard it. She could have picked it out of a thousand. Hadn't she listened to it just this way often enough? Hadn't she listened with her head on his chest, and heard it slow down after they had made love? It was like a little secret she knew about his body, and it had always made her smile to know the effect she had on him (p. 62).

The hour she spends listening to Samuel's heart in Mr. Pope's chest does indeed heal her – Selzer writes that she leaves with "the certainty that she had at last been retrieved from the shadows and set down once more upon the bright lip of her life" (p. 62).

Selzer's story explores organ transplantation as giving rise to a new set of meanings that are bound up with intimacy and renewal. The transplantation of Samuel's organs has changed his relationship to his wife in a way that his death alone would not; it has put her in a kind of intimate relationship with strangers that she otherwise would not have, and which she must acknowledge in an act of intimacy – an act that allows her life to go on, as her husband's post mortem intimacy with Mr. Pope allowed his life to go on. His story makes tolerably plain that there are dimensions to organ transplantation not quite captured by the easy rescue model.

Aaron Ridley has tried to turn an intuition like the one that seems to be driving Hannah into an argument. His target is the proposal that the dead should be seen as a source of organs for the needy living, without requiring anything in the way of explicit permission from an advance directive executed by the now-dead person, or even the consent of the family. I note that this is not the same position being advocated here: it is possible that a person could have a duty to do something, while it is yet wrong for others to make her do it. But there is enough contact between what Ridley wants to attack and I to defend to make a consideration of his view appropriate.

Although the dead are, Ridley admits, strictly speaking beyond harm, to treat them as though they were on that basis simply resources for the living is to misunderstand in a very general way just what human beings are. It is to see us as owning, rather than being, our bodies. Ridley thinks that if we take the "no harm can come to the dead" view as justifying routinely retrieving organs, then we have accepted a justification that would allow any kind of use of dead bodies. He imagines using human organs as targets in a shooting gallery set up to promote a charity, quite understandably refers to such a practice as "in appalling taste" and "vile," and intimates that the considerations that show why we properly respond to the shooting gallery notion with repugnance shows too, that routine harvesting of human organs would also fail to acknowledge the respect appropriately due to people (Ridley, 1998, p. 257–258.)

It is important that Ridley takes himself to be describing, not just an understanding one might reasonably have of the significance of one's body, but a view that *must* be held, on pain of having otherwise a confused understanding of what human beings are and why they matter; one gets the impression that he is concerned that any other view flirts with a sort of dualism. However, there are a number of possible attitudes one can have toward one's body without being clearly confused, either metaphysically or morally. You can reasonably think of the matter as Ridley does: we are our bodies. Or, you might reasonably think that we are our *living* bodies, and when we die, we are no longer to be identified with the non-living body. On such a view, at death we do not start existing as a corpse; we simply no longer exist. Our corpse is a kind of property then, a part of the estate we leave behind us.

There are no doubts other reasonable contenders. But a single alternative will do to counter Ridley's claim to uniquely accommodate our intuitions regarding the shooting gallery scenario. Using parts of dead human bodies as targets, even for charity, may be appalling because human bodies deserve respect due to their tight correlations with living human beings, and because to use them as targets is to use them as we use cheap, disposable artifacts. If parts of human corpses are someone's property, this conclusion is not invalidated: flags, first editions, and Flemish masterpieces are all property, and yet many people would have a similar response if the Stars and Stripes, a Gutenberg Bible, or Rembrandt's *Night Watch* were to be used for target practice.

Further, the kind of good that transplantation pursues is of deep moral significance and, generally, not available otherwise. Human organs are not being used in roles for which we might as well as use paper bullseyes or clay pigeons. Nor has transplantation the kinds of emotional or symbolic resonances as has the practice of plunging bullets into parts of human bodies.

But rather than push these points further, I want to acknowledge the power in Selzer's story, and to accept that a plausible way of accounting for that power is Ridley's contention that human organs are and continue to be part of the human beings they originally helped to constitute. Would such an understanding provide a person with good reason to withhold her organs from someone who is likely to die if they are withheld?

This, I think, depends on the general stance we take concerning the relationship between ourselves and others, what we might call the "default attitude." There are, as I have already suggested, powerful cultural norms that install the attitude that our separateness is a greatly important feature about human beings, taken to be closely connected conceptually to integrity and dignity, and causally bolstered by its association with masculinity as a culturally normative notion. Intimacy with others, in part because it imperils certain notions of "normative masculinity," is seen as something of a threat to us, or to many of us. But I do not believe that the only way we can acknowledge or cherish the significance of our distinctiveness or of our intimate relationships is by means of attitudes that have as a consequence that thousands die what are in effect untimely deaths.

The fact that we can give vital parts of ourselves to others, sustaining their ability to act and to experience even after our own is gone, can be seen as a highly concrete affirmation of our continuing interest, and indeed, participation of a kind, in the weal of our communities after our own deaths. The connection to pregnancy, and more broadly, to parenthood, is patent: if one of the ways in which people tend to see parenthood is as a way of continuing their own influence and interests into a future they will not experience, and if part of what inclines us to see the matter this way is our physical connection to our children, we should be able to see organ transplantation in something of the same way.

Indeed, this is not merely a way in which some people might come to see organ donation – a new advertising strategy that might be used after the impact of the Michael Jordan campaign is over – but rather a construction of the practice of organ sharing that is not only possible, but which we have strong moral reason to accept, precisely since it avoids any cheapening of the significance of human beings, their parts and their relationships, while extending human lives. I will now argue that the task of accepting this sort of view is not only a personal challenge, but a matter of public interest as well.

ORGAN PROCUREMENT AND POLITICAL PHILOSOPHY

I take it that "easy rescue" type considerations provide us with strong presumptive reasons to provide organs for people who need them, even given an appropriate understanding of the significance of human organs and human intimacy; accepting Ridley's view of the relationship of human selves and human bodies does not derail this conclusion. We have available and should take seriously a way of thinking about ourselves and our relationships that endorses our metaphoric pregnability – that is, the ability of our bodies to sustain lives other than our own, and the affiliated notion that such an ability fosters moral attitudes that elevate connection over discreteness as the distinguishing way in which we think about ourselves as morally worthy beings. We have reason to accept such a view, at least because it is not inconsistent with any demonstrably correct understanding of who and what we are, and because it allows us to recognize and discharge duties of easy rescue, saving lives that other understandings squander.

Hence, I am inclined to think that people typically have duties to provide organs to others, should the opportunity arise, and indeed, duties to reconsider and possibly to refigure their attitudes about themselves and others insofar as those attitudes threaten their inclinations to act in accordance with this duty. It could be argued against this conclusion, however, that the very need to revamp attitudes may make the duty in question no longer one of easy rescue, at least for many people; recalcitrant attitudes, difficult to shift, would not threaten our performance of our duty, but rather excuse us from it.

It is not immediately clear how serious this objection is. Ridley hoped to argue that seeing dead human bodies as a standing reserve of organs was inconsistent not simply with certain attitudes, but with attitudes backed by an appropriate understanding of what humans are and why they matter. But this view, I have argued, is mistaken; we can properly regard and honor ourselves while at the same time acknowledging the possibility and importance of the kind of intimate relationship with other people that transplantation involves, and the greater possibility of saving lives with such an attitude itself provides us with strong reason to endorse it. Imagine someone coming upon the drowning child who has a strong view about the importance of a carefully crafted appearance. She feels that her own dignity is importantly caught up with the way she and her surroundings look, and pays careful attention to maintaining the appearances. Pulling the child out of the pond can threaten the integrity of her look; rather than *chic*, she'll be soggy. Does this give her sufficient grounds to let the child drown?

This example has some analogies to the case at hand. Just as the feelings about the self Ridley describes are morally open to people, so there is nothing intrinsically wrong with the notion that human dignity can be effectively conveyed through careful attention to order and appearance; it is not as though the person's reluctance to rescue is a matter of prejudice against the ethnicity of the drowning child. But neither is the analogy perfect. The kind of individualistic understandings of self-and-body boundaries that drive the reluctance to donate organs being considered here are tolerably widespread and entrenched. What I think it does show is that our moral intuitions are not satisfied with an understanding of easy rescue in which "easy" means roughly the same as "costless." More particularly, it suggests that, if we harbor attitudes that make otherwise easy rescues difficult, we have moral reason to wish things were different in our own psychic economies. In the light of easy rescue opportunities blocked by patterns of attitudes that seem themselves in some sense optional, such as a passion for order and style, we should desire that such attitudes would in the right circumstances be temporarily silenced. In the case at hand, we have reason to wish that a sense of violated boundaries might be transfigured into a more accommodating notion of ourselves and our relationships.

This consideration brings into play the social aspect of the question of organ retrieval, since social practices and understandings can do a great deal to install and nurture certain patterns of feeling. The question I now want to consider is whether we can regard providing organs to others as a practice that should form part of a collection of duties recognized socially, and facilitated through public policy and law. Could a good society enforce an organ provision duty, in a way at least weakly analogous to how conscription is enforced, or to take what is perhaps a better example, to how service on juries is mandatory? If a certain conception of human relationships facilitates that duty, may such a society foster it?

Proposing the details of a revised system of organ procurement is not part of my present ambition, but certain features of the policy I have in mind do need to be mentioned. I proposed a weak analogy between organ provision and such standing social duties as jury duty or the draft here in part because the standard for exemption from providing organs should, as I see it, be entirely subjective; if you want "conscientious objector" status, you can get it simply by self-proclamation. No review board nor judge need concur that your reasons are adequate, nor that you are sincere. So "opting out" would be an easy matter.

But it is important to be clear that a "presumed consent" policy is not what's on the table. The policy in question does not rest on the assumption that most people would consent to be organ donors. The animating principle, rather, is that, should the correct circumstances arise, people are obligated to provide organs, unless excusing conditions are present, and that is no abuse of state power to aid citizens in the exercise of this duty.

This last point might be thought to take some showing. In particular, it might be thought that justifying a communitarian understanding of the citizen-polity relationship would be required, particularly as I have suggested that fostering certain images of the nature and significance of human relatedness may well be a crucial role for the state to play. For it will surely strike many that liberal political philosophy will be inhospitable to such a role, or to a political recognition of this duty at all. Even if the moral arguments in support of a presumptive duty to provide organs were strong enough to do the job without the need for ideas about organ provision as making people in general metaphorically pregnable, they should not be countenanced at the political level. To do so would require relying on arguments drawing on specific, contestable understandings of the good. But that is precisely what liberalism abhors. This is true even if it could be shown that an understanding of beneficence strong enough to generate a duty to provide organs is very broadly recognized in a polity. The arguments purporting to show that there is a duty of beneficence are surely not so strong as to make a person flat-out irrational if she does not accept them. Further, if many of us would need to refashion our understanding of intimacy and of how to mark the significance of our bodies to remove barriers to appreciating the call of beneficence here, that would seem even more reason to expect a liberal political order to reject the notion that any such moral duty, involving not only a contestable notion of the good, but also the need to adopt new forms of self-understanding, could have political countenance.

Communitarianism, on the other hand, seems much more hospitable to recognizing a duty of organ provision. Communitarians don't, after all, have to worry about justificatory neutrality: if the value of providing organs is inseparable from some (set of) visions of the good, or if certain understandings of intimacy facilitate people's appreciation of the duty, that's not an in-principle problem. Cherishing the notion that people ought to see their own good as complexly intertwined with the good of others, and hence that we should do more for each other might well be part of the conception of the good that a political community sees as part of its point to promote. Indeed, this might seem more than just a notional possibility: socially promoting beneficence seems to cohere with communitarianism's spirit, since communitarian theories of the self underscore the significance of "encumbrance," of identification with significant features of one's community, including its moral commitments, as an essential feature of a person's identity. A person's relationship to the community and its values is not, as it is on the liberal vision, ultimately a matter of choice exerted from some more or less nominal perspective; the relationship between community and self-understanding, to what provides us with the "why" of our choices and actions, is much tighter, in part at least constitutive rather than elective.

If the analysis so far is on track, we're left with these questions: is the ability to accommodate politically the conclusions for which powerful moral arguments can be made a mark in favor of a given political conception? If communitarianism is superior to liberalism in this respect, is that is a reason to suppose it may be superior *tout court*?

It would seem that if tolerance is indeed as important a personal and political virtue as we generally assume (and as centuries of violence in the name of certain conceptions of the good would seem to demonstrate) then any such inferences would seem much too quick – or at least the operative sense of "reason to suppose" would have to be extremely weak. What would at least need to be shown to provide this political philosophy with any real support is that communitarianism – or, more precisely, some version of communitarianism – not only accommodates a significant moral conclusion that liberalism cannot, but that the form of communitarianism in question is no more likely to lead to disrespect, coercion or violence toward dissenters than its liberal rival, such tolerance of pluralism standing as the significant moral conclusion that liberalism prides itself on accommodating.

The typical moves against liberalism include maintaining that liberalism's vaunted neutrality is overstated – i.e. that its justificatory strategies are not altogether innocent of certain contentious assumptions about what has value – while also averring that the kind of neutrality to which liberalism aspires in principle would render it practically ineffective if achieved. This has been argued effectively, to choose but one example, in Ezeckiel Emanuel's *The Ends of Human Life* (1991), where he focuses on medical ethical case studies to show that only specific, contestable constellations of values can put sufficient content into bioethical principles and policies for them to have a practical impact on deliberation and action.

Such criticisms speak to whether liberalism, as a viable political philosophy, has a unique claim to tolerance and respect for value pluralism. If they are warranted, and liberalism is unable to function absent commitment to, in principle, reasonably contestable values, then it becomes one substantive political philosophy among others, not a referee for contending conceptions of the good, floating on a cloud of purely procedural justice above the fray. Seen as itself a conception of the good, it still has an important contributions to make to political life. We might reasonably assign it the job of vigilantly warning rival views about the dangers inherent in uncritically enacting policies that are justified by, and help entrench, richly contentful conceptions of the good, particularly (though not solely) on people whose normative commitments are other than those endorsed by the view in question. Such warning, however, along with appropriate responses, must proceed without pretending that public policy could altogether avoid drawing on such conceptions.

The liberal warning could be taken to heart by exposing policy proposals to various kinds of questions. One might be called the *convergence question*: is the moral goal in view, and the practices, virtues and understandings that facilitate its attainment, reasonable from a variety of normative perspectives? Justifying a goal or practice simply by avowing, "this is our way," may make sense within certain communities, but it is not the best ground for putting the power of a modern state embedded in a pluralistic culture behind a policy. To the extent that a given policy suggestion can be motivated by a variety of viable moral and political perspectives, we have reason to suppose that enacting it does not constitute wrongdoing.

A second query might be called the *fallibilism question*. A social policy that involves marshaling common resources in service of a certain conception of the good needs to strike a balance between a sincere endorsement of its characteristic constellation of values, and fallibilism, the recognition that the animating conception of the good could be mistaken in its views about what is most worth pursuing, or that the policy might be mistaken about how the good is best to be pursued. This goes beyond merely recognizing the durability of value pluralism. The point is not merely that, despite whatever a state might choose to do, not every inhabitant will accept the schedule of values reflected in its actions. Nor is it solely the moral conviction that respecting a person's conception of the good is caught up with respecting that person herself, important as such respect is. It is, rather, the epistemic point that, however good the considerations that speak in favor of a given ranking of goods, or in support of particular strategies for attaining them, it is possible that other considerations may come to show that this ranking or those strategies are mistaken. In honoring dissent, a community provides itself with an important resource for the continual renewal of its own moral visions.

A third concern might be called *least infringement*. It is surely reasonable to prefer those policies that expose dissenters to the least significant intrusions upon their way of life consistent with progress toward the goal.

In terms of these considerations, social policies designed to increase the availability of transplantable organs, and to foster a notion of human interrelationship that emphasizes what connects rather than what separates us, fare well. There's clearly much more than "this is our way" to be said for the goal of increasing the availability of transplantable organs, and what there is to be said can be heard from a great many moral locations.

But what of the means to this end that have been suggested here? Is there not something more controversial in trying to get state backing for a particular vision of how people are related to one another? The answer to this sort of question depends, in part, on the extent to which one believes that neutrality about such matters is possible. If modern states willy-nilly endorse and promulgate certain visions of human relationships, then the issue is not, may the state do so, but what are the appropriate constraints on which visions it chooses and which means it employs to install them. For issues of means, it seems that the same questions are pertinent as for issues about ends: To the extent that the means are reasonable, in that they do not impose heavy burdens on dissenters, and that dissent is both possible and honored – in that, for example, the means are promulgated in ways that do not by-pass rational agency and are themselves open for review and debate – the view should pass muster.

How might government power facilitate a wider appreciation of other ways of looking at human relationships? In large part, such shifts require much in the way of cultural, rather than political support, and "mediating structures" would no doubt have a good bit to do in reorienting the way people think about themselves and others. Organ procurement might well serve as a useful lever for unsettling the current view. Imagine, for example, religious leaders discussing organ procurement in terms that stress duty and relationship, rather than gift and discretion, imaginative writers and other artists exploring the pregnability metaphor. But the very movement by government authorities toward an "opt-out" system – including the political debates that would no doubt occur – could make available to people the thought that there are alternatives to thinking about transplantation as gifts, and that, although those alternatives require specific conceptions of the good and of the significance of human relationship, such conceptions have much to be said for them.

Reasonable forms of communitarianism – by which I mean those that appreciate the epistemic and moral consequences of pluralism – have this advantage over prevailing understandings of liberalism, I believe: they allow for, and even encourage the possibility of political discourse about ends, and not just means, about the kind of people we should be, and the kind of communities in which we should live. It seems to me possible to engage in such discourse, and even to come to certain practical conclusions as a result of deliberation, that are not essentially oppressive or alienating; indeed, quite the contrary. If organ provision, and similar easy rescues are to be acknowledged as duties in U.S. public policy, we will need to reflect about what kind of people we are, what kind of people we want to be, and how we might move, both individually and as a community, from where we are to where we would like to be. Neither pluralism nor fallibilism entails that large-scale polities are either morally or practically barred from discussing ends, and from using commodious conceptions of the good, emerging from appropriately structured forms of reasoning, as the basis of social policy – so long as appropriate provisions for dissenters are in place.

And finally, while I don't regard seeing the provision of organs as a duty, rather than as a choice, as inherently illiberal (easy rescue arguments, with ample accommodation for dissenters, probably are justifiable in the kinds of liberal polities that allow any form of presumptively mandatory contribution, such as service on juries, to the community), it seems to me that it is more likely to be a part of the social policy of a country that sees connectedness, or as it is more ordinarily called, solidarity as social value along with liberty, and can engage in political discussion about how such goods relate to each other. In fact, organ procurement policy as an expression of solidarity does not merely facilitate the scope of easy rescue arguments, but constitutes the basis of an argument for the provision duty which is motivationally and conceptually distinct from easy rescue, lacking the calculations of benefit to others versus harms to self that easy rescue suggests. Given communitarian understandings of the relationship between people and the groups in which they live, understanding organ procurement through the lens of the pregnability metaphor can turn the availability of these life-extending resources from a "convergent" to a "common" good, to use a distinction of Charles Taylor's (1989) – that is, from something we all happen to value from the perspective of its contribution to our own ends, to something we value because it represents our acknowledgment of each other's worth. Taylor has argued that the availability of common goods actually enhances rather than threatens the legitimacy of political orders.

Many individual fates have been touched by organ transplantation, and many more might be. But there are other benefits lying latent in this nexus of technology and social practices, benefits not just to individuals, but to communities: a deepened appreciation of our interdependence, desire for common weal, and not only individual prospering. Ironically, to obtain a richer helping of the individual benefits, we may need to think more creatively about a topic that high tech medical innovation is not much associated with, in fact has often been presented as inimical to – the fate we share.

ACKNOWLEDGMENTS

As is usually the case, I am indebted to Hilde Lindemann Nelson for a close reading of an earlier draft. A remote ancestor of this article was given as a contribution to a panel discussion on communitarianism and bioethics at the American Society for Bioethics and Humanities held on October 30, 1999. The panel was ably organized by Professor Mark Kuczewski of the Medical College of Wisconsin, and I am thankful to have been invited to participate.

REFERENCES

Calabresi, G., & Bobbit, P. (1978). *Tragic Choices*. New York: W. W. Norton.

Calhoun, C. (1989). Justice, care, gender bias. *J. Philosophy, 85*, 451–463.

Emanuel, E. (1991). *The Ends of Human Life*. Cambridge, MA: Harvard University Press.

Gilligan, C. (1982). *In a Different Voice*. Cambridge MA: Harvard University Press.

Lloyd, E. (1993). *The Man of Reason: "Male" and "Female" in Western Philosophy*. (2nd ed.). New York: Routledge.

Nelson, J. L. (2000). Ethics and embryos. *Forum for Applied Research and Public Policy, 15*, 40–53.

Purdy, L. (1999). Should we put the 'xeno' in transplant? (unpublished, on file with the author).

Rachels, J. (1999). *The Elements of Moral Philosophy*. New York: Mc-Graw Hill.

Ridley, A. (1998). *Beginning Bioethics*. New York: St. Martin's.

Rosenbaum, S. (1989). *Liberalism and the Moral Life*. Cambridge, MA: Harvard University Press.

Selzer, R. (1990). Follow your heart. Redbook, September.

Taylor, C. (1989). Cross purposes: the liberal-communitarian debate. In: S. Rosenbaum (1989).

3. SHOULD WE ADOPT A MARKET STRATEGY TO ORGAN DONATION?

Julia D. Mahoney

INTRODUCTION

Over the past three decades, technological advances have transformed organ transplantation from an experimental procedure into a highly effective therapy, resulting in an ever-increasing need for transplantable organs. Regrettably, the supply of suitable organs has failed to keep pace with the demand and, as a consequence, each year thousands of patients die while awaiting organ transplants (Porter, 1997). To date, efforts to secure an adequate supply of life-saving organs have relied on appeals to altruism, but the results of this system have proved disappointing. While studies indicate widespread public support for the idea of organ transplantation, in practice a large number of individuals exhibit reluctance or unwillingness to donate their own organs or those of their deceased family members (Marshall et al., 1996; Siminoff et al., 1995).

The acute shortage of transplantable organs has sparked a fierce and impassioned debate over what measures ought to be taken to increase the available supply. Of the options under consideration, among the most controversial is the use of financial incentives, enabling the sources of organs (or, in some instances, their surviving family members) to receive valuable consideration in exchange for consenting to organ removal. Although the notion of paying individuals money for body parts triggers revulsion and disgust (Kass, 1992), the need for more organs has convinced medical, legal

The Ethics of Organ Transplantation, Volume 7, pages 65–88.
2001 by Elsevier Science Ltd.
ISBN: 0-7623-0764-1

and ethical experts that financial incentives merit careful consideration (Hansmann, 1989).

The argument advanced by proponents of financial incentives is simple: If the price offered for a particular good is raised, basic economic theory enables us to predict with a high degree of confidence that the available supply of that good will increase. In other words, potential donors of transplantable organs can be expected to respond positively to the prospect of financial rewards (Cohen, 1995). Opponents of financial incentives, by contrast, question the assertion that making compensation available will prove an effective strategy for increasing the supply of transplantable organs, on the grounds that offers of payment might provoke outrage, thereby causing potential organ providers to refuse to make organs available under any circumstances (Prottas, 1992). Moreover, opponents fear that payments for organs would make society as a whole worse off by causing human beings and their usable parts to be viewed as nothing more than saleable commodities and reducing or eliminating altruistically motivated gifts (Caplan et al., 1993).

This chapter examines the controversy over financial incentives for organ donors, and discusses how compensation arrangements for organ sources might function. I argue that while the rhetoric of the debate over financial incentives suggests that the adherents and opponents of financial incentives have sharply contrasting views on legal and ethical issues relating to organ transplantation, in reality the two sides are in substantial agreement on a number of key issues. Understanding the areas of consensus brings into focus the points of actual disagreement, and provides a foundation for thinking about which forms of market compensation are likely to prove both acceptable and effective.

I begin by surveying what I see as the three most important points of (often unacknowledged) agreement. First and foremost, transplantable organs are already the subject of market activity, for human organs are continually exchanged for valuable consideration. Although the most important issue in the debate over financial incentives is often described as *whether* transplantable organs will become market commodities, in fact human organs are already bought and sold every day as part of the provision of transplant services, albeit under highly regulated conditions. Contrary to the claims of a number of opponents of financial incentives, compensating organ sources would not transform organ transplantation from a system based on generosity to one based on the pursuit of self-interest. Instead, such payments would simply expand the group of individuals who are eligible to share in the substantial financial returns generated by organ transplantation. The second point of tacit agreement is that some regulation of commerce in human organs is necessary, for both fervent supporters and determined opponents of payments to organ sources recognize the need for reasonable and appropriate regulation in order to protect the health of the public and the safety of organ providers and transplant recipients. Finally, all participants in the debate over financial incentives concur that although human components are, in many instances, now worth considerable sums of money, the value of a human being can never be equated with the economic value of her constituent parts.

After reviewing the points on which widespread agreement prevails, this chapter turns to the areas of genuine controversy. Supporters and opponents of financial incentives disagree, often bitterly, on two key issues. One is the importance of insisting that organ sources make transplantable organs available out of altruism, rather than self-interest. The other is whether financial incentives would actually work. Resolution of the first issue demands careful consideration of the circumstances under which members of society ought to be encouraged to perform altruistic acts for others. So far, supporters of altruism have failed to provide convincing justifications for the purported superiority of altruism. As to the second issue, whether financial incentives would prove effective is an empirical question, and although it is impossible to provide a definitive answer to that question, available evidence indicates that compensating organ sources has the potential to alleviate the organ shortage.

THE EXISTENCE OF MARKETS IN TRANSPLANTABLE ORGANS

At present, federal law, as well as the laws of many states, prohibits payments to organ sources for any organ to be used for transplantation purposes (Cohen, 1995). The National Organ Transplantation Act (NOTA), passed in 1984, states, "it shall be unlawful for any person to knowingly acquire, receive, or otherwise transfer any human organ for valuable consideration for use in human transplantation if the transfer affects interstate commerce." Under the terms of the statute, the definition of "human organ" includes hearts, livers, kidneys, pancreases, and corneas. The restriction on payments to organ sources contained in NOTA was enacted in haste, without extensive legislative debate, in the wake of press reports that a former physician intended to establish a brokerage firm that would buy organs from third world residents for resale to transplant patients in the United States (Joralemon, 1995; Cohen, 1995).

NOTA's prohibition on payments for organs used in transplantation does not extend to all transactions. Although it is commonplace to state that the effect of NOTA is to make markets in transplantable organs illegal, NOTA contains exceptions for "reasonable payments associated with removal and transportation" made by transplant centers to Organ Procurement Organizations (OPOs), the non-profit firms that distribute organs under the system administered by the United Network for Organ Sharing (UNOS). Moreover, NOTA does not restrict the ability of transplant programs to sell these organs to patients as part of a comprehensive package of transplant services. Transplantable organs are scarce and desirable resources and rights to their possession and use carry substantial economic value (Childress, 1997). NOTA does not prevent these precious rights to transplantable organs from *ever* being exchanged for valuable consideration. Rather, the practical impact of NOTA is to prohibit payments at the initial stage, when the organ is collected from its human source.

This distinction is critical, because the failure to comprehend the existence of markets in organs has distorted the debate over compensating organ sources. A great deal of the unease over payments to organ donors is rooted in the conviction that human body parts are incompatible with functioning markets, and that organs should never be the subject of bargained-for exchanges (Murray, 1996). The language that accompanies such protestations creates the misleading impression that transplantable organs are given away, not sold, and that the forces of altruism alone, unsullied by the desire for financial reward, are responsible for guiding transplantable organs from the original possessor to the final recipient. Organ transplantation is said to belong to the world of the gift, which is frequently contrasted with the world of the market (Murray, 1996). Speaking of human organs as gifts creates the impression that OPOs and transplant programs function as mere intermediaries, charged with delivering the organs from donors to transplant patients.

The truth is more complicated: while the initial transfer of a transplantable organ is gratuitous, subsequent transfers are the result, at least in part, of institutions pursuing their financial self-interest. Moreover, in most instances transplant *recipients* can obtain needed replacement organs only if they are covered by Medicare, Medicaid, private medical insurance or are otherwise in a position to pay for the transplant (Evans, 1989). This means that desperately ill transplant patients obtain new organs only if they or a third party acting on their behalf are willing and able to *purchase* such organs. The cruel reality, then, is that ability to pay is an important component of the organ allocation system, for only those who clear the financial hurdle are eligible to obtain organs.

Although transplant programs frequently assert that patients are charged not for the organ itself, but only for transplant services, this distinction is nonsensical. Transplant services are worthless without an accompanying organ, in the same way that transplantable organs are devoid of value without transplantation services. The notion that transplant programs charge only for medical services, but provide the organ at no charge, is akin to an assertion that restaurants charge for "dining services," while the food itself is not a commodity (Mahoney, 2000). However soothing to public sentiment the assertion that organs are not the subject of bargained-for exchanges may be, the fact remains that the rights to possess and use transplantable organs are exchanged for valuable consideration at several points in the distribution process. While organ providers and their relatives are not permitted to exchange transplantable organs for valuable consideration, other participants in the transplantation process are. As a result, the debate over compensating organ sources and their survivors does not turn on whether transplantable organs will be bought and sold, but on the permissible terms and conditions of market activity.

The acceptance of the existence of markets in human organs presents, at first glance, a perplexing puzzle. If the idea of markets in human organs sparks such horror, why have no proposals been advanced to eliminate all market activity in organs? Why do self-identified opponents of markets confuse payments to organ sources with commercial activity in organs, and conclude that if organ sources go uncompensated then, by definition, markets have been eliminated? If commerce in human organs is genuinely repugnant, one could argue, then surely the opponents of markets ought to be insisting that organs be donated at every stage, for only if rights to possess or use transplantable organs are never exchanged for anything of value can organs be regarded as not commodified. Yet instead of insisting that the ban on commerce be extended to all transactions involving organs, even the fiercest opponents of compensation nevertheless accept a régime under which rights to transplantable organs are, in effect, sold.

The answer to this conundrum illustrates that the opponents of financial incentives are not, in practice, intractable foes of commerce in transplantable organs. Proposals that would have the effect of ending commerce in transplantable organs are not under consideration for the simple reason that the present system would collapse if financial returns were made unavailable at each and every stage of the transplantation process. No one thinks that the current level of organ transplantation services would be maintained if transplant programs were prohibited from collecting payments for transplanting new organs into their patients. To articulate such a possibility is to reveal its absurdity, for everyone understands that many transplant centers would close if they were forced to depend, in whole, on charitable donations and public funding to meet their operating expenses. Insisting on a purely altruistic system would lead to a sharp increase in human suffering, as the number of transplants plummeted.

One might argue that the present system amounts to an ideal compromise: limited market activity in human organs is permitted but the popular image of the human body as not for sale remains intact. Insisting that organ sources not be compensated fosters the impression that transplantation is based on altruism, and that the institutions involved in organ transplantation are engaged in a wholly charitable enterprise, one with no business overtones. The misunderstandings about the extent of markets in transplantable organs, unfortunately, have had a detrimental impact on deliberations over the desirability of financial compensation for organ sources. A great deal of energy has been expended debating *whether* human organs ought to be exchanged for valuable consideration, when in fact that question was answered long ago in the affirmative. Discussions of the merits of commodifying human organs have distracted public focus from the real controversies, which amount to disputes over what the extent of the market in transplantable organs should be.

The conclusion that some level of market activity is inevitable does not, of course, suggest that all transfers of organs ought to be sales rather than donations, or that extending the operation of markets by offering financial incentives to organ sources is *necessarily* a good idea. Rather, comprehending that transplantable organs are already, for all practical purposes, bought and sold provides a solid foundation for thinking about how markets in human organs might be organized and regulated. The scarcity and economic value of transplantable organs means that rights to possess and transfer these materials – in short, "property rights" in transplantable organs – will be sought after, regardless of whether the sources of organs are permitted to receive financial compensation. At issue in the debate over organ transplantation is what the precise contours of property rights in human organs will be, not whether property rights in human organs exist.

THE NEED FOR MARKET REGULATION

Markets in human organs are subject to extensive regulation, and no proposals to implement a system of unregulated exchanges are under serious deliberation. As with the acceptability of markets in human organs, the consensus on this point is so broad as to have gone virtually unnoticed. The issue of what the contours of such restrictions should be engenders considerable controversy, but both proponents and opponents of financial incentives agree that prudent regulations should, at a minimum, protect the lives and health of organ sources, transplant recipients and the general public (Cohen, 1995). The dispute over financial incentives, then, is not about whether individuals will be permitted to auction their kidneys over the Internet, or whether United States transplant programs should begin purchasing organs abroad from high-risk populations for resale to their patients.

Commerce in transplantable organs is by no means unique in being subject to a variety of restrictions. Markets in many goods and services are extensively regulated by governmental entities. Although the term "market" may evoke images of an open-air bazaar, unhampered by regulatory oversight, it is important not to lose sight of the fact that "market" simply denotes a network of mutually agreed-upon, bargained-for exchanges, the terms and conditions of which are frequently circumscribed by law and custom. Markets in financial products, rental properties, and food, to list but three prominent examples, are governed by detailed regulatory régimes, and no one suggests that markets in these important goods are non-existent because they are regulated.

THE IMPORTANCE OF RESPECT FOR THE HUMAN SOURCES OF TRANSPLANTABLE ORGANS

Allowing payments to organ sources might be risky, it is feared, because the availability of compensation could have the effect of putting a price on a part of an individual, thereby causing humans to think of each other as economic commodities, not unique human beings (Radin, 1996). If the sum of the economic worth of organs procured from a cadaveric donor is, for example, $200,000, then the total value of the deceased individual may be viewed as "only" $200,000. Such a bald economic calculus is, to some, reminiscent of other "sales of the body," such as prostitution or even slavery, and accounts for a significant share of the widespread horror elicited by the thought of commerce in organs (Kass, 1992).

Uneasiness over the potential equation of specific monetary sums with portions of human beings is compounded by the ambivalent attitude of a large percentage of the general public toward the practice of organ transplantation. The knowledge that human components can be transferred from one body to another inevitably stirs feelings of anxiety, for transplantation dissolves the physical boundaries that have separated humans from one another for millennia. Until this century, procedures for grafting parts of one body onto another were the province of myth, not science (Doniger, 1996; Barkan, 1996). These marvelous advances in medicine bring with them a danger that human beings will be regarded as a collection of spare parts, and that the special nature of each individual might be obscured, even in the absence of compensation paid directly to the sources of human organs (Fox & Swazey, 1992).

The danger that organ sources might be viewed as compilations of raw materials to be harvested and distributed, rather than as unique human beings worthy of profound respect, is a serious one, and the prospect of humans being regarded as mere instruments in pursuit of an end should cause concern. But the sense of urgency that accompanies the collection of transplantable organs, leading to the risk that respect for the dignity of each and every organ source might be eroded, exists independent of any compensation scheme for the organ sources themselves. Callous attitudes toward organ donors can flourish, regrettably, in the absence of financial incentives paid to organ sources (Fox, 1996). The utility of transplantable organs apart from the body of their original human source is what gives rights to their use and possession value, and creates incentives for organ procurement agencies and transplant centers to attempt to gain access to these organs.

The late twentieth century revolution in medical technology has led to a dramatic increase in the value (both economic and otherwise) of human body parts, as advances in medical technology have rendered a number of parts of one human being useful to others (Andrews & Nelkin, 1998). Regardless of whether financial incentives for organ sources (or other human sources of usable human materials, such as the sperm and ova necessary for many reproductive technologies) are available, the medical community and general public will be forced to confront the issue of how to collect and use portions of human beings while exhibiting respectful attitudes toward individuals. An interdiction on payments for organs at the first stage of the distribution chain – when the organ is transferred from the organ source to the organ procurement agency – cannot guarantee protection against the diminished reverence that may spring from new technologies. Only an attitude of mindful respect toward each individual can ensure that human uniqueness will not be forgotten as human parts become interchangeable to a degree unfathomable even a few decades ago.

COMPENSATING THE SOURCES OF ORGANS: IS ALTRUISM SUPERIOR TO SELF-INTEREST?

Supporters and opponents of the use of financial incentives are in ferocious disagreement on the merits of insisting that organs be made available for transplantation out of altruistic motivations rather than economic self-interest. As noted earlier in this chapter, the legal prohibition on payments to organ sources was enacted almost two decades ago, without measured consideration of the advantages and drawbacks of providing compensation to organ sources. At the time, the shortage of transplantable organs was less acute than it is today, and the transplant community was optimistic that appeals to altruism would prove an effective strategy for alleviating this shortage. In addition, the use of financial incentives in medicine was in many quarters regarded as inappropriate (Blumstein, 1993).

The legal and regulatory climate at the beginning of the twenty-first century differs significantly from the environment in which NOTA became law. The introduction of sophisticated immunosuppressive drugs has led to greater success in transplantation, fueling demand for additional usable organs and lengthening the list of transplant patients in dire need of organs. Efforts to secure a sufficient supply of organs through appeals to generosity have met with failure, or at best limited success. Numerous commentators have lamented the fact that informational and educational campaigns, along with "required request" policies that obligate hospitals to ask survivors of eligible donors to agree to organ retrieval, have not adequately increased the organ supply (Cohen, 1995). Perhaps the most important change of the past two decades is the attitude toward the role of financial incentives in health care. Making medical decisions – at least in part – on the basis of financial considerations is no longer regarded as inimical to the ethical provision of medical services, but is instead accepted as an inevitable aspect of modern health care (Blumstein, 1993).

Against this backdrop, it makes sense to revisit the proscription of payments to organ sources, and to consider the possibility that the legislation passed by the United States Congress in 1984 has outlasted whatever usefulness it may once have had. In discussions of financial incentives as a means to increase the supply of transplantable organs, medical and legal experts often assume that the payment of compensation represents a course of last resort, one to be tried only in the event that alternative measures for augmenting available organs fail (Childress, 1997). The notion that a system of organ procurement based on the altruism of potential organ sources is *necessarily* superior to one that relies on appeals to financial self-interest deserves careful scrutiny, not automatic acceptance. So far the rhetoric of altruism has been notable for its lack of nuance, with generosity regarded as an unqualified good and no attention devoted to the practical consequences of altruistic acts. A more balanced view would recognize the importance of altruism but temper praise with concern for its real world impact on prospective organ sources, their friends and families, and transplant recipients.

The Assumed Superiority of Altruistic Donations

The persistence of the idea that altruistic strategies for increasing the supply of transplantable organs are preferable to appeals to economic self-interest presents something of a puzzle. It is far from clear, upon reflection, why donated organs should be inherently superior to purchased ones. The arguments commonly advanced in support of this proposition are unpersuasive. As noted earlier in this chapter, the requirement that organ sources and their survivors act out of generosity does not remove human organs from the commercial realm, but merely delays market activity until later stages in the distribution process. Consequently, denying payment to organ sources cannot be justified on the grounds that such prohibitions ensure that organs remain non-commercial goods. Advocates of altruism may argue that to allow organ sources or their survivors to receive valuable consideration for body parts is unseemly, as these transactions can be viewed as putting a price on one's own life or the life of a family member. But such objections ignore the fact that in other contexts – most notably, when purchasing life insurance – individuals habitually determine the economic worth of the lives most precious to them. Indeed, it is interesting to note that when life insurance was first introduced, public acceptance was slow to occur, in part due to widespread reluctance to assign monetary sums to human lives (Zelizer, 1979). Moreover, interdictions on compensation for organs will not prevent individuals from marketing their own body components, for compensation is already available for the human sources of a number of types of usable tissue, including non-replenishable tissue such as ova (Andrews & Nelkin, 1998).

It may be that prohibiting payments for organs can be defended on the grounds that altruism is always preferable to self-interest, and that both law and social norms should encourage altruism whenever possible. That argument is a curious one, however, because it fails to explain why, out of all the opportunities for society to require or encourage individuals to act out of altruism instead of self-interest, organ procurement should be singled out for special treatment. The usual means of acquiring goods in our society is to offer payments to the individuals and institutions in possession of the desired goods, not to exhort others to be generous.

The assumption that gifts of organs are preferable to sales has potentially detrimental consequences, for supporters of organ donation rarely consider either the magnitude of the burdens of relying on altruistic behavior or whether these burdens are distributed equitably. In assessing the desirability of uncompensated transfers, it makes sense to ask who is giving and who is receiving, in order to figure out the impact of generosity on the distribution of both health and wealth. Asking the less affluent to perform acts of generosity that benefit the better off may not be desirable social policy, especially given the financial barriers that limit access to transplantation services. The fact that transplants are often unavailable to the poor and uninsured means that some individuals who are asked to give would be unlikely to receive organs if they were potential recipients instead of potential donors.

The burdens of altruism include the emotional strain of being asked to agree to consent to organ removal. In the case of cadaveric donors, this burden is shouldered by individuals who may not be emotionally equipped to be generous. The critical need to harvest organs as soon as practicable after death obligates organ procurement personnel to urge the recently bereaved to undertake an act of tremendous generosity at a moment of great vulnerability. Asking individuals who have just suffered a terrible loss to make a significant gift runs counter to the traditional treatment of surviving family members, who are normally the *recipients* of generosity (Epstein, 1997).

In evaluating the desirability of altruistic acts, it also makes sense to determine whether the altruism under consideration is necessary. If the prohibition on compensation for cadaveric organs has caused or exacerbated the organ shortage, then the sacrifices of living organ donors can be regarded as noble but tragic, given that the health risks assumed are avoidable. However laudable altruism may be in theory, it seems perverse to have in place transplantation laws and regulations that increase the need for friends and family of transplant patients to demonstrate their unselfish natures by undergoing major surgery. No doubt numerous relatives and friends of transplant recipients are delighted to serve as living donors, but the risks of serving as a living donor are not zero. Adherents of altruism need to explain why subjecting living donors to surgery is preferable to purchasing cadaveric organs.

Moreover, the prohibition on payments for organs has another worrisome but little noted effect: it forces potential donors to choose between giving and not giving, but prohibits all intermediate options. Every human being is confronted with the task of balancing concerns for the welfare of others with the pursuit of self-interest. While a life completely devoid of altruistic projects is unimaginable, so is an existence devoted exclusively to the flourishing of others. Consequently, each individual is compelled to make difficult choices, at times sacrificing the interests of family, friends and wider community for the sake of her own needs and desires (Hampton, 1993). Precisely how that delicate balance is to be struck is a deeply personal matter, and will vary depending on each person's ethical and religious commitments, as well as her life circumstances. With respect to most charitable projects, an altruist can elect to donate greater and lesser quantities of time and money, adjusting her level of generosity as her personal and professional circumstances dictate. A physician, for example, might elect to donate one hour of her time per week to a local clinic for indigents, or fifty hours, or some amount in between. But in the case of transplantable organs, a potential donor faces a stark choice, for she may not elect to receive partial payment. In consequence, she may be forced to choose between giving more than she would prefer or not giving at all.

The idea of lifesaving gifts exerts a strong appeal, but the enthusiastic approbation accorded to the idea of altruism needs to be tempered by a recognition that altruism is a complex and mysterious phenomenon. In practice, the forces of generosity have proven difficult to harness. Although an impressive quantity of empirical evidence indicates that human beings are, under certain limited circumstances, willing and eager to engage in uncompensated transfers (Batson & Shaw, 1991), and a number of researchers have asserted that generosity toward others is an essential component of human nature (Piliavin & Charng, 1990), efforts to inculcate altruism have met with limited success at best. As noted earlier in this chapter, campaigns to augment the number of available organs through public appeals to generosity have failed to provide a solution to the organ shortage crisis (DeJong et al., 1995). The use of individual self-interest to shape human behavior is far better understood than the use of altruism. To point out this disparity is not to argue that appeals to altruism have no role in ensuring an adequate supply of needed organs, but only to suggest that appeals to self-interest are more likely to yield predictable results.

The Effect of Financial Compensation on the Cost of Transplants

Not allowing organ sources to be compensated monetarily is often defended on instrumental grounds, with the claim that payments to organ sources and their families would increase the total costs of transplantation. According to this theory, payments to organ sources represent an additional expense associated with organ transplantation, one that will be borne by the transplant patient and therefore lead to an increase in the total costs of transplants for the recipients (Evans, 1993). Organ transplants, already among the most expensive of medical procedures, could – so the reasoning goes – become even more inaccessible for patients who lack good medical insurance and whose operations and follow-up services are not covered by any governmental program.

Given what we know about how markets function, however, the effect of payments to organ sources is likely to be the opposite, with financial incentives resulting in an increase in the number of usable organs. When the supply of a particular good increases, the price of that good will fall, all other things being equal (Barney & Reynolds, 1989). As several economists have observed, one reason that organ transplants are so expensive is that the organ shortage permits transplant programs to charge extremely high prices for their packages of goods and services (Blair & Kaserman, 1991). Alleviating the organ shortage would increase competition among transplant programs, as patients are able to choose among transplantation providers. In addition, greater numbers of transplantable organs will permit transplant programs to operate at enhanced levels of efficiency, and it is possible that savings achieved from improved operations would be passed on to patients, if programs are competing with one another.

Even if payments to organ sources fail to increase the supply of usable organs, payments to organ sources may represent a less expensive means of collecting transplantable organs than the present system, at least in some instances. Right now, the financial cost of procuring each suitable organ exceeds zero. Even though Organ Procurement Organizations do not pay the survivors of organ sources, to collect organs they must spend money on public education initiatives, the education of health care professionals, and key personnel such as organ recovery coordinators (Thorne, 1996). While some of these expenditures represent costs that OPOs would incur regardless of whether payments were offered, a substantial portion of the monies spent by OPOs represent "exhortation" costs, or funds devoted to persuading potential donors to donate (Thorne, 1998). Depending on the respective magnitudes of the "exhortation" costs and the payments that would be required to achieve a comparable number of available organs, financial incentives may turn out to be a cheaper means of obtaining organs. The issue of which method of collecting organs – financial incentives, soliciting donations, or a combination of the two – is the most cost effective deserves careful attention.

Lack of Compensation as a Reliable Proxy for Safety

Human biological materials derived from uncompensated sources are frequently assumed to be safer than similar materials from paid sources. The conviction that payments for organ donors would pose a threat to the health of transplant recipients gained currency in the 1960s, in the wake of research that demonstrated that the blood supply of the United States, which depended in large part on paid sources, was of lower quality than the blood used for transfusions in the United Kingdom, where blood was collected from altruistic donors (Titmuss, 1971). There is no evidence, however, that donated organs *necessarily* pose fewer dangers to transplant recipients than purchased ones, for the safety of human biological materials, including blood, depends largely on the safety measures taken by institutions that collect and distribute such materials, as well as the populations the human sources are drawn from

(Kessel, 1974). Indeed, the problems with hepatitis and HIV viruses in the blood supply experienced by the United States, France and other nations illustrates the hazards of equating donated human biological materials with safe materials.

Most important, financial incentives for organ sources have the potential to lead to a safer organ supply. If compensation results in a larger number of usable organs, transplant professionals will be in a position to exercise greater selectivity in choosing which organs to transplant. As a result, the average quality of transplanted organs could increase (Barnett et al., 1993). Whether financial incentives would in fact promote a safer organ supply is, obviously, an empirical question. At this stage, all that can be said with confidence is that neither purchased nor donated organs would have a monopoly on safety, and any system of financial incentives would have to be designed with safety as a paramount consideration.

Regardless of whether organs are donated or sold by their sources, transplant programs have every incentive to take steps to ensure that transplanted organs meet strict safety requirements. Not only do transplant programs face fears of liability, but they also have a substantial interest in maintaining good professional reputations.

A Note on "Presumed Consent"

A possible strategy for increasing the organ supply without resorting to financial incentives is to enact "presumed consent" laws, which would authorize Organ Procurement Organizations to harvest organs in the event that the decedent has failed to register any objections to serving as an organ donor. In essence, under a system of "presumed consent" individuals are assumed to be altruistic, absent evidence to the contrary. Proponents of presumed consent schemes note that the disparity between the supply of and demand for usable organs can be traced, in large part, to the difficulties procurement organizations have experienced in obtaining permission to recover organs (Futterman, 1998). Instituting a policy under which organ donors would no longer be required to take affirmative steps to "opt in" might help close this gap.

Presumed consent proposals raise many of the concerns discussed earlier in this section. The choices available to potential organ sources would still be limited to donating or not donating, albeit with a different default rule. The distributional impact of presumed consent régimes might be to collect organs from the poor – without compensation to survivors – for the use of the affluent and adequately insured. In addition, critics of presumed consent proposals question whether consent to organ removal can really be presumed, observing that empirical evidence that potential donors would consent if actually asked is sparse (Veatch & Pitt, 1995).

Presumed consent also triggers alarm on the grounds that a rule that the state has a claim to the organs of its citizens serves to expand governmental property rights in human bodies (Cohen, 1995). Permitting the government to assert property rights in cadavers of individuals who have neglected to "opt out" of the presumed consent régime may prove politically unacceptable. The debate over government ownership of rights to possess and use cadaveric organs under a presumed consent régime, however, highlights the reality that property rights in transplantable organs are inevitable, and that the real issue at stake is which individuals or institutions will be permitted to exercise these property rights, not whether the property rights will exist at all.

THE EFFECTIVENESS OF FINANCIAL INCENTIVES

The unanswered question about financial incentives, of course, is whether they would prove an effective means of augmenting the supply of transplantable organs. This question is not new, for proposals to compensate the sources of organs are by no means a recent phenomenon. Since the adoption of NOTA in 1984, several serious proposals have been advanced, but discussions of their respective advantages and disadvantages have been hampered by the fact that participants in the debate have opposite instincts regarding the probable efficacy of payments for organs. Supporters of financial incentives note, correctly, that as a general rule offering compensation for a scarce resource leads to more of it, as individuals respond to opportunities to increase their wealth. Viewed from this perspective, the solution to the organ shortage is readily apparent: offer potential organ donors money or other valuable consideration in exchange for organs, and watch the number of usable organs climb (Blair & Kaserman, 1991).

Opponents of financial incentives are quick to rejoin that the problem may not be so simple. Transplantable organs differ from the average market good, and prospective donors may be unwilling to think of pieces of their own bodies (or those of their family members) as exchangeable for valuable consideration. Even though transplantable organs are, in fact if not in rhetoric, market goods, in the popular imagination human body parts are not commodities. Compensation schemes could backfire, critics point out, if prospective organs donors perceive offers of valuable consideration as insults and refuse to make organs available for transplant under any circumstances (Pelligrino, 1991; Prottas, 1992). Opponents of financial incentives might also worry that offers to exchange valuable consideration for organs could undermine public support of organ transplantation, already perceived as fragile, by highlighting the role that money plays in the collection and distribution of organs.

It bears emphasis that proponents of financial incentives are not committed to the idea that all organ sources *should demand* payments for organs. The availability of financial incentives may lead to a system in which some organ sources are compensated, while others continue to donate. A mixed system of donation and compensation would have the powerful advantage of offering distinct sets of incentives, for as economist Kenneth Arrow has observed, altruists may not respond to financial incentives, and non-altruists cannot be expected to respond to pleas for generosity (Arrow, 1971). The availability of financial incentives, then, could have the positive effect of tapping into the population that fails to respond to altruistic appeals, without affecting the behavior of altruistically motivated donors. While the availability of remuneration might conceivably discourage some potential altruists from agreeing to donate, charitable donations and commercial sales coexist in many institutional settings. The existence of markets for artwork, for example, has not led art patrons to stop giving paintings to museums, even though donors understand that museums acquire objects through both gifts and purchases.

Whether financial incentives would prove an effective method of eliminating or reducing the shortage of transplantable organs is, in the final analysis, an empirical question, and one that is impossible to answer at present, given the legal prohibitions that have been in place in the United States for the past sixteen years (Adams et al., 1999). In assessing the desirability of financial incentives in organ transplantation, however, it should be recalled that twenty years ago similar doubts were expressed regarding the potential efficacy of financial incentives in medicine in general, and the intervening decades have proved the doubters wrong (Blumstein, 1993). More important, available evidence from abroad suggests that financial incentives for living kidney providers have the effect of increasing the supply of available kidneys, and that small payments to survivors of cadaveric donors, earmarked for burial expenses, have succeeded in increasing the organ supply of Spain (Cohen, 1995). In sum, there is reason to conclude that financial incentives have promise as a strategy for increasing the organ supply.

The results of several public opinion polls provide limited support for the conclusion that the judicious use of financial incentives may lead to more organs becoming available for transplant. In two recent studies, approximately one-half of respondents expressed approval for at least one form of compensation (Nelson et al., 1993). Moreover, results from a recent survey of undergraduates suggests that the prices demanded for agreeing to donate organs at death might be relatively modest (Adams et al., 1999). Of course, responses to survey questions do not necessarily predict with accuracy the behavior of individuals in real life situations. Nonetheless, the results of survey research deserve measured consideration, particularly in light of the dearth of other empirical evidence. At the very least, the level of acceptance of prospective financial incentives suggests that a non-trivial percentage of the population is likely to consider seriously exchanging rights to possess organs for money.

It is entirely possible – even probable – that the effectiveness of various financial incentive plans will vary substantially, depending on the terms and conditions of the bargain. Opponents of financial incentives carry a heavy burden if they maintain that no system of compensation, under any circumstances, can result in an overall increase in the supply of transplantable organs, for the claim that financial incentives for organ sources can *never* lead to increases in the supply of organs strains credulity. Proposals to compensate organ sources, after all, range from modest stipends for burial expenses to significant cash payments to surviving relatives. (The leading proposals are discussed in the next section of this chapter.) Right now, it is impossible to determine which proposals would prove the most efficacious, and both supporters and opponents of financial incentives should admit that the present state of knowledge is severely limited. Instead of wasting precious time in arguing, those involved in this debate should marshal resources and attempt to provide answers to questions concerning the circumstances under which financial incentives are likely to meet with public acceptance or rejection, with the goal of tailoring compensation arrangements in response to concrete findings.

Above all, experts in medicine, law and ethics should recognize that their attitudes and conclusions may be factors in shaping public responses to various financial incentive plans. If prominent members of the transplant community oppose financial incentives, news of their negative response could reduce the chances of success of experimental programs. While individual preferences with regard to organ collection are notoriously difficult to shape and predict, the debate over financial incentives should at least acknowledge the possibility that prognostications of failure might turn out to be self-fulfilling prophecies. This does not mean, of course, that participants in the debate should feel obliged to be anything less than honest. Rather, discussions of the efficacy of financial incentives should be characterized by open-mindedness and flexibility.

HOW FINANCIAL INCENTIVES MIGHT BE STRUCTURED

Financial compensation for the sources of transplantable organs and their survivors can take a variety of forms. This section discusses the advantages and drawbacks of several leading proposals. The examples discussed below by no means exhaust the ways that compensation arrangements might be structured, but instead describe the most widely discussed alternatives.

Payments to the Survivors of Cadaveric Donors

The simplest and most straightforward means of purchasing cadaveric organs would be for Organ Procurement Organizations to augment their solicitations of organs with offers to pay compensation to the survivors of organ sources. Under this scheme, the existing organ collection protocols, whereby procurement organizations furnish information and emotional support to the survivors of eligible donors, could remain unchanged, except that offers to pay would supplement requests for donation. The amount of payment could be uniform within each organ category or could fluctuate, depending on the characteristics of each particular organ. Applicable law could provide that compensation for organs be paid directly to surviving relatives, or, alternatively, to the estate of the decedent, to be distributed pursuant to the decedent's last will and testament or state intestacy statutes. A variation of this option would be to permit different organ procurement institutions to compete to acquire transplantable organs. Instead of restricting the operations of each Organ Procurement Organization to its particular area, the law governing transplants could authorize survivors of organ sources to sell organs to any licensed procurement organization. Under this scheme, survivors could select the highest compensation available, leading rival organ collection firms to compete on the basis of price and other terms.

Of all the proposed compensation arrangements, payments to survivors is the most likely to provoke controversy, due to its explicit character. In addition, direct payments negotiated at or shortly after death raise several of the same concerns as requests for donation at that difficult time: survivors are usually in shock, and, arguably, not in an ideal frame of mind to decide how to dispose of organs. Nevertheless, direct payment schemes offer several advantages. One is expanding the range of available options for the relatives of potential organ sources, for as a general rule more choices are preferable to fewer. Another is remedying what might be termed the unfairness of refusing to permit the surviving relatives of organ sources to share in the significant financial returns available from organ transplantation. Finally, the explicit character of direct, above-board payments would guarantee that the general public is aware of the opportunity to exchange rights to transplantable organs for valuable consideration, which might increase the program's chances of success.

Advance Sales by Cadaveric Donors: the Benefits of an Options Market

Another means of expanding the market in human organs would be to allow living individuals to sell organ procurement firms the rights to harvest their organs in the event they become suitable cadaveric donors. As Lloyd Cohen, the principal architect of this proposal, points out, such a market would represent a variation of the current practice of asking citizens to agree to be organ donors upon death (Cohen, 1995). The principal departure from the present system, besides financial remuneration, would be that family members would not be permitted to veto the organ provider's decision after death has occurred.

Rights to harvest organs could be sold in a variety of circumstances. Cohen envisions an organ sales campaign that is "extensive rather than intensive," one that informs organ sources of their choices without exerting pressure to agree to sell. As examples of situations in which individuals could execute organ sales contracts, Cohen lists driver's license renewals, filing tax returns and purchasing insurance. Payments for organ options could be remitted at the time the agreement is reached, upon the death of the seller, or when and if usable organs are successfully harvested, with money being paid to designees of the organ seller. Cohen strongly favors the final alternative, on the grounds that transaction costs would be far lower (Cohen, 1995).

The advance sales option would afford potential organ providers the chance to decide whether or not to sell their organs in the course of their lifetimes, at a time and place of their own choosing. Instead of two choices – to agree or decline to serve as a donor – organ sources would have three, including the option to exchange organs for valuable consideration. Choosing to sell rather than donate organs would not necessarily represent a decision not to be altruistic: Organ sellers could always designate a charitable organization as the recipient of sale proceeds, or stipulate that the money be divided between their survivors and their chosen charitable cause. This flexibility would enable organ sources to select the beneficiaries of their altruism as well as their desired quantity of altruism.

Contributions to Designated Charities

Beneficiaries of organ sales could be limited to charitable organizations. Under this plan, sources of organs would have the power to designate which charity would receive the proceeds from organ sales, but neither they nor their families would be eligible to realize financial gains from the decision to donate. To those whose disapproval of financial compensation is rooted in a belief that organs should be made available for transplantation out of altruistic motivations, this option presents an attractive alternative. Transplantable organs would be a result of altruism, but the organ donor would be accorded power to apportion the benefits. However, it is uncertain whether this option would measurably increase the supply of usable organs. The number of potential organ sources who would refuse to donate organs under the current system, but would agree if a charity of their choice would receive a cash donation, may not be large.

Reductions in Health Insurance Premiums

Offering individuals reductions in their health insurance premiums in exchange for agreeing to furnish organs has been proposed as a possible method for increasing the supply of available organs (Hansmann, 1989). As Henry Hansmann observes, health insurance companies have expertise in actuarial calculations and would therefore be in a good position to calculate the economic value of the insured's pledge to allow any usable organs to be harvested. The administration of a such a system would be fairly uncomplicated: insurance companies could simply submit the names of declared organ sources to a central registry, which hospitals could consult to determine whether or not a decedent is a declared organ provider. Individuals who agree to be listed on the registry would be able to spend the money they save on themselves, their families, or various charitable projects.

The appeal of a health insurance premium reduction scheme lies in its ease of administration (at least in theory) and the fact that the financial rewards would be distributed in a subtle way, obviating any need for an explicit exchange of valuable consideration for transplantable organs. The amount saved by each self-identified organ provider, however, would be modest, given the small probability of any particular individual turning out to be an eligible organ donor. Such a small financial incentive might fail to have a significant impact on an individual's decision to make his or her organs available for transplant.

Stipends for Funeral Expenses

In 1999, the State of Pennsylvania's Department of Health announced that it was considering a pilot program that would authorize the state to pay a "funeral benefit" of $300 to be used for funeral and burial expenses. Supporters of the program insist that the money represents a gesture of appreciation to the survivors of the organ donor, not a payment for organs. Opponents, by contrast, characterize the program as a naked attempt to evade the ban on compensation dictated by federal law (The Lancet, 1999). Although what label to affix to financial compensation – payment or "gesture of appreciation" – is from one perspective a silly quibble, avoiding commercial language might increase the chances of public acceptance of the scheme. Of course, gaining public approval through the use of nomenclature that is arguably misleading raises its own troubling issues.

Whether payments toward funeral expenses are likely to meet with a higher level of popular approval or prove more efficacious than other compensation arrangements is an open question. Requiring proceeds from organ sales to be spent for the decedent's benefit might make survivors more comfortable with accepting the money, in part by defusing public disapproval of the transaction. The $300 stipend may not be enough money to affect the decisions of survivors, but the willingness of Pennsylvania to experiment with such a program underscores the importance of addressing the question of whether financial incentives are acceptable to the medical and legal communities, as well as the public at large.

Compensation for Living Organ Donors

Proposals that living organ sources be eligible to collect payments in exchange for surrendering a kidney (or, far more rarely, a portion of a liver or lung) trigger impassioned reactions. The most common objection raised is that allowing individuals to sell parts of their bodies could lead them to assume excessive risks to their life and health. The protection of the health of living organ sources is, of course, of great importance, but this is true regardless of whether the living organ source is donating or selling his organ (Radcliffe-Richards et al., 1998). In any event, sales of organs by living donors can and should be regulated to ensure that a reasonable level of safety is achieved, in the same way that construction work and other potentially hazardous occupations are regulated.

Regulation of organ sales by living individuals could include requirements that all pertinent health risks, both long and short term, be fully disclosed in advance of the organ retrieval procedure. In addition, organ sellers could be required to purchase adequate health insurance before being permitted to offer organs for sale. The sales program could be structured so as to require all living organ sellers to sell only to OPOs or transplant centers. In the alternative, buyers and seller could simply bargain directly. Although the idea of buyers and sellers of organs interacting with one another may be startling, such an innovation can hardly be characterized as radical. Direct dealing already takes place in the context of ova used for fertility services: prospective parents frequently advertise for eligible ova providers, without the use of an intermediary fertility clinic.

CONCLUSION

In the final analysis, the arguments advanced in opposition to payments to organ sources are not convincing. Refusals to pay organ sources cannot be justified on the grounds that organs should not become commodities, for that particular Rubicon was crossed long ago. Assertions that organ sources must act out of altruism, not self-interest, are nonsensical, given the economic returns that are available to others involved in organ transplantation and the fact that, as a general rule, individuals are not expected to give away valuable items they possess. It is true that selling organs may, in the case of living organ sources, carry certain health risks, but those risks are present for *donors* of organs as well, and it is unclear why uncompensated sources of organs should be allowed to assume greater risks than compensated ones. In any event, appropriate regulation can address a number of the perceived dangers of such payments. For example, liability rules can be designed to promote the safety of the organ pool, and health and safety regulations can ensure that living organ sources do not undertake excessive health risks. As for empirical objections, claims that financial incentives are unlikely to work are not supported by the available evidence. At the very least, opponents of financial incentives should acknowledge that they cannot demonstrate that all compensation schemes are doomed to failure.

The disagreement over the use of financial incentives to increase the supply of transplantable organs is frequently characterized as a choice between a system of organ transplantation founded on altruism and a system based on the principles of the market. That characterization is wrong, for markets in transplantable organs already exist, and will continue to operate for the foreseeable future. So far, society has demanded that organ donors (or their survivors) make organs available out of altruism, not financial motivations, but has failed to insist upon similar renunciations of financial self-interest on the part of other individuals and institutions involved in transplantation. Not compensating organ sources and their survivors helps foster the impression that organ transplants are unrelated to commerce, but at the cost of diverting attention from important questions concerning how commercial activity in human organs should proceed. The ongoing loss of life caused by the lack of transplantable organs demands that experts in medicine, law and ethics devote serious attention to designing effective compensation schemes for the sources of organs.

REFERENCES

Adams, F. A., Barnett, A. H., & Kaserman, D. L. (1999). Markets for Organs: the Question of Supply. *Contemporary Economic Policy, 17*(2), 147–155.

Andrews, L., & Nelkin, D. (1998). Whose Body Is It Anyway?: Disputes Over Body Tissue in a Biotechnology Age. *The Lancet, 53*, 51–57.

Arrow, K. (1972). Gifts and Exchanges. *Phil. and Pub. Affairs, 1*, 343–362.

Barkan, L. (1996). Cosmas and Damian: Of Medicine, Miracles and the Economies of the Body. In: S. Youngner, R. Fox & J. Swazey (Eds), *Organ Transplantation: Meanings and Realities* (pp. 221–250).

Barnett, A. H., Blair, R. D., & Kaserman, D. L. (1992). Improving Organ Donation: Compensation Versus Markets. *Inquiry, 29*, 372–378.

Barney, L. D., & Reynolds, R. L. (1989). An Economic Analysis of Transplant Organs. *Atlantic Economic Journal, 17*(3), 12–20.

Batson, C. D., & Shaw, L. (1991). Evidence for Altruism: Toward a Pluralism of Prosocial Motives. *Psychological Inquiry, 2*, 107–122.

Blair, R. D., & Kaserman, D. L. (1991). The Economics and Ethics of Alternative Cadaveric Organ Procurement Policies. *Yale Journal on Regulation, 8*, 403–452.

Blumstein, J. F. (1993). The Use of Financial Incentives in Medical Care: the Case of Transplantable Organs. *Health Matrix, 3*(1), 1–30.

Caplan et al. (1993). Financial Compensation for Organ Donation: Good Idea or Anathema? *Transplantation Proceedings, 25*, 2740–2742.

Childress, J. (1997). *Practical Reasoning in Bioethics.*

Cohen, L. (1995). *Increasing the Supply of Transplant Organs: the Virtues of an Options Market.*

DeJong et al. (1995). Options for Increasing Organ Donation: The Potential Role of Financial Incentives, Standardized Hospital Procedures, and Public Education to Promote Family Discussion. *The Milbank Quarterly, 73*, 463–479.

Doniger, W. (1996). Transplanting Myths of Organs Transplants. In: S. Youngner, R. Fox & J. Swazey (Eds), *Organ Transplantation: Meanings and Realities* (pp. 194–220).

Epstein, R. (1997). *Mortal Peril: Our Inalienable Right to Health Care?*

Evans, R. (1989). Money Matters: Should Ability to Pay Ever Be a Consideration in Gaining Access to Transplantation? *Transplantation Proceedings, 21*, 3419–3423.

Evans, R. (1993). Organ Procurement Expenditures and the Role of Financial Incentives. *Journal of the American Medical Association, 269*, 3113–3118.

Fox, R., & Swazey, J. (1992). *Spare Parts: Organ Replacement in American Society.*

Fox, R. (1996). Afterthoughts. In: S. Youngner, R. Fox & J. Swazey (Eds), *Organ Transplantation: Meanings and Realities* (pp. 252–272).

Futterman, L. G. (1998). Presumed Consent: The Solution to the Critical Donor Shortage? In: A. L. Caplan & D. H. Coelho (Eds), *The Ethics of Organ Transplants: the Current Debate* (pp. 161–172).

Hampton, J. (1993). Selflessness and the Loss of Self. In: E. F. Paul, F. Miller & J. Paul (Eds), *Altruism* (pp. 135–165).

Hansmann, H. (1989). The Economics and Ethics of Markets for Human Organs. In: J. F. Blumstein & F. Sloan, *Organ Transplantation Policy: Issues and Prospects*, 57–86.

Joralemon, D. (1995). Organ Wars: the Battle for Body Parts. *Medical Anthropology Quarterly*, *9*, 335–356.

Kass, L. (1992). Organs for Sale? Propriety, Property, and the Price of Progress. *The Public Interest*, *107*, 65–86.

Kessel, R. (1974). Transfused Blood, Serum Hepatitis and the Coase Theorem. *J. Law and Economics*, *17*, 265–289.

The Lancet (1999). Paying Respect to Organs, *353*, 2085.

Mahoney, J. D. (2000). The Market for Human Tissue. *Virginia Law Review*, *86*, 163–223.

Marshall et al. (1996). Marketing Human Organs: the Autonomy Paradox. *Theoretical Medicine*, *17*, 1–18.

Murray, T. (1996). Organ Vendors, Families, and the Gift of Life. In: S. Youngner, R. Fox & J. Swazey (Eds), *Organ Transplantation: Meanings and Realities* (pp. 101–125).

Nelson et al. (1993). Financial Incentives for Organ Donation: a Report of the UNOS Ethics Committee Payment Subcommittee. United Network for Organ Sharing White Paper (available at www.unos.org/Resources/bioethics_whitepapers_finance.htm).

Pelligrino, E. D. (1991). Families' Self-Interest and the Cadaver's Organs. *Journal of the American Medical Association*, *265*, 1305–1306.

Peters, T. G. (1991). Life or Death: the Issue of Payment in Cadaveric Organs. *Journal of the American Medical Association*, *265*, 1302–1305.

Piliavin, J. A., & Charng, H. (1990). Altruism: A Review of Recent Theory and Research. *Ann. Rev. of Soc.*, *16*, 27–65.

Porter, R. (1997). *The Greatest Benefit to Mankind: A Medical History of Humanity.*

Prottas, J. (1992). Buying Human Organs: Evidence that Money Doesn't Change Everything. *Transplantation*, *53*, 1371–1373.

Radcliffe-Richards, J. et al. (1998). The Case for Allowing Kidney Sales (Letter). *The Lancet*, *351*, 1950–1952.

Radin, M. J. (1996). *Contested Commodities.*

Siminoff, L. A., Arnold, R. M., Caplan, A. L., Virnig, B. A., & Seltzer, D. L. (1995). Public Policy Governing Organ and Tissue Procurement in the United States: Results from the National Organ and Tissue Procurement Study. *Ann. Int. Med.*, *123*(1), 10–17.

Thorne, E. D. (1996). The Cost of Procuring Market-Inalienable Human Organs. *J. of Regulatory Economics*, *10*, 191–200.

Thorne, E. D. (1998). When Private Parts Are Made Public Goods: The Economics of Market-Inalienability. Yale. *J. on Regulation*, *15*, 149–175.

Titmuss, R. (1971). *The Gift Relationship: From Human Blood to Social Policy.*

Veatch, R. M., & Pitt, J. B. (1995). The Myth of Presumed Consent: Ethical Problems in New Organ Procurement Strategies. *Transplantation Proceedings*, *27*, 1888–1892.

Zelizer, V. A. R. (1979). *Markets and Morals: The Development of Life Insurance in the United States.*

4. ETHICAL ISSUES IN LIVING RELATED DONORS

Aaron Spital

INTRODUCTION

Few issues in medicine have generated as much controversy as has living organ donation. Despite years of experience and increasing use of living donors, this practice continues to be debated today. In this chapter, I will review relevant ethical concerns. I will argue that these concerns notwithstanding, when practised with care, organ donation by related and even unrelated volunteers is a valuable and acceptable procedure that should continue at least until there is an adequate supply of cadaveric organs (Spital, 1998a). My discussion will be aimed primarily at competent altruistic volunteers; the complicated question of commercialism in transplantation will be touched upon only briefly. I begin with a historical overview of living kidney donation because kidneys were the first organs successfully transplanted and because a historical perspective is necessary to understand the evolution of the ethical issues involved.

HISTORICAL OVERVIEW

Before the availability of renal replacement therapies, the diagnosis of end-stage renal disease (ESRD) was the equivalent of a death sentence (Kreis, 1985; Land, 1989). The desperate predicament of ESRD patients led to sporadic attempts to transplant kidneys from animals and cadavers, as well as

The Ethics of Organ Transplantation, Volume 7, pages 89–123.

ISBN: 0-7623-0764-1

"free kidneys" removed from living people for therapeutic purposes. None of these early transplants functioned more than a few months and many never functioned at all (Hume et al., 1955; Groth, 1972).

By the early 1950s it was recognized that graft rejection, resulting from biological incompatibility between the donor and recipient, was a major barrier to successful transplantation (Hume et al., 1955; Merrill et al., 1956; Groth, 1972; Murray, 1982). In an attempt to overcome this serious obstacle, Michon and his colleagues at the Necker Hospital in Paris performed the world's first living related donor renal transplant in December 1952; a healthy mother donated one of her kidneys to her 16 year old son (Hume et al., 1955; Groth, 1972; Eurotold Project, 1997). The graft functioned well initially but was rejected after only three weeks. Based on this dismal experience, including failures of their own, Hume and his colleagues concluded in the Spring of 1954: "Renal homotransplantation has no place in the therapy of human patients at this time" (Hume et al., 1955). It is ironic that success would finally occur only a few months later at Dr. Hume's own institution.

In the early 1950s, Dr. Joseph Murray, a plastic surgeon at the Peter Bent Brigham Hospital in Boston with an interest in skin grafting, turned his attention to renal transplantation (Murray, 1982). Murray recognized the importance of immunological compatibility to transplantation; he knew that while skin grafts from unrelated donors were rejected, grafts from identical twins survived. Armed with this knowledge, Murray performed renal autotransplantation experiments in dogs (in which there is no immunological barrier) and was able to achieve lasting success (Murray, 1982).

Drawing upon this experience, on December 23, 1954, Dr. Murray and his colleagues took the courageous step of transplanting a kidney from a young man, Ronald Herrick, to his identical twin brother Richard, who was suffering from ESRD (Merrill et al., 1956; Murray, 1982). The kidney functioned immediately and the recipient made a rapid and complete recovery. He married his recovery room nurse and fathered two children before dying of a myocardial infarction eight years later (Murray, 1982). This was the world's first successful human renal transplant and stands as a landmark in medical history.

Encouraged by this dramatic success, over the next few years more identical twin renal transplants were performed with excellent results (Murray, 1982; Tilney, 1986). Many lessons were learned from the identical twin experience, the most important being that successful human renal transplantation was possible. This stimulated research aimed at finding ways to make this lifesaving procedure available to a broader range of potential recipients, most of whom are not fortunate enough to have an identical twin willing to donate. With the introduction of effective immunosuppression in the early 1960s, this goal became a reality and reports of successful transplantation of kidneys from non-twin living relatives and cadavers began to appear (Murray et al., 1963; Starzl et al., 1963). However, because the results of kidney transplantation from living donors were much better than those obtained with cadaveric donors (Advisory Committee to the Renal Transplant Registry, 1972), living relatives became the preferred source of transplanted kidneys. Recent data indicate that at many centers this is still the case today (Spital, 2000).

ETHICAL CONCERNS ABOUT LIVING ORGAN DONATION

The preceding historical review demonstrates that living donors were instrumental to the development of successful clinical transplantation. However, since its inception, this practice was beset by ethical concerns, the most troubling of which was summarized in 1964 by Dr. Francis Moore, then surgeon-in-chief at the Peter Bent Brigham Hospital: "Thus, for the first time in the history of medicine a procedure is being adopted in which a perfectly healthy person is injured permanently in order to improve the well-being [not of himself but] of another. Some laboratories have viewed this matter with such misgivings that under no circumstances have they used tissues from volunteer human donors" (Moore, 1964). In addition to concerns about harming the donor and the redefinition of an acceptable surgical procedure, there were also concerns about the donor's motivation and ability to provide valid consent when the life of a relative was at stake (Hamburger & Crosnier, 1968; McGeown, 1968; Fellner & Schwartz, 1971; Fox & Swazey, 1992). Nevertheless, because of the very low operative risk of uninephrectomy for a healthy person, the lack of effective alternative therapies for ESRD patients, and the recognition that the desire to save a loved one is a powerful and admirable motivating force, living related kidney donation became an accepted practice even though the long term risks were unknown (Eisendrath et al., 1969; Merrill, 1971; Spital, 1998b).

Since the early days of renal transplantation the situation has changed dramatically. In developed countries, dialysis became increasingly available and the results of cadaveric transplantation improved greatly. No longer was ESRD equivalent to a death sentence, even in the absence of a living donor transplant (Kreis, 1985). Furthermore, rare postoperative donor deaths were reported (Starzl, 1987; Najarian et al., 1992) and a few follow-up studies raised concerns about long term risks as well (Hakim et al., 1984; Provoost & Brenner, 1993). As a result of these developments, the debate about the propriety of using living donors reemerged with heightened vigor. While some experts continued to support living organ donation (Sutherland, 1985; Rapaport, 1987; Spital, 1988a; Daar, 1995), others began to suggest that this practice should only be used as a last resort or not at all (Kreis, 1985; Starzl, 1987; Kleinman & Lowy, 1992; Michielsen, 1995). Not surprisingly, there is a wide variation in the rate of acceptance of living donors among transplant centers around the world (Chugh & Jha, 1995; Eurotold Project, 1997; USRDS Report, 1999).

In view of persisting concerns about the use of living organ donors (Kleinman & Lowy, 1992; Russell & Jacob, 1993; Michielsen, 1995; Elliott, 1995; Isoniemi, 1997) it is worthwhile asking whether this practice should continue. In order to answer this question we must first address several others:

(1) do we still need living donors?
(2) what is the major ethical dilemma in living organ donation? and
(3) what are the relevant ethical principles and where do they lead us?

DO WE STILL NEED LIVING DONORS?

The answer to this question is undoubtedly yes. Renal transplantation is the best and most cost-effective therapy available for eligible ESRD patients (de Charro & de Wit, 1996; Price & Akveld, 1998; USRDS Report, 1999; Neylan et al., 1999; Smith et al., 2000; Wolfe et al., 1999) and is therefore the preferred form of renal replacement from the point of view of the recipient and society (Daar et al., 1997). However, despite devoting much effort toward increasing the pool of available cadaveric organs, there remains a severe and steadily worsening worldwide shortage of organs (Siminoff et al., 1995; Daar et al., 1997; Cohen & Wight, 1999; Neylan et al., 1999). For example, as of October 31,1999, 66,175 people in the United States were waiting for an organ transplant and a new name is added to the waiting list every 16 minutes (Fig. 1) (UNOS, 1999). Tragically, many of these people will die before a suitable organ can be found. Because of this desperate situation, healthy people have recently been called upon to donate non-renal organ segments as well (Singer et al., 1989; Shaw et al., 1991; Kramer & Sprung, 1995; Gruessner et al., 1997).

Another reason to continue using living donors is that they still provide superior results when compared with cadaveric ones, at least in the case of kidneys (Fig. 2) (Cecka & Terasaki, 1997; Terasaki et al., 1997; Lin et al., 1998; Hariharan et al., 2000). However, the obvious benefits of living organ donation cannot alone justify this practice. Before recommending that it be continued, we must also believe that it is ethically acceptable (Spital, 1998b).

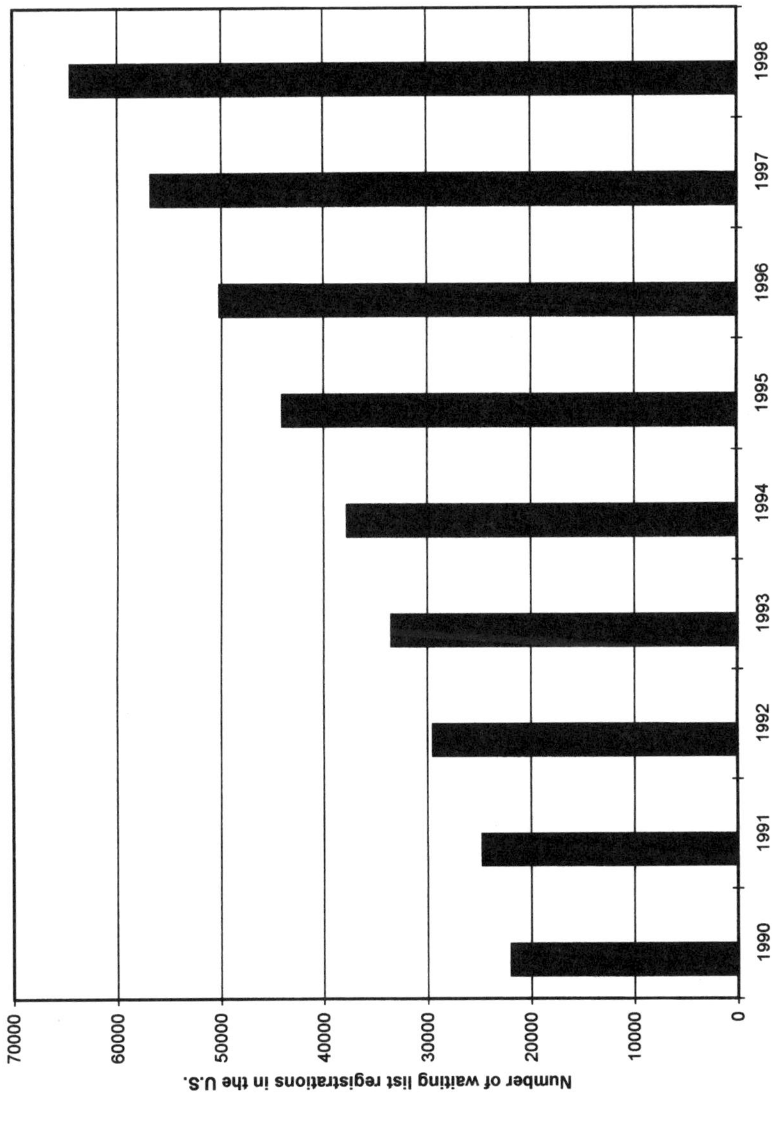

Fig. 1. Rapid growth in the total number of registrations on the U.S. organ transplant waiting list at year end between 1990 and 1998. Drawn from data obtained from UNOS (1999).

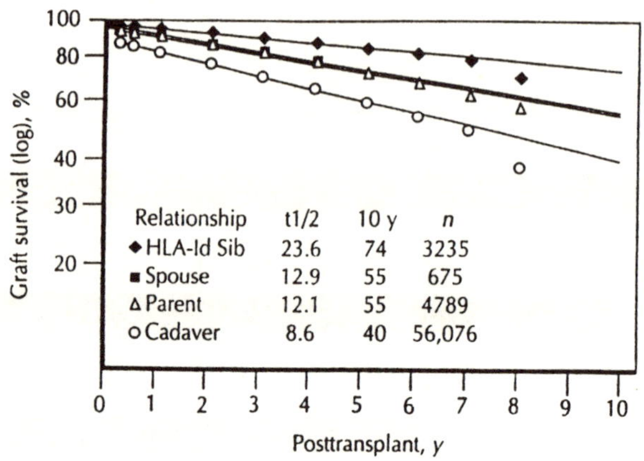

Fig. 2. Survival of kidney transplants reported to the University of California, Los Angeles Kidney Transplant Registry. Reprinted from Terasaki et al. (1997) with permission.

THE MAJOR ETHICAL DILEMMA IN LIVING ORGAN DONATION

Over thirty years ago, MFA Woodruff suggested that living kidney donation is analogous to heroic rescue (Woodruff, 1966): "The opportunity of saving a life by pulling someone out of a fire, or rescuing them from drowning, is comparable to the situation of the kidney donor, with just the difference that the kidney donor has a little longer to make his mind up." If this were the whole story, respect for autonomy would suggest that the wishes of potential donors regarding organ donation should be controlling (Elliott, 1995). In his book on the ethics of biotechnology, Harris (1992) supports this view: "If I decide that I would like to donate one of my kidneys and run the risks of the procedure and the risk that I might subsequently have kidney failure, then it seems that this is a matter for me. Like all other risks that I choose to run . . . these are matters of personal choice."

But while respect for donor autonomy is necessary, I believe that it is not sufficient for determining the suitability of a particular volunteer. What is missing from Harris's analysis is the recognition that there is a fundamental difference between a heroic deed carried out by a single individual and one which requires the help of others. It is one thing for a mother to choose to jump in front of a car to save her child (Whitington, 1996), but quite another for the mother to ask someone to push her into the car's path to help her accomplish her noble goal (Elliott, 1995; Spital, 1998b). Clearly, living organ donation is more analogous to the latter situation.

Recognizing the need for physician involvement is vital to the ethical assessment of living organ donation. As Elliott (1995) points out: "the doctor is not a mere instrument of the patient's wishes . . . [he] is also a moral agent who should be held accountable for his actions." Thus from the perspective of the transplant team, the major ethical dilemma in living organ donation is "deciding not simply whether a subject's choice is reasonable . . . but whether [the transplant team] is morally justified in helping the subject accomplish it" (Elliott, 1995). Others have reached a similar conclusion (Woodruff, 1964; Singer & Siegler, 1988; Strong & Lynch, 1996; Spital, 1998b).

ETHICAL PRINCIPLES RELEVANT TO LIVING ORGAN DONATION

When transplant professionals evaluate the acceptability of a potential living donor, several ethical principles should be considered. These include: (1) respect for autonomy; (2) non-maleficence; and (3) beneficence (UNOS Ethics Committee, 1992; Beauchamp & Childress, 1994; Eurotold Project, 1997; Spital, 1998b). Justice is another important ethical principle, but it is less relevant to living organ donation and will be considered only briefly (de Ortuzar et al., 1997; Eurotold, 1997). Although "principlism" has been criticized as inadequate to guide assessments of the suitability of potential living donors (de Ortuzar et al., 1997), I believe it is a reasonable place to start.

Respect for Autonomy

Autonomy refers to self-rule and means that "a person chooses and acts freely and rationally out of her own life plan, however ill-defined" (Childress, 1982). "Respect for the autonomous choices of other persons runs as deep in common morality as any principle" (Beauchamp & Childress, 1994). One justification of voluntary living organ donation is that it is an expression of individual autonomy (Caplan, 1993a). But how can transplant professionals be sure that a potential donor is acting autonomously? The requirement for informed consent is designed to achieve this goal (Beauchamp & Childress, 1994; Kasiske et al., 1996; Majeske et al., 1996; Daar et al., 1997).

Informed consent has several elements (Beauchamp & Childress, 1994): (1) competence to understand and decide; (2) disclosure of all relevant information; (3) understanding of the information disclosed; (4) ability to choose freely; and (5) reasoned consent. Questions have been raised about the validity of consent given by living donors primarily because of concerns about freedom of choice and the level of understanding among these volunteers (Fox & Swazey, 1992; Caplan, 1993a, b, 1997; Russell & Jacob, 1993; Michielsen, 1995; Eurotold Project, 1997; Spital, 1998b). Fears about inadequate disclosure of information resulting from a conflict of interest for the transplant team (Caplan, 1997) can be assuaged by appointing a donor physician who is not involved in the care of the potential recipient (UNOS Ethics Committee, 1992; Price & Akveld, 1998).

Concerns About Voluntarism

One of the arguments against living organ donation is the fear that some offers may not be truly voluntary (McGeown, 1968; Kleinman & Lowy, 1992; Caplan, 1993a, b, 1997; Russell & Jacob, 1993; Michielsen, 1995; Isoniemi, 1997). Many potential donors, who are almost always emotionally (and usually genetically) related to their recipients, may feel obligated to donate and that they have no real choice (Adams, 1987; Fox & Swazey, 1992; Caplan, 1993b; Majeske et al., 1996; Superina et al., 1999). Pressure to donate may take two forms: it can be external, in which case pressure is brought to bear by another person such as a family member, or it can be internal arising out of a sense of duty or guilt (Adams, 1987; Singer et al., 1989; Kleinman & Lowy, 1992; Majeske et al., 1996; Sells, 1997).

Several studies have shown that while external pressure occurs in some cases, such pressure is unusual (Smith et al., 1986; Stiller et al., 1985; Morris et al., 1987; Simmons et al., 1987; Schover et al., 1997; Karrfelt et al., 1998; Toronyi et al., 1998). In those cases in which external pressure does occur (usually from family or friends), it seems to be more often against donation than in favor of it (Fellner, 1970; Smith et al., 1986; Schover et al., 1997). Nevertheless, it is important to carefully screen volunteers since those who have been pressured to donate are often ambivalent – a feature that may correlate with donor regret posttransplant (Smith et al., 1986; Simmons et al., 1987). To avoid a conflict of interest, such screening should be performed by a skilled professional not involved in the care of the recipient (UNOS Ethics Committee, 1992; Price & Akveld, 1998).

Internal pressure has been more concerning and almost certainly more common. However, when it occurs, it would be wrong to conclude automatically that the decision to donate is not voluntary. Faden and Beauchamp point out that even when people feel "tightly constrained by circumstances . . . it does not follow . . . that persons in such 'coercive situations' do not act *autonomously* . . . [For example] a great many consenting surgery candidates of all types are persons left without meaningful choices . . . But this loss of freedom cannot be equated with a loss of autonomy . . . In a true situation of coercion, what *controls*, and thus deprives one of autonomy, is the [forced] will of another person, substituted for one's own will or desire . . ." (Faden & Beauchamp, 1986).

Viewed in this light, internal pressure to donate does not eliminate the ability to make a voluntary choice. Sells (1991, 1997) agrees: "The donor is compelled to make [a] decision . . . He is not compelled to donate. Voluntariness survives" (Sells, 1991). Crouch and Elliott (1999) point out that even close relationships do not eliminate freedom to choose: "If we are ever to get straight about the nature of voluntariness, we must recognize that moral and emotional commitments are not exceptional, are not constraints on freedom, but rather part of ordinary human life." Similarly, Singer et al. (1989) conclude: "[Although internal] pressure is unavoidable . . . the need to balance selfishness and altruism is a universal feature of family relationships. We do not think that it invalidates voluntary consent." And Price points out (Eurotold Project, 1997): "the mere fact that a person feels bound to donate does not, in itself, render the consent given involuntary . . . the very people who feel such responsibility most keenly, i.e. parents of sick children, are the most willing, determined donors and the least ambivalent of all."

The conclusion of these authors, that strong emotional bonds need not compromise voluntarism among living organ donors, seems reasonable but needs more justification and will be considered further below (see *Autonomous choices without informed consent* and *An ethic of care as an alternative to informed consent in living related organ donation).* However, first I wish to review the other major perceived threat to donor autonomy: consent without full understanding.

Concerns About Understanding

In addition to worries about voluntarism, there has long been concern that living organ donors may not fully understand what they are agreeing to do. The elements of informed consent would suggest that potential living donors reach a decision only after collecting and carefully considering information about the risks and benefits of donation. However, over thirty years ago, Fellner and Marshall discovered that many donors make an immediate decision that precedes information gathering and clarification (Fellner & Marshall, 1968, 1970). Furthermore, none of their donors changed their minds after receiving information from the transplant team. These observations were confirmed in the classic studies of Simmons et al. (1987) in which 78% of the donors interviewed said they knew right away they would donate and 62% were classified by the investigators as having made an immediate choice; only 25% used a classic model of reasoned decision making. They concluded that "the majority of donors *volunteer immediately upon hearing of the need* without any time delay or any period of deliberation" (Simmons et al., 1987). These data show that decisions of potential donors are often made in the face of limited understanding of risks and benefits, an observation that led Fellner and Marshall (1970) to conclude that for many donors informed consent is a myth. Under these circumstances, should offers of donation be accepted as expressions of autonomous choice?

Autonomous Choices Without Informed Consent

It is important to remember that autonomy and informed consent are not the same. It is respect for autonomy we seek to protect and informed consent is but one way to accomplish this. Consent that is not fully informed may still be valid as long as it expresses a competent person's free choice. In its review of this issue, The Nuffield Council on Bioethics (1995) concluded: "The ethically significant requirement is not that consent be **complete**, but that it be **genuine**." But without informed consent how can we be sure that one's choice is truly her own?

Fellner and Marshall have suggested that many people use another acceptable process (probably unknowingly) to decide about organ donation: moral decision making (Fellner & Marshall, 1970). The three components of this process are (Fellner & Marshall, 1970; Simmons et al., 1987): (1) awareness of the consequences of one's actions for another; (2) ascription of responsibility to oneself; and (3) acceptance of moral norms. The fact that this information is immediately available to many potential donors may explain and justify their seemingly instantaneous decisions. For example, consider the parents of a child doing poorly on dialysis. The potential benefits of a transplant are immediately apparent, most parents feel deeply responsible for the welfare of their children, and it is a widely accepted moral norm for parents to make major sacrifices for their children (Caplan, 1993b; Jacobs et al., 1998; Spital, 1998b).

This analysis suggests that in some cases, informed consent may not be necessary to protect donor autonomy. Informed consent is designed to protect vulnerable people from exploitation by physicians and investigators who may not share the same values as their patients or may not consider the welfare of research subjects to be paramount (Beauchamp & Childress, 1994; Nuffield Council, 1995). But while the risk of exploitation is an important concern in impersonal relationships, in personal ones there may be little or no such risk at all. In a discussion of this issue, Hardwig (1989) said: "we don't need an ethics to protect us from those who understand us and care about our interests." Consider the parents of a dying child who desperately wish to save their child's life and are willing to do whatever is necessary to accomplish this goal. When they offer to donate an organ to save their child, regardless of the risk for themselves, few would question the voluntary nature of their choice. There is no risk of exploitation here that must be guarded against by requiring that the parents provide informed consent. Such considerations led Majeske et al. (1996) to conclude: "The traditional requirements of informed consent do not appear well suited to evaluations of living related donors' decision making . . . informed consent is based on an impartialist understanding of the requirements of autonomy that de-emphasizes personal relationships so that each decision maker is conceived as being free to pursue autonomous goals. In living related [organ] donation, however, partiality and personal relationships frequently play essential roles because personal relationships importantly influence or even constitute potential donors' personal goals. Thus, in order to evaluate donors' decisions . . . it seems plausible to use a theoretical ethical framework that recognizes interrelatedness [which informed consent does not]." An ethic of care may provide such a framework (Majeske et al., 1996).

An Ethic of Care as an Alternative to Informed Consent in Living Related Organ Donation

As alluded to in the previous discussion, traditional ethical theory, with its emphasis on rules, rights, and obligations, is designed for impartial impersonal situations and does not adequately describe the ethics of personal relationships (Hardwig, 1989; Houlgate, 1993; Majeske et al., 1996; Crouch & Elliott, 1999). Living organ donation usually involves such relationships because the potential donor and intended recipient are often members of the same family. In their discussion of this subject, Crouch and Elliott (1999) point out: "the picture of the independent and self-interested agent [promulgated by traditional ethical theory] is inappropriate in the context of the family . . . In families, the important factor is that family members cherish each other simply for each other's sake . . . being devoted to 'the family' and its members is a source of deep meaning and value in our lives and the lives of those around us."

In contrast to traditional ethical theory, an ethic of care is designed to guide and explain behavior in personal relationships. It stresses the value of emotional attachments, instructs us to work to strengthen these bonds, and points to them as justification for action (Majeske et al., 1996). In their discussion of this issue, Majeske et al. (1996) have said: "Our actions are not a result of fixed rules or some sort of decision-making calculus but of affection and regard for the related other." Similarly, Hardwig (1989) concludes: "the appropriate motive for action in personal relationships [is not duty or responsibility but rather] is simply that we want to do these things. Persons pursue whatever *ends* they have simply because they want to . . . And in a personal relationship, I and my well-being are ends of yours . . . [and you and] your ends are my ends too." These concepts were vividly illustrated by a set of parents, each of whom had donated a kidney to their daughter (Pierce & Pierce, 1973): "In our case, with our daughter's life at stake, possible future risks to the donor were not a consideration. There was no question as to 'whether'. Suzy needed, and that was all there was to it." The feeling and actions of these parents are highly commendable, but they are neither surprising nor unique. If confronted with a similar situation, it is very likely that most caring parents would respond the same way (Spital & Spital, 1988; Whitington, 1996).

Because most living organ donors are emotionally related to their recipients, an ethic of care would seem to be an appropriate framework in which to consider the offers of related volunteers. Majeske et al. (1996) point out: "The responses of living donors most frequently cited as seeming to violate the voluntariness requirements of informed consent initially appear to be more comprehensible within an ethical framework of care than from the perspective of traditional impartialist ethics . . . The quick decision making and lack of detailed consideration of risks and benefits by living donors seem to parallel the natural caring responses and the lack of rules or calculus for moral decisions regarding related others described in much of the ethic of care literature."

While pointing out that an ethic of care seems to explain the behavior of donors who are closely related to their recipients, Majeske et al. (1996) have criticized this concept on several grounds: (1) an ethic of care suggests that there is an obligation to donate without providing a method for defining the limits of that obligation; (2) it is unclear which relationships are sufficiently close to conclude that an ethic of care is an appropriate framework in which to consider them; and (3) this ethical construct gives no guidance about how to prioritize when there are conflicting obligations to care.

While these criticisms appear valid, I believe that an ethic of care is still a valuable framework in which to consider offers of organ donation by close relatives. When transplant centers are approached by a volunteer, what they are concerned with is not whether that person is obligated to donate but rather whether or not her consent is a valid expression of her autonomy. Consideration of an ethic of care reminds us that when the welfare of a cherished loved one is at stake, many people choose to donate simply because the person they wish to help is of such great importance to them (Stiller et al., 1985); to them, the risks are immaterial. This explains why for many donors the decision to donate is not a difficult one and why they often decide so quickly and are so committed to donating (Fellner & Marshall, 1968; Hamburger & Crosnier, 1968; Fellner & Marshall, 1970; Smith et al., 1986; Simmons et al., 1987; Goldman, 1993; Schover et al., 1997; Toronyi et al., 1998). This also explains the predictable observation that most people would be willing to accept a great deal of added risk to donate a kidney to their children (Spital & Spital, 1988b).

When living organ donation is considered in the light of an ethic of care, it becomes clear that the requirement for informed consent may not always make sense. While all potential donors have the right to make an informed choice, they also have the right to waive this claim (Beauchamp & Childress, 1994) and many close relatives appear to do just this. Instead of carefully weighing risks and benefits, some individuals base their decisions primarily on care and concern. Despite incomplete understanding and the possibility of internal pressure, consent which emanates from deep affection should be looked upon as an expression of autonomy and considered just as valid as consent which is fully informed. As noted by Crouch & Elliott (1999): "it should not strike one as ethically problematic that a mother might *naturally* want to donate part of her liver to her dying child. Neither love nor conscience constrains the mother's autonomy; rather, they give voice to her autonomy and say something about the kind of agent she is . . .".

The observations that the vast majority of donors are glad they donated and would do it again (Eisendrath et al., 1969; Marshall & Fellner, 1977; Smith et al., 1986; Morris et al., 1987; Simmons et al., 1987; Gouge et al., 1990; Bunzendahl, 1991; Westlie et al., 1993; Sterneck et al., 1995; Whitington, 1996; Jakobsen, 1997; Schover et al., 1997; Jacobs et al., 1998; Toronyi et al., 1998; Johnson et al., 1999) and that a significant number of family members refuse to donate (Renz et al., 1995), strongly support the premise that offers of organ donation by close-caring relatives, even when made immediately, are indeed autonomous choices. Furthermore, the fact that transplant centers accept organs from close relatives but are usually unwilling to accept offers from altruistic strangers (who are able to give truly informed consent) (Spital, 2000), indicates that many centers recognize the importance of personal relationships (Majeske et al., 1996) and agree that fully informed consent is not always necessary nor sufficient for determining the acceptability of a potential living donor.

The above discussion assumes strong emotional bonds between the donor and recipient, e.g. between parents and their children. But of course, the strength of personal relationships varies greatly. Among those that are not as strong, e.g. between some siblings, consent may derive less from an ethic of care than from a fear of family ostracism or lifelong guilt. Some of these potential donors may be extremely ambivalent, which is a risk factor for a negative reaction after donation (Simmons & Anderson, 1982; Simmons et al., 1987; Switzer et al., 1996). To reduce the risk of accepting such individuals, several protective practices should be a routine part of the donor evaluation (Fellner, 1973; Singer et al., 1989; Shaw et al., 1991; UNOS Ethics Committee, 1992; Fox & Swazey, 1992; Caplan, 1993a; Kasiske et al., 1996; Eurotold Project, 1997; Schover et al., 1997; Price & Akveld, 1998; Spital, 1998a; Casas et al., 1999). These include: (1) a careful psychosocial assessment of prospective donors to be sure they are competent and really want to donate; (2) insistence that this assessment be made by an experienced professional not involved in the care of the recipient; (3) provision of clear verbal and written information regarding the risks and benefits of donation during a volunteer's first visit to the transplant center; (4) exercising great care to avoid exerting pressure to donate; (5) asking for consent twice: first for the evaluation, and later for the donor operation (assuming the volunteer is acceptable); and (6) informing potential donors that the center is prepared to offer a medical excuse for not donating even when none exists. When these safeguards are employed, decisions of potential related donors should be considered autonomous. In agreement with this conclusion, Elliott has said: "The most worrying part of living organ donation is not freedom of choice . . . The worrying part is the chance of harm to a healthy donor" (Elliott, 1995). Let us now consider this other major concern about using living donors.

Non-Maleficence

The ethical principle of non-maleficence asserts that one should not inflict harm intentionally (Beauchamp, 1994). This principle is expressed in the Hippocratic oath and is thus deeply ingrained in the minds of physicians. In living organ donation physical harm is unavoidable and is therefore seen by some physicians as a violation of this fundamental principle they have promised to uphold (Land, 1989; Fox & Swazey, 1992; Kleinman & Lowy, 1992; Strong & Lynch, 1996; Spital, 1998b). This is perhaps the strongest argument for abandoning this practice (Starzl, 1987; Elliott, 1995; Isoniemi, 1997). However, the principle of non-maleficence is not absolute and may be justifiably overridden when the benefit of an action exceeds the harm inflicted, e.g. amputating a gangrenous limb to save a patient's life (Beauchamp, 1994; Nuffield Council, 1995; Daar et al., 1997; Eurotold Project, 1997; Spital, 1998b). As Dr. Moore pointed out over 10 years ago: "The ancient dogma of 'first, do no harm' appears simple and obvious. But on closer examination, it seems to have been mere window dressing for the necessary hurt that has accompanied much of medical practice over the centuries" (Moore, 1988).

Of course, while most surgical procedures are performed primarily to benefit the person undergoing surgery, this is not true of donor nephrectomy. However, even this does not present an insurmountable ethical barrier to living organ donation (Spital, 1998b). There are other accepted medical procedures designed to help someone other than the person who is physically harmed, e.g. Cesarean section (Moore, 1988). Such action may be justified if the person operated upon derives enough benefit to justify the risk, even though this was not the primary purpose of the procedure, the person freely agrees and the procedure helps that person accomplish a morally good act (Spital, 1998b). Clearly, altruistic living organ donation meets the latter criterion. To see whether it satisfies the first, we must carefully consider its risks, its possible benefits (for the donor as well as the recipient), and the balance of the two. I will focus on kidney donation since there is much more experience with this organ than with any other.

Risks of Donor Nephrectomy

Donor nephrectomy is a major surgical procedure and postoperative complications are inevitable (Tufveson et al., 1998). A review of relevant studies reported an average postoperative complication rate of 32% (Kasiske et al., 1996). However, most of these were minor and recent reports indicate that this rate is now much lower (Johnson et al., 1997; Shaffer et al., 1998). Studies from the 1970s and 80s reported major complication rates of between 2 and 4% (Bay & Hebert, 1987; Kasiske et al., 1996). More recent data from the University of Minnesota (Johnson et al., 1997) and from a survey of 173 U.S. transplant centers (Bia et al., 1995) indicate that as is true of the overall rate, the rate of major complications has also declined, although reported rates depend on how 'major' is defined; e.g. compare the reports of Johnson (1997) and Shaffer (1998).

Of course, the most dreaded complication of kidney donation is donor death and such deaths have occurred (Starzl, 1987). Fortunately, this tragic event is very rare. Based on the results of a survey of members of the American Society of Transplant Surgeons, Najarian et al. (1992) estimated the perioperative mortality of donor nephrectomy to be 0.03%. A survey of United Network for Organ Sharing (UNOS)-approved U.S. transplant centers led to an identical estimate (Bia et al., 1995). To put this risk in perspective, the Patient Care and Education Committee of the American Society of Transplant Physicians (ASTP) pointed out (Kasiske et al., 1996): "the risk of dying as a result of donor surgery is of a similar order of magnitude as the risk of dying as a result of a motor vehicle accident in one year in the United States."

Psychological complications, especially depression, have also been reported (Kemph, 1966; Eisendrath et al., 1969; Bennett & Harrison, 1974; Hirvas et al., 1976; Morris et al., 1987; Simmons et al., 1987; Weizer et al., 1989; Kasiske et al., 1996; Schover et al., 1997; Johnson et al., 1999). However, such reactions affect only a minority of donors and are rarely severe (Fellner & Marshall, 1968, 1970; Bennett et al., 1974; Smith et al., 1986; Morris et al., 1987; Sharma & Enoch, 1987; Simmons et al., 1987; Bonomini, 1991; Kasiske et al., 1996; Schover et al., 1997). In fact, one study found that non-donor parents had more psychosomatic and psychiatric symptoms than did donor parents after their child was transplanted (Karrfelt et al., 1998). Even when the transplant is unsuccessful, very few donors regret donating; although regret is more common in these cases, most donors are still glad they did all they could to help their loved one (Hamburger & Crosnier, 1968; Marshall & Fellner, 1977; Simmons & Anderson, 1982; Sharma & Enoch, 1987; Schover et al., 1997). A generally benign psychological course has also been reported among liver donors (Goldman, 1993).

What about the long term outlook for kidney donors? A few studies suggested that kidney donors may be at increased risk for developing proteinuria, hypertension, and renal failure years after nephrectomy (Hakim et al., 1984) and there are rare reports of donors who developed ESRD (Said & Soyannwo, 1996). However, most studies have found that the risk of a healthy kidney donor developing renal failure is very small (Najarian et al., 1992; Kasiske et al., 1995, 1996; Saran et al., 1997). Indeed, the previously referred to ASTP survey estimated that the risk of ESRD among kidney donors is no greater and may actually be lower than it is among the general population (Bia et al., 1995). And most reassuring is the recent study from Sweden which found that the survival rate among 430 people who had donated a kidney between 1964 and 1994 was actually better than that of the general population (Fig. 3), probably because only healthy people were permitted to donate (Fehrman-Ekholm et al., 1997).

This discussion indicates that while the probability of a serious donor complication is very small, it is not zero. Therefore, as previously mentioned, justification of living organ donation requires that this risk be balanced by benefit, a concept which leads us to consider another important ethical principle: beneficence.

Beneficence

This ethical principle instructs us to do good for others, especially when there is little or no risk to ourselves (Beauchamp & Childress, 1994). This raises the

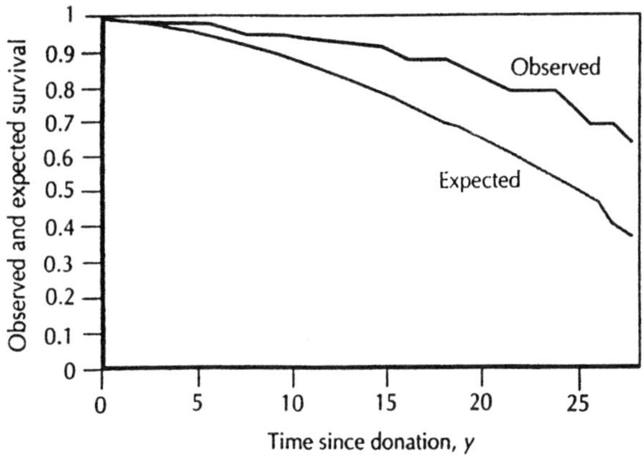

Fig. 3. Observed and expected survival rates of 430 living kidney donors who underwent nephrectomy in Sweden between 1964 and 1994. Reprinted from Fehrman-Ekholm et al. (1997) with permission.

interesting question of whether people are obligated to donate organs to loved ones. However, what I wish to focus on here is another aspect of beneficence, namely that achieving good provides strong prima facie justification for action and, if large enough, may even justify inflicting harm. To see if this is true of living organ donation, we must carefully consider its benefits.

Benefits of Living Kidney Donation

In view of the superior results achieved with living donors and the shortage of cadaveric organs, it is clear that living donors may provide enormous benefits for recipients. Living organ donation may therefore be considered a heroic and morally good act (Bonomini, 1991; Caplan, 1993a). This is an important consideration. However, because there is some risk for the donor, the high likelihood of recipient benefit does not provide sufficient justification for accepting a living donor. Remember that the issue here is not whether the potential donor's choice is reasonable but rather whether the physician should help that person accomplish it (Elliott, 1995). When making this determination, the potential donor's physician must consider the donor's welfare first and foremost (Merrill, 1971). (It is for precisely this reason that separate donor and recipient physicians are recommended). From this vantage point, justification for exposing a person to the risks of donor nephrectomy requires that these risks be balanced by potential benefits for the *donor* (Land, 1989; UNOS Ethics Committee, 1992). Often this appears to be the case.

There is much evidence that many living related kidney donors benefit psychologically through an improved quality of life (Westlie et al., 1993; Jacobs et al., 1998; Johnson et al., 1999) and lasting increases in self-esteem resulting from the knowledge that they have made a major sacrifice to help save a life (Fellner & Marshall, 1968, 1970; Eisendrath et al., 1969; Marshall & Fellner, 1977; Simmons & Anderson, 1982; Simmons et al., 1987; Brunzendahl et al., 1991; Simforoosh et al., 1991; Kasiske et al., 1996; Jacobs, 1998; Karrfelt, 1998). While not all investigators have found these psychological rewards among kidney donors (Gouge et al., 1990), few if any would question the enormous benefit to the donor of seeing a cherished loved one resurrected (Spital, 1998b). As one set of parental donors put it six years after seeing their daughter restored to health (Pierce & Pierce, 1973): "There is no doubt in our minds that we, as kidney donors, have gained much more than we lost." For donors such as these, the psychological benefit derived from donating greatly exceeds the physical harm incurred (Spital, 1998b). Surprisingly, some potential donors may also benefit physically when treatable health problems are detected during the donor evaluation (Jones et al., 1993); in fact, Daar et al. (1997) have suggested that more lives may have been saved as a result of this screening process than have been lost through donation. The fact that the vast majority of donors are glad they donated and would do it again (Eisendrath et al., 1969; Marshall & Fellner, 1977; Smith et al., 1986; Morris et al., 1987; Simmons et al., 1987; Gouge et al., 1990; Bunzendahl et al., 1991; Westlie et al., 1993; Jakobsen, 1997; Schover et al., 1997; Jacobs et al., 1998; Toronyi et al., 1998) strongly supports the view that kidney donation usually benefits the donor as well as the recipient.

The large psychological benefits experienced by closely related voluntary kidney donors (e.g. parents) provide justification for exposing such individuals to the small risk of donor nephrectomy. This was suggested by Dr. Schreiner over thirty years ago: "If giving a kidney is for [the donor's] spiritual or psychiatric good, and this is recognized as part of the total person, it seems to me that the [physical harm resulting from donation] becomes quite permissible . . ." (Schreiner 1966).

Justice

The final ethical principle to consider is justice. This refers to "fair, equitable, and appropriate treatment in light of what is due or owed persons" (Beauchamp & Childress, 1994). Justice is an important issue in transplantation because of the goal of equitably distributing an insufficient supply of cadaveric organs.

Although justice is less relevant to living organ donation, it is worth noting that policies regulating this practice indirectly impact all potential recipients. By removing patients from the recipient pool, living donors increase the likelihood that a cadaveric organ will become available for a particular individual. Any unnecessary restrictions on living organ donation would needlessly worsen the severe organ shortage (Evans, 1989).

SHOULD WE CONTINUE TO USE LIVING RELATED ORGAN DONORS?

Let us now return to the question we began with: should we continue to use living related donors? The previous analysis indicates that at least for kidneys, when the potential donor is healthy, free to choose, and emotionally close to the recipient, the answer to this question is "yes" (Spital, 1998b). This conclusion is based on the following: (1) there is a severe shortage of cadaveric organs and living donors provide excellent results for recipients; (2) the risk of kidney donation for a healthy person is very low; (3) the likelihood that the donor as well as the recipient will benefit is high; (4) offers by competent genuine volunteers deserve respect as expressions of individual autonomy; and (5) organ donation is a morally good act. Similar considerations apply to emotionally invested donors of some non-renal organs as well (Singer et al., 1989; Shaw et al., 1991; Kramer & Sprung, 1995; Strong & Lynch, 1996; Whitington, 1996). For example, despite posing higher risks than kidney donation (Mayer, 1996), at experienced centers living liver donation by devoted healthy parents is justified when, as is often the case, the prognosis for their child after transplantation is reasonably good (Singer et al., 1989; Sterneck et al., 1995; Strong & Lynch, 1996; Whitington, 1996; Grewal et al., 1998; Casas et al., 1999). Under these circumstances, the potential benefit for both the donor and recipient is enormous since a liver transplant is the beloved child's only hope for survival (Casas et al., 1999).

It appears that when practised with care, some types of living related organ donation are ethically acceptable and valuable practices that should continue at least until there is an adequate supply of high quality cadaveric organs (Bonomini, 1991; UNOS Ethics Committee, 1992; Caplan, 1993a, 1997; Daar et al., 1997; Eurotold Project, 1997; Jakobsen, 1997; Spital, 1998a, b; Tufveson et al., 1998). Surveys suggest that most of the public would agree (Fellner & Schwartz, 1971; Stiller et al., 1985; Spital et al., 1988; Shanteau & Skowronski, 1991; Caplan, 1993a).

SHOULD THE RANGE OF ACCEPTABLE LIVING DONORS BE EXPANDED BEYOND GENETIC RELATIVES?

Because of the very favorable risk benefit ratio, most U.S. transplant centers accept living kidney donors (Spital, 2000). Until recently, almost all of these donors have been genetically related to their recipients. Although a few unrelated donors were used in the earliest days of renal transplantation (Advisory Committee to the Renal Transplant Registry, 1972), this practice was soon abandoned because of poor results, increasing availability of dialysis, and concern about the donor's motivation and the risk involved (McGeown, 1968; Burley & Stiller, 1985; Levey et al., 1986; Blake & Cardella, 1989; Spital, 1998c). As recently as 1991, the World Health Organization (1991) stated in its "Guiding principles on human organ transplantation" that "adult living persons may donate organs, but in general such donors should be genetically related to the recipients."

Nevertheless, over the past 15 years, interest in unrelated living kidney donors has increased tremendously because of the severe organ shortage, the improving ability to successfully transplant poorly matched donor recipient pairs, evidence that the risk of donor nephrectomy for a healthy person is very low, and the belief that transplantation is the optimal therapy for patients with ESRD (Spital, 1998c). It has been estimated that spouses could provide functioning kidneys for as many as 25% of all adult potential renal transplant recipients (Terasaki et al., 1995). Not surprisingly, experience with unrelated living donor kidney transplantation is growing. The results of these transplants have been excellent and superior to those obtained with cadaver donors (Fig. 2) (Squifflet et al., 1990; Ploeg et al., 1993; D'Alessandro et al., 1995, 1998; Terasaki et al., 1995, 1997; Lowell et al., 1996; Alfani et al., 1997; Binet et al., 1997; Foss et al., 1998; Said & Curtis, 1998; Cecka, 1999; Gjertson & Cecka, 2000; Humar et al., 2000).

Genetically unrelated living donor renal transplantation is clearly effective, but efficacy is not sufficient to recommend this practice. Desirable ends alone do not justify the means of achieving them. Before accepting genetically unrelated living donors, we must first be sure that this practice is ethically appropriate (Spital 1998c). As I attempt to answer this question, I will consider emotionally (but not genetically) related potential donors and completely unrelated volunteers separately because of important differences between them.

Emotionally Related Living Organ Donors

If, as I have argued, it is ethically acceptable for genetic relatives to donate organs to loved ones, then people who are related to a recipient through emotional ties alone (e.g. spouses, friends, in-laws) should also be considered ethically acceptable (Lawton, 1978; Newton, 1979; Burley & Stiller, 1985; Levey et al., 1986; Blake & Cardella, 1989; Spital, 1991, 1992, 1998c; Binet et al., 1997; Daar, 1999). Several considerations support this view. The physical risk to the donor is independent of her relationship to the recipient. Psychological pressure to donate should be no greater, and may actually be less, for emotionally related than for genetically related volunteers (Newton, 1979; Burley & Stiller, 1985; Evans, 1989; Jacobs et al., 1998; Spital, 1998c). When the donor is emotionally related to her recipient, commercialism is not an issue. Love and partnership are the main reasons for donating and the bonds motivating emotionally related donors may be as strong or stronger than those motivating genetically related ones (Squifflet et al., 1990; Binet et al., 1997; Thiel et al., 1997; Foss et al., 1998; Jacobs et al., 1998; Spital, 1998c). Thiel (1997) recently provided a vivid example of the very strong bonds that may exist between spouses: "When we informed the first non-blood-related Swiss donor in 1991 that we would accept her as a donor for her brother or sister only but not for her husband, she answered spontaneously, 'You cannot imagine how much I would rather donate a kidney to my husband than to one of my brothers or sisters. I share the fate of his illness with him every day.' " As indicated by this statement, like genetically related donors, spousal donors may benefit greatly from the restored health of the recipient (Binet et al., 1997; Jakobsen, 1997; Foss et al., 1998; Jacobs et al., 1998; Daar, 1999; Mathieson et al., 1999); they may also experience increased self-esteem (Sadler et al., 1971; Squifflet, 1990; Jacobs et al., 1998). Similar benefits may accrue to other types of emotionally related donors (Sadler et al., 1971; Simforoosh et al., 1991). During adulthood, spouses (not parents, children, or siblings) are considered our closest relatives (Fox & Swazey, 1992). Although some opponents of spousal donation are concerned about the high rate of divorce (Isoniemi, 1997), preliminary observations indicate that the relationships of spousal donors and their recipients remain the same or improve after transplantation, even when the graft fails (Binet et al., 1997); furthermore, even if the partners eventually separate, this would have no bearing on the morality of donating. Like genetically related donors, most emotionally related donors have no regrets about donating and would donate again if they could (Sadler et al., 1971; Simforoosh et al., 1991; Binet et al., 1997). Finally, several studies suggest that the vast majority of the public would donate a kidney to their spouses and a smaller majority would likely donate to a close friend (Lawton, 1978; Stiller et al., 1985; Spital, 1988b; Toronyi et al., 1998).

Based on these considerations it appears that the use of emotionally related donors is ethically acceptable, provided the safeguards recommended for the evaluation of genetically related volunteers are employed. Consistent with this conclusion is the observation that over the past 15 years, attitudes of transplant centers toward emotionally related donors have become very positive (Spital, 1986, 1989, 1994, 1996, 2000; Bia et al., 1995), and the vast majority of U.S. centers are now willing to accept emotionally related volunteers (Fig. 4) (Spital, 1996, 2000). While these donors accounted for less than 10% of all kidneys transplanted in the United States in 1998, their use has been steadily increasing (Fig. 5) (HCFA 1999, Shaffer et al., 1998).

Altruistic Strangers as Living Organ Donors

Though not likely to ever be the source of large numbers of organs, from time to time strangers step forward and offer to donate to someone they do not know (Sadler et al., 1971; Simforoosh et al., 1991; Matas et al., 2000). Instead of offering praise and admiration, the medical community has long greeted these remarkable people with distrust and suspicion (Hamburger & Crosnier, 1968; Fellner & Schwartz, 1971; Sadler et al., 1971; Fellner, 1973). Drs. Hamburger and Crosnier (1968) provided part of the rationale for this view: "individuals who [offer] to donate a kidney to a prospective recipient to whom they are not connected by any kind of emotional tie are frequently pathologic by psychiatric criteria." However, this conclusion was reached before any formal study of this issue had been done.

In 1971, Sadler and his colleagues published the results of their careful psychological study of 18 actual genetically unrelated kidney donors, nine of whom were completely unknown to their recipients (Sadler et al., 1971). The investigators found that these volunteers shared many features with living related donors: the decision to give was almost immediate, none of them felt coerced by physicians or recipients, there were no regrets or psychological complications after donating, and all experienced lasting increases in self-esteem (Sadler et al., 1971). Most remarkable were the observations regarding the strangers. They " 'knew' their response was wholesome . . . They were the most cooperative and helpful and were the kind of patients the ward nurses 'liked to have around.' The relationship with their living recipients continues to be wholesome and friendly" (Sadler et al., 1971). The authors also studied 22 people who offered to donate a kidney to a stranger in response to a public appeal. "Of these [donor] candidates, 80% were stable, self-supporting,

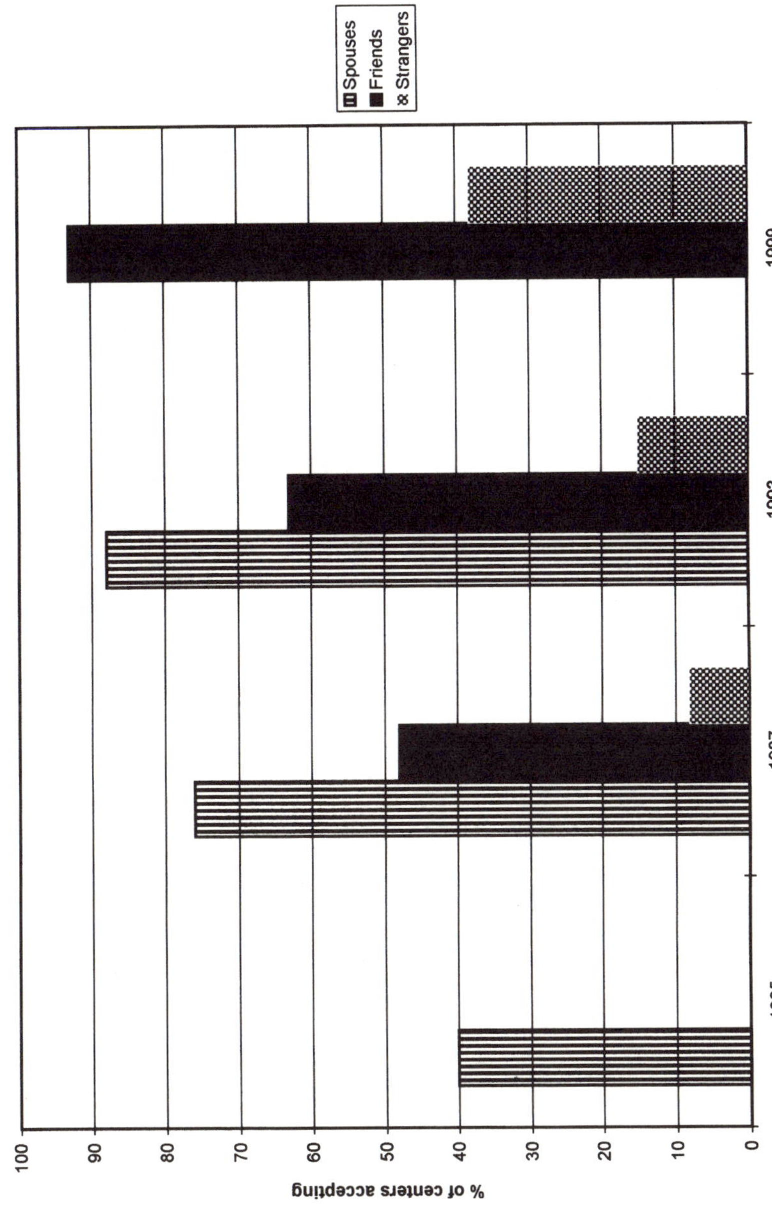

Fig. 4. Evolution of attitudes toward various types of genetically unrelated living kidney donors at U.S. transplant centers. Drawn from data from Spital (1986, 1989, 1994, 2000).

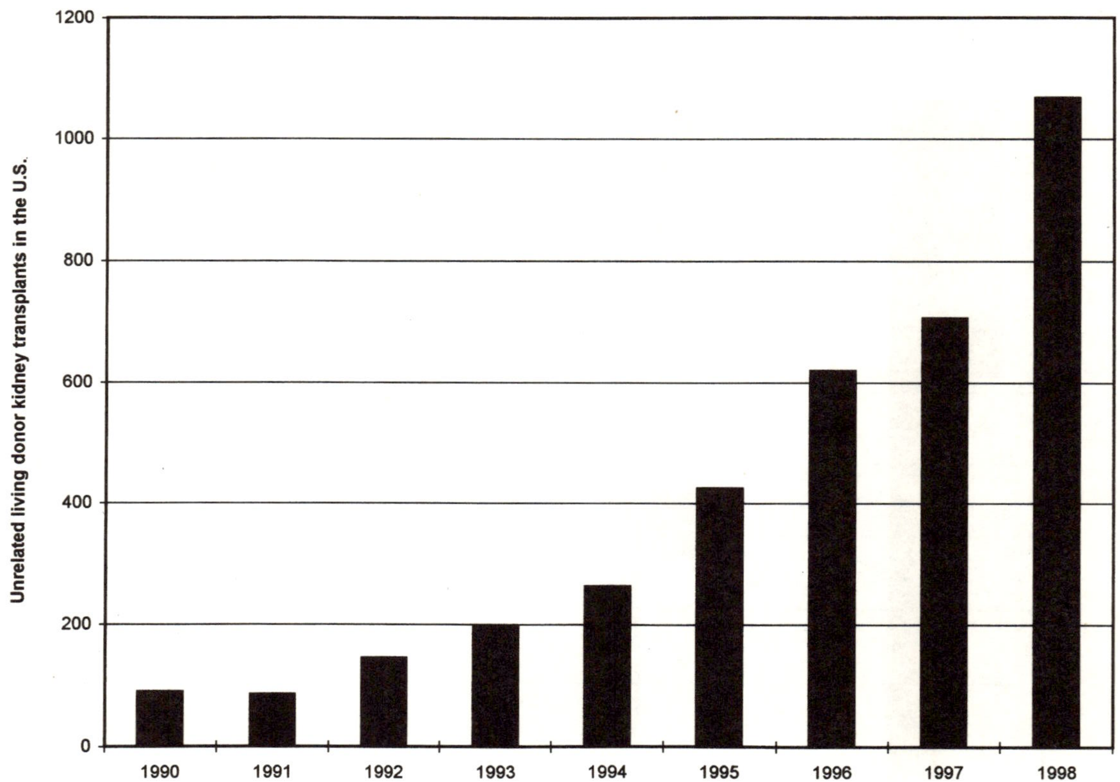

Fig. 5. Steady growth in the annual number of unrelated living donor kidney transplantations performed in the U.S. between 1990 and 1998. Drawn from data obtained from HCFA (1999).

middle-class citizens . . . 75% were well educated . . . The overwhelming reason for wanting to give an organ was to help someone in distress . . . [this was a group] of remarkable social and personal stability" (Sadler et al., 1971). Two years later Dr. Sadler reported an update of this study in which he succinctly characterized these unrelated volunteers: "Here, then, were a group of very fine human beings" (Sadler, 1973).

Sadler and his colleagues also surveyed 450 members of the general public and found that 19% said they would donate to a stranger in dire need of a kidney and 33% were unsure (Sadler et al., 1971). In another public survey, 11% of 116 respondents said they would definitely donate a kidney to a stranger and 43% said they probably would donate (Fellner & Schwartz, 1971). Similarly, two small studies of related donors found that 26% in one (Stiller et al., 1985) and 47% in the other (Toronyi et al., 1998) would have considered donating a kidney to a stranger. And a survey of college students also found some willingness to donate organs to strangers (Shanteau & Skowronski, 1991).

These results probably overestimate public altruism because participants were selected for willingness to respond and some belonged to special groups (donors and college students); furthermore, some respondents may have given what they perceived to be socially desirable answers which did not reflect what they would really have done (Siminoff et al., 1995; Spital, 1998c). It is likely that only a small minority of people would actually donate a kidney to a stranger. Nevertheless, the impressive success of the National Marrow Donor Program, which now has over 3 million people registered as potential bone marrow donors, indicates that there are many individuals who are willing to take risks to help people they do not know (Walker, 1999). Furthermore, whatever the percentage of people who would really donate an organ to a stranger, about 70% of a random sample of the U.S. public believe that kidney donation by strangers is an acceptable practice (Spital & Spital, 1988b).

The fact that many people would consider donating a kidney to a stranger, that most of those who would not would likely still find this practice acceptable, and that the few who have done so had little evidence of psychopathology, argue strongly that the desire to donate to a stranger may be a sign of healthy altruism rather than mental illness (Fellner & Schwartz, 1971; Sadler et al., 1971; Sadler, 1973; Lawton, 1978; Spital, 1998b, c). In an editorial on this subject published over 25 years ago, Fellner (1973) concluded: "No doubt there are [emotionally disturbed individuals among unrelated volunteers], but there are many sane people who, for reasons of their own that are not crazy reasons, want to donate part of themselves to a stranger in need."

A poignant example is the recent donation of a kidney by a renowned German transplant surgeon to a recipient he did not know (Karcher, 1996).

Another major concern about allowing strangers to donate organs is that this would open the door to commercialism in transplantation (Broyer & Affleck, 2000). While this possibility is abhorrent to some people, others, including the members of the International Forum for Transplant Ethics, have argued that carefully regulated organ sales may be ethically acceptable and should be reconsidered (Radcliffe-Richards et al., 1998; Cameron & Hoffenberg, 1999). But even for those who remain strongly opposed to this practice, the fear of commercialism does not justify excluding organ donations by altruistic strangers. The possibility of abuse is not sufficient to ban what would otherwise be an acceptable and valuable practice (Daar, 1991; Ploeg et al., 1993). For example, we do not ban driving even though some people endanger the safety of others by drinking before they drive; instead we try to prevent drunken driving and punish offenders (Spital, 1998c). In agreement with this approach, Evans (1989) points out: "The moral evil in trafficking stems, not from the donation of organs by a non-relative, but from the profit-directed commercial arrangements . . . Thus the proper response is to attack the exploitation of the act of donation, not the act itself." It should also be noted that risk of commercialism could be nearly eliminated by establishing a registry of potential unrelated living organ donors, which would protect the identity of the volunteers, as has been done for potential marrow donors (Levey et al., 1986; UNOS Ethics Committee, 1992).

Based on the previous discussion, it is concluded that the desire to donate an organ to a stranger need not be a sign of psychopathology and that the fear of commercialism is not sufficient to ban this practice. If these premises are accepted, it becomes difficult to categorically exclude altruistic strangers from donating organs for several reasons. At reputable centers, the outcome of transplantation with genetically unrelated donors is excellent (Cecka, 1999). As previously noted, the physical risk to the donor is independent of her relationship to the recipient. Because there is no sense of obligation, altruistic strangers should be able to provide fully informed consent and therefore may be considered to be true volunteers (Sadler et al., 1971; Lawton, 1978; Fellner, 1973; Burley & Stiller, 1985; Caplan, 1997; Spital, 1998b, 1998c). Like related donors, unrelated donors may benefit as a result of lasting increases in self-esteem and the knowledge of their magnificent deed (Sadler et al., 1971; Sadler, 1973; Butterworth et al., 1993); in fact, some data suggest that when compared with related donors, unrelated donors may derive more personal satisfaction from donating, perhaps because they have gone even further 'beyond the call of duty' (Butterworth et al., 1993; Chang et al., 1998). As discussed above, surveys suggest that the majority of the public believe that organ donation by altruistic strangers is acceptable (Spital & Spital, 1988b) and a significant minority would consider making such a donation themselves (Sadler et al., 1971; Fellner & Schwartz, 1971; Stiller et al., 1985; Toronyi et al., 1998). Despite similar potential for abuse, unrelated bone marrow donation is a widely accepted practice even though there are risks for the donor (Evans, 1989). Finally, organ donation by an altruistic stranger is a morally praiseworthy act. As Evans (1989) points out: "altruism receives its highest expression in the absence of personal relationships . . . The gift of an organ to a complete stranger . . . seems worthy of the highest respect." He also argues convincingly: "It seems . . . perverse to emphasize [the importance of] altruism [in living donor transplantation] and then grossly to circumscribe its opportunities for expression [by restricting donation to relatives]" (Evans, 1989).

These considerations suggest that organ donation by altruistic strangers is ethically acceptable provided the same safeguards recommended for protecting the autonomy of related donors (see *Respect for Autonomy*) are employed. Most important are careful psychosocial and medical evaluations by skilled professionals (with experience evaluating potential organ donors) who are not involved in the care of the recipient and can therefore act as donor advocates. In addition, because there are no personal bonds between completely unrelated potential donors and their intended recipients, an ethic of personal relationships does not apply (see *An ethic of care as an alternative to informed consent in living related organ donation*). In such cases it is essential to obtain fully informed consent. To help accomplish this, it is recommended that the medical evaluation of the potential donor and the transplant be delayed for several weeks to give the volunteer ample time to gather information and reach a carefully reasoned decision (Sadler, 1973; Singer et al., 1989; Spital, 1998b).

Consistent with the favorable medical and ethical considerations discussed above, attitudes at transplant centers toward organ donation by altruistic strangers have gradually become more liberal (Daar et al., 1997; Spital, 2000). A recent survey found that a large minority of U.S. centers would now consider such donors (Spital, 2000) whereas very few of them would have done so in the past (Fig. 4) (Spital, 1989, 1994). On the other hand, these transplants remain rare. While this is partially explained by the rarity of unrelated volunteers, it is also likely that even liberal centers are uncomfortable with this practice, do not encourage it, and are reluctant to proceed when faced with an actual volunteer (Spital, 2000).

SUMMARY AND CONCLUSIONS

When practiced with care, the use of living organ donors remains a valuable and ethically acceptable practice. This conclusion is based on the dire need for organs, the very low risk for a healthy donor (at least for kidneys), the high likelihood that the donor as well as the recipient will benefit from transplantation, and the fact that organ donation by a competent volunteer is a morally good act and an expression of individual autonomy (Spital, 1998b). While fuly informed consent is essential to protect the autonomy of unrelated volunteers, it may not always be necessary for relatives whose offers of organ donation emanate primarily from love and concern. However, safeguards should be employed during the evaluation of all volunteers so that unacceptable individuals can be detected and excluded. These include people at high surgical risk, people who are incompetent or very ambivalent about donating, volunteers motivated by psychopathology or unrealistic expectations, and people who are being pressured to donate. When the recommended safeguards are followed, the pool of ethically acceptable living donors may be expanded beyond traditional genetic relatives to include emotionally related individuals and even completely unrelated volunteers.

REFERENCES

Adams, R. K. (1987). Live organ donors and informed consent: a difficult minuet. *J. Legal Medicine*, *8*, 555–586.

Advisory Committee to the Renal Transplant Registry. (1972). The Ninth Report of the Human Renal Transplant Registry. *JAMA*, *220*, 253–260.

Alfani et al. (1997). Analysis of 160 consecutive living unrelated kidney transplants: 1983–1997. *Transplant. Proc.*, *29*, 3399–3401.

Bay, W. H., & Hebert, L. A. (1987). The living donor in kidney transplantation. *Ann. Intern. Med.*, *106*, 719–727.

Beauchamp, T. L., & Childress, J. F. (1994). *Principles of Biomedical Ethics*. New York, Oxford University Press.

Bennett, A. H., & Harrison, J. H. (1974). Experience with living familial renal donors. *Surg. Gyn. Obs.*, *139*, 894–898.

Bia et al. (1995). Evaluation of living renal donors. The current practice of U.S. transplant centers. *Transplantation*, *60*, 322–327.

Binet et al. (1997). Outcome in emotionally related living kidney donor transplantation. *Nephrol. Dial. Transplant.*, *12*, 1940–1948.

Blake, P. G., & Cardella, C. J. (1989). Kidney donation by living unrelated donors. *CMAJ*, *141*, 773–775.

Bonomini, V. (1991). Ethical aspects of living donation. *Transplant. Proc.*, *23*, 2497–2499.

Broyer, M., & Affleck, J. (2000). In defense of altruistic kidney donation by strangers: a commentary. *Pediatr Nephrol.*, *14*, 523–524.

Bunzendahl et al. (1991). Retrospective evaluation of psychosocial factors in former living related kidney donors. In: W. Land & J. B. Dossetor (Eds), *Organ Replacement Therapy: Ethics, Justice, Commerce* (pp. 57–59). Berlin, Springer-Verlag.

Burley, J. A., & Stiller, C. R. (1985). Emotionally related donors and renal transplantation. *Transplant. Proc., 17* (Suppl 3), 123–127.

Butterworth et al. (1993). Psychosocial effects of unrelated bone marrow donation: experiences of the National Marrow Donor Program. *Blood, 81*, 1947–1959.

Cameron, J. S., & Hoffenberg, R. (1999). The ethics of organ transplantation reconsidered: paid organ donation and the use of executed prisoners as donors. *Kidney Intern., 55*, 724–732.

Caplan, A. (1993a). Must I be my brother's keeper? Ethical issues in the use of living donors as sources of liver and other solid organs. *Transplant. Proc., 25*, 1997–2000.

Caplan, A. L. (1993b). Am I my brother's keeper? *Suffolk University Law Review, 27*, 901–914.

Caplan, A. L. (1997). Am I my brother's keeper? Ethics and the use of living donors (chapter 11). In: *Am I My Brother's Keeper?* (pp. 115–126). Bloomington, Indiana University Press.

Casas et al. (1999). Living donor liver transplantation in critically ill children. *Pediatr. Transplantation, 3*, 104–108.

Cecka, J. M., & Terasaki, P. I. (1997). Living donor kidney transplants: superior success rates despite histoincompatibilities. *Transplant. Proc., 29*, 203.

Cecka, J. M. (1999). Results of more than 1000 recent living-unrelated donor transplants in the United States. *Transplant. Proc., 31*, 234.

Chang et al. (1998). A comparison of related and unrelated marrow donors. *Psychosomatic Medicine, 60*, 163–167.

Childress, J. F. (1982). *Who Should Decide? Paternalism in Health Care*. New York, Oxford University Press. p. 60.

Chugh, K. S., & Jha, V. (1995). Differences in the care of ESRD patients worldwide: Required resources and future outlook. *Kidney Intern., 48* (Suppl. 50), S7-S13.

Cohen, B., & Wight, C. (1999). A European perspective on organ procurement. *Transplantation, 68*, 985–990.

Crouch, R. A., & Elliott, C. (1999). Moral agency and the family: the case of living related organ transplantation. *Cambridge Quarterly of Healthcare Ethics, 8*, 275–287.

D'Alessandro et al. (1995). Living related and unrelated donors for kidney transplantation: a 28-year experience. *Ann. Surg., 222*, 353–364.

D'Alessandro et al. (1998). Living unrelated renal donation: The University of Wisconsin experience. *Surgery, 124*, 604–611.

Daar, A. S. (1991). The case for using living non-related donors to alleviate the worldwide shortage of cadaver kidneys for transplantation. *Ann. Acad. Med. Singapore, 20*, 443–452.

Daar, A. S. (1995). Living organ donation: Time for a donor charter. *Clin. Transplant 1994*. 376–380.

Daar et al. (1997). Living-donor renal transplantation: evidence-based justification for an ethical option. *Transplant. Rev., 11*, 95–109.

Daar, A. S. (1999). Living non-related kidney transplantation: time to be taken seriously. *Transplant. Proc., 31*, 1769–1771.

de Charro, F. & de Witt, A. (1996). An appraisal of living donor kidney transplantation. *Transplant. Proc., 28*, 3559–3561.

de Ortuzar et al. (1997). Bioethics and organ transplantation. *Transplant. Proc., 29*, 3627–3630.

Eisendrath et al. (1969). Psychologic considerations in the selection of kidney transplant donors. *Surg. Gyn. Obs., 129*, 243–248.

Elliott, C. (1995). Doing harm: living organ donors, clinical research and The Tenth Man. *J. Med. Ethics*, *21*, 91–96.

Eurotold Project Management Group (1997). Donnelly, P. K. & Price, D. (Eds), *Questioning Attitudes to Living Donor Transplantation* (pp. v, 50–64). Leicester, U.K.

Evans, M. (1989). Organ donations should not be restricted to relatives. *J. Med. Ethics*, *15*, 17–20.

Faden, R. R., & Beauchamp, T. L. (1986). *A History and Theory of Informed Consent* (pp. 344–346). New York, Oxford University Press.

Fehrman-Ekholm et al. (1997). Kidney donors live longer. *Transplantation*, *64*, 976–978.

Fellner, C. H., & Marshall, J. R. (1968). Twelve kidney donors. *JAMA*, *206*, 2703–2707.

Fellner, C. H., & Marshall, J. R. (1970). Kidney donors-The myth of informed consent. *Amer. J. Psychiat.*, *126*, 1245–1251.

Fellner, C. H., & Schwartz, S. H. (1971). Altruism in disrepute. Medical versus public attitudes toward the living organ donor. *N. Engl. J. Med.*, *284*, 582–585.

Fellner, C. H. (1973). Organ donation: for whose sake? *Ann. Intern. Med.*, *79*, 589–592.

Foss et al. (1998). Unrelated living donors in 141 kidney transplantations. *Transplantation*, *66*, 49–52.

Fox, R. C., & Swazey, J. P. (1992). *Spare Parts. Organ Replacement in American Society* (pp. 31–42). New York, Oxford University Press.

Gjertson, D. W., & Cecka, J. M. (2000). Living unrelated donor kidney transplantation. *Kidney Intern.*, *58*, 491–499.

Goldman, L. S. (1993). Liver transplantation using living donors. Preliminary donor psychiatric outcomes. *Psychosomatics*, *34*, 235–240.

Gouge et al. (1990). The quality of life of donors, potential donors, and recipients of living-related donor renal transplantation. *Transplant. Proc.*, *22*, 2409–2413.

Grewal et al. (1998). Complications in 100 living-liver donors. *Ann. Surg.*, *228*, 214–219.

Groth, C. G. (1972). Landmarks in clinical renal transplantation. *Surg. Gyn. Obs.*, *134*, 323–328.

Gruessner et al. (1997). Simultaneous pancreas-kidney transplantation from live donors. *Ann. Surg.*, *226*, 471–482.

Hakim et al. (1984). Hypertension and proteinuria: long-term sequelae of uninephrectomy in humans. *Kidney Intern.*, *25*, 930–936.

Hamburger, J., & Crosnier, J. (1968). Moral and ethical problems in transplantation. In: F. Rapaport & J. Daussert (Eds), *Human Transplantation* (pp. 37–44). New York: Grune and Stratton.

Hardwig, J. (1989). In search of an ethics of personal relationships. In: G. Graham & H. LaFollette (Eds), *Person to Person* (pp. 63–81). Philadelphia, Temple University Press.

Hariharan et al. (2000). Improved graft survival after renal transplantation in the United States, 1988 to 1996. *N. Engl. J. Med.*, *342*, 605–612.

Harris, J. (1992). *Wonderwoman and Superman. The Ethics of Human Biotechnology* (p. 113). Oxford, Oxford University Press.

Health Care Financing Administration (HCFA) (1999). *End stage renal disease, Program Highlights.*

Hirvas et al. (1976). Psychological and social problems encountered in active treatment of chronic uremia. II. The living donor. *Acta. Med. Scand.*, *200*, 17–20.

Houlgate, L. D. (1993). Ethical theory and the family. In: D. T. Meyers, K. Kipnis & C. F. Murphy (Eds), *Kindred Matters. Rethinking the Philosophy of the Family.* (pp. 59–73). Ithaca, Cornell University Press.

Humar et al. (2000). Living unrelated donors in kidney transplants. *Transplantation, 69*, 1942–1945.

Hume et al. (1955). Experiences with renal homotransplantation in the human: report of nine cases. *J. Clin. Invest., 34*, 327–382.

Isoniemi, H. (1997). Living kidney donation; a surgeon's opinion. *Nephrol. Dial. Transplant., 12*, 1828–1829.

Jacobs et al. (1998). Kidney transplants from living donors: how donation affects family dynamics. *Adv. Renal Replacement Therapy, 5*, 89–97.

Jakobsen, A. (1997). Living renal transplantation – the Oslo experience. *Nephrol. Dial. Transplant., 12*, 1825–1827.

Johnson et al. (1997). Complications and risks of living donor nephrectomy. *Transplantation, 64*, 1124–1128.

Johnson et al. (1999). Long-term follow-up of living kidney donors: quality of life after donation. *Transplantation, 67*, 717–721.

Jones et al. (1993). Unrecognized health problems diagnosed during living donor evaluation: a potential benefit. *Transplant. Proc., 25*, 3083–3084.

Karcher, H. (1996). German doctor donates kidney. *Br. Med. J., 313*, 443.

Karrfelt et al. (1998). To be or not to be a living donor. *Transplantation, 65*, 915–918.

Kasiske et al. (1995). Long-term effects of reduced renal mass in humans. *Kidney Intern., 48*, 814–819.

Kasiske et al. (1996). The evaluation of living renal transplant donors: clinical practice guidelines. *J. Am. Soc. Nephrol., 11*, 2288–2313.

Kemph, J. P. (1966). Renal failure, artificial kidney and kidney transplant. *Am. J. Psychiat., 122*, 1270–1274.

Kleinman, I., & Lowy, F. H. (1992). Ethical considerations in living organ donation and a new approach. *Arch. Intern. Med., 152*, 1484–1488.

Kramer, M. R., & Sprung, C. L. (1995). Living related donation in lung transplantation. Ethical considerations. *Arch. Intern. Med., 155*, 1734–1738.

Kreis, H. (1985). Why living related donors should not be used whenever possible. *Transplant. Proc., 17*, 1510–1514.

Land, W. (1989). The problem of living organ donation: facts, thoughts, and reflections. *Transplant Int., 2*, 168–179.

Lawton, R. L. (1978). Living non-related donors for transplantation. *Proc. Dialysis Transplant Forum, 8*, 30–34.

Levey et al. (1986). Kidney transplantation from unrelated living donors. Time to reclaim a discarded opportunity. *N. Engl. J. Med., 314*, 914–916.

Lin et al. (1998). Center-specific graft and patient survival rates. 1997 United Network for Organ Sharing (UNOS) Report. *JAMA, 280*, 1153–1160.

Lowell et al. (1996). Living-unrelated renal transplantation provides comparable results to living-related renal transplantation: a 12-year single-center experience. *Surgery, 119*, 538–543.

Majeske et al. (1996). In search of an ethical framework for consideration of decisions regarding live donation. In: B. Spielman (Ed.), *Organ and Tissue Donation. Ethical, Legal, and Policy Issues* (pp. 89–101). Carbondale, Southern Illinois University Press.

Marshall, J. R., & Fellner, C. H. (1997). Kidney donors revisited. *Am. J. Psychiat., 134*, 575–576.

Matas et al. (2000). Non-directed donation of kidneys from living donors. *N. Engl. J. Med., 343*, 433–436.

Mathieson et al. (1999). The spouse as a kidney donor: ethically sound? *Nephrol. Dial. Transplant.*, *14*, 46–48.

Mayer, A. D. (1996). The argument against live-donor liver transplantation. *J. Hepatology*, *24*, 628–630.

McGeown, M. G. (1968). Ethics for the use of live donors in kidney transplantation. *Am. Heart J.*, *75*, 711–714.

Merrill et al. (1956). Successful homotransplantation of the human kidney between identical twins. *JAMA*, *160*, 277–282.

Merrill, J. P. (1971). Statement of the Committee on Morals and Ethics of the Transplantation Society. *Ann. Intern. Med.*, *75*, 631–633.

Michielsen, P. (1995). More or less living donation? *Clin. Transplant 1994*, 344–347.

Moore, F. D. (1964). New problems for surgery. *Science*, *144*, 388–392.

Moore, F. D.(1988). Three ethical revolutions: ancient assumptions remodeled under pressure of transplantation. *Transplant. Proc.*, *20* (Suppl. 1), 1061–1067.

Morris et al. (1987). Psychosocial complications in living related kidney donors: and Australian experience. *Transplant. Proc.*, *19*, 2840–2844.

Murray et al. (1963). Prolonged survival of human-kidney homografts by immunosuppressive drug therapy. *N. Engl. J. Med.*, *268*, 1315–1323.

Murray, J. E. (1982). Reflections on the first successful kidney transplantation. *World J. Surg.*, *6*, 372–376.

Najarian et al. (1992). Twenty years or more of follow-up of living kidney donors. *Lancet*, *340*, 807–810.

Newton, W. T. (1979). Who is the brother that I should keep? *Arch. Surg.*, *114*, 992–993.

Neylan et al. (1999). The allocation of cadaver kidneys for transplantation in the United States: consensus and controversy. *J. Am. Soc. Nephrol.*, *10*, 2237–2243.

Nuffield Council on Bioethics. (1995). *Human Tissue Ethical and Legal Issues* (p. 45). London

Pierce, E. G., & Pierce, R. A. (1973). The Agony and the Ecstasy. *Transplant. Proc.*, *5*, 1067–1068.

Ploeg et al. (1993). Living unrelated kidney donation: an underutilized resource? *Transplant. Proc.*, *25*, 1532–1534.

Price, D., & Akveld, H. (1998). Living donor organ transplantation in Europe: re-evaluating its role. *European J. Health Law*, *5*, 19–44.

Provoost, A. P., & Brenner, B. M. (1993). Long-term follow-up of humans with single kidneys: the need for longitudinal studies to assess true changes in renal function. *Curr. Opin. Nephrol. Hypertension*, *2*, 521–526.

Radcliffe-Richards et al. (1998). The case for allowing kidney sales. *Lancet*, *351*, 1950–1952.

Rapaport, F. T. (1987). Living donor kidney transplantation. *Transplant. Proc.*, *19*, 169–173.

Renz et al. (1995). Donor selection limits use of living-related liver transplantation. *Hepatology*, *22*, 1122–1126.

Russell, S., & Jacob, R. G. (1993). Living-related organ donation: the donor's dilemma. *Patient Education Counseling*, *21*, 89–99.

Sadler et al. (1971). The living, genetically unrelated, kidney donor. *Semin Psychiat.*, *3*, 86–101.

Sadler, H. H. (1973). The motivation of living donors. *Transplant. Proc.*, *5*, 1121–1123.

Said, R., & Soyannwo, M. (1996). Renal failure in a living-related kidney donor: case report and review of the literature. *Am. J. Nephrol.*, *16*, 334–338.

Said, M. R., & Curtis, J. J. (1998). Living unrelated renal transplantation: progress and potential. *J. Am. Soc. Nephrol.*, *9*, 2148–2152.

Saran et al. (1997). Long-term follow-up of kidney donors: a longitudinal study. *Nephrol. Dial. Transplant.*, *12*, 1615–1621.
Schover et al. (1997). The psychosocial impact of donating a kidney: long-term followup from a urology based center. *J. Urol.*, *157*, 1596–1601.
Schreiner, G. E. (1966). Dialysis and transplantation: ethical problems. In: G. E. W. Wolstenholme & M. O'Connor (Eds), *Ethics in Medical Progress: With Special Reference to Transplantation* (pp. 130–131). Ciba Foundation Symposium. Boston, Little Brown.
Sells, R. A. (1991). Voluntarism of consent in both related and unrelated living organ donors. In: W. Land & J. B. Dossetor (Eds), *Organ Replacement Therapy: Ethics, Justice, Commerce* (pp. 18–24). Berlin, Springer-Verlag.
Sells, R. A. (1997). Voluntarism and coercion in living organ donation. In: G. M. Collins, J. M. Dubernard, W. Land & G. G. Persijn (Eds), *Procurement, Preservation, and Allocation of Vascularized Organs* (pp. 295–300). Dordrecht, Kluwer Academic Publishers.
Shaffer et al. (1998). Two hundred and one consecutive living-donor nephrectomies. *Arch. Surg.*, *133*, 426–431.
Shanteau, J., & Skowronski, J. J. (1991). The decision to donate organs: an information-integration analysis. In: J. Shanteau & J. Harris (Eds), *Organ Donation and Transplantation: Psychological and Behavioral Factors*. pp. 59–67.
Sharma, V. K., & Enoch, M. D. (1987). Psychological sequelae of kidney donation. A 5–10 year follow up study. *Acta Psychiat. Scand.*, *75*, 264–267.
Shaw et al. (1991). Ethics of lung transplantation with live donors. *Lancet*, *338*, 678–681.
Simforoosh et al. (1991). Social aspects of kidney donations in 300 living related and unrelated renal transplantations. In: W. Land & J. B. Dossetor (Eds), *Organ Replacement Therapy: Ethics, Justice, Commerce* (pp 77–82). Berlin, Springer-Verlag.
Siminoff et al. (1995). Public policy governing organ and tissue procurement in the United States. Results from the National Organ and Tissue Procurement Study. *Ann. Intern. Med.*, *123*, 10–17.
Simmons, R. G., & Anderson, C. R. (1982). Related donors and recipients: five to nine years post-transplant. *Transplant. Proc.*, *14*, 9–12.
Simmons et al. (1987). *Gift of Life. The Effect of Organ Transplantation on Individual, Family, and Societal Dynamics*. New Brunswick, Transaction Books.
Singer, P. A., & Siegler, M. (1988). Whose kidney is it anyway? Ethical considerations in living kidney donation. *American Kidney Fund Nephrology Letter*, *5*, 16–20.
Singer et al. (1989). Ethics of liver transplantation with living donors. *N. Engl. J. Med.*, *321*, 620–622.
Smith et al. (1986). Living-related kidney donors: a multicenter study of donor education, socioeconomic adjustment, and rehabilitation. *Am. J. Kid. Dis.*, *8*, 223–233.
Smith et al. (2000). Cadaveric versus living donor kidney transplantation. A Medicare payment analysis. *Transplantation*, *69*, 311–314.
Spital et al. (1986). The living kidney donor: alive and well. *Arch. Intern. Med.*, *146*, 1993–1996.
Spital, A. (1988a). Living kidney donation: still worth the risk. *Transplant. Proc.*, *20*, 1051–1058.
Spital, A., & Spital, M. (1988b). Living kidney donation. Attitudes outside the transplant center. *Arch. Intern. Med.*, *148*, 1077–1080.
Spital, A. (1989). Unconventional living kidney donors – attitudes and use among transplant centers. *Transplantation*, *48*, 243–248.
Spital, A. (1991). The ethics of unconventional living organ donation. *Clin. Transplant.*, *5*, 322–326.

Spital, A. L. (1992). Unrelated living donors: should they be used? *Transplant. Proc.*, *24*, 2215–2217.

Spital, A. (1994). Unrelated living kidney donors. An update of attitudes and use among U.S. transplant centers. *Transplantation*, *57*, 1722–1726.

Spital, A. (1996) Do U.S. transplant centers encourage emotionally related kidney donation? *Transplantation*, *61*, 374–377.

Spital, A. (1998a). Living kidney donors: still a valuable resource. *Curr. Opin. Organ Transplantation*, *3*, 205–211.

Spital, A. (1998b). When a stranger offers a kidney: ethical issues in living organ donation. *Am. J. Kid. Dis.*, *32*, 676–691.

Spital, A. (1998c). Unconventional living kidney donors. In: J. L. Touraine, J. Traeger & H. Betuel et al. (Eds), *Organ Allocation* (pp. 297–309). London, Kluwer Academic Publishers.

Spital, A. (2000). Evolution of attitudes at U.S. transplant centers toward kidney donation by friends and altruistic strangers. *Transplantation*, *69*, 1728–1731.

Squifflet et al. (1990). Unrelated living donor kidney transplantation. *Transplant Int.*, *3*, 32–35.

Starzl et al. (1963). The reversal of rejection in human renal homografts with the subsequent development of homograft tolerance. *Surg. Gyn. Obs.*, *117*, 385–395.

Starzl, T. E. (1987). Living donors: con. *Transplant. Proc.*, *19*, 174–176.

Sterneck et al. (1995). Selection of the living liver donor. *Transplantation*, *60*, 667–671.

Stiller et al. (1985). Living related donation. *Transplant. Proc.*, *17* (Suppl. 3), 85–100.

Strong, R. W. & Lynch, S. V. (1996). Ethical issues in living related donor liver transplantation. *Transplant. Proc.*, *28*, 2366–2369.

Superina et al. (1999). Ethical issues in pediatric liver transplantation. *Transplant. Proc.*, *31*, 1342–1344.

Sutherland, D. E. R. (1985). Living related donors should be used whenever possible. *Transplant. Proc. 17*, 3–10.

Switzer et al. (1996). Helping unrelated strangers: physical and psychological reactions to the bone marrow donation process among anonymous donors. *J. Appl. Social Psychol.*, *26*, 469–490.

Terasaki et al. (1995). High survival rates of kidney transplants from spousal and living unrelated donors. *N. Engl. J. Med.*, *333*, 333–336.

Terasaki et al. (1997). Risk rate and long-term kidney transplant survival. *Clin. Transplant 1996*, 443–458.

Thiel, G. (1997). Emotionally related living kidney donation: pro and contra. *Nephrol. Dial. Transplant.*, *12*, 1820–1824.

Tilney, N. L. (1986). Renal transplantation between identical twins: a review. *World J. Surg.*, *10*, 381–388.

Toronyi et al. (1998). Attitudes of donors toward organ transplantation in living related kidney transplantations. *Transplant. Int.*, *11* (Suppl.1), S481-S483.

Tufveson et al. (1998). Live donor transplantation in Sweden and other Nordic countries with emphasis on the benefits of the procedure. In: Touraine et al. (Eds), *Organ Allocation* (pp. 273–284). London, Kluwer Academic Publishers.

UNOS Ethics Committee. (1992). Ethics of organ transplantation from living donors. *Transplant. Proc.*, *24*, 2236–2237.

UNOS (1999). www.unos.org/Newsroom/critdata_wait.htm

U.S. Renal Data System (USRDS) 1999 Annual Data Report. (1999). *Am. J. Kid. Dis.*, *34* (Suppl. 1), S132, S148.

Walker, T. (1999). The National Marrow Donor Program. *Minn. Med.*, *82*, 26–28.

Weizer et al. (1989). Suicide by related kidney donors following the recipients' death. *Psychother. Psychosom.*, *51*, 216–219.

Westlie et al. (1993). Quality of life in Norwegian kidney donors. *Nephrol. Dial. Transplant.*, *8*, 1146–1150.

Whitington, P. F. (1996). Living donor liver transplantation: ethical considerations. *J. Hepatology*, *24*, 625–627.

Wolfe et al. (1999). Comparison of mortality in all patients on dialysis, patients on dialysis awaiting transplantation, and recipients of a first cadaveric transplant. *N. Engl. J. Med.*, *341*, 1725–1730.

Woodruff, M. F. A. (1964). Ethical problems in organ transplantation. *Br. Med. J.*, *1*, 1457–1460.

Woodruff, M. F. A. (1966). Transplantation: the clinical problem. In: G. E. W. Wolstenholme & M. O'Connor (Eds), *Ethics in Medical Progress: With Special Reference to Transplantation* (pp. 15). Ciba Foundation Symposium. Boston, Little Brown.

World Health Organisation. (1991). Guiding principles on human organ transplantation. *Lancet*, *337*, 1470–1471.

5. WHO SHOULD RECEIVE DONOR ORGANS?

Erich H. Loewy

INTRODUCTION

This chapter will address the question of who should receive donor organs. Such a question can be interpreted on an individual basis: that is which particular patient should, since organs are in short supply, receive such organs a question of micro-allocation. Or, and on the other hand, it can be interpreted on a basis of who (which transplant program, region, etc.) should receive a donated organ a question of macro-allocation. Both of these are questions which have been hotly debated and for which no satisfactory answer has ever been found.

Organs to be transplanted are scarce resources. But they differ from other scarce resources in that they are (no matter how much one might be willing to spend) not renewable: in many cases the decision to give to one precludes giving to another, another who may by that decision very well be doomed to death. They are also different in that they were once a part of another being and, therefore, have not only a material but very important symbolic value.(Loewy, 1987)

In writing this chapter certain assumptions have been made and will not be argued for. The first is that organ transplantation is an ethically legitimate medical practice and that it does not materially differ from other medical practice. The second perhaps more serious assumption is that organ transplantation in our current health-care system in the United States remains a viable medical practice which should be available to all who qualify. In a

The Ethics of Organ Transplantation, Volume 7, pages 125–147.
2001 by Elsevier Science Ltd.
ISBN: 0-7623-0764-1

society where over forty million have no health-care coverage such an assumption is perhaps more troublesome. I am not suggesting that we should discontinue the practice of transplanting organs I am suggesting that basic care for all is logically prior to far more exotic care for some. Further, I claim that our society – like all other industrialized societies – can well afford a reasonable amount of both kinds of health-care for all.

First of all, we need to be clear: transplanting a kidney differs materially from transplanting a liver, a heart or a heart and lungs. There are methods for substituting for kidney (dialysis) or pancreatic (insulin) function for a considerable length of time; that is not the case for heart, liver and lungs. Furthermore, paired organs may be transplanted from live donors; there is consensus (another assumption that I will not argue for or against) that live donor donation for non-paired organs such as hearts or hearts and lungs is not acceptable. Although we readily accept the sacrifice of one life for another in war, we fail to condone such practices when it comes to donating organs. In terms of being obtainable from live donors, livers are more akin to kidneys than to hearts. Parts of a liver may be transplanted from donor to recipient because regeneration of an adequate liver in both donor and recipient is most likely to result. Again there is a difference here: the short-term risk to the donor of harvesting a kidney is minimal; the long-term risk may be a bit greater. In liver transplantation the opposite pertains: the immediate risk to the donor is by no means trivial but the long-term risk is extremely negligible. Such background information is essential.

In addressing any ethical problem (whether it is at the bedside or whether it is about policy issues) we tend to ask what shall we do? I would suggest that this, as a first question, is the wrong question. It presumes that we who are concerned about the proper answer are entitled to make such decisions. In truth, the proper first question is procedural: not what should we decide but who, in a given set of circumstances is entitled to decide and how shall such a decision be translated into praxis. We have generally evaded this question and have tended to fall back on expertise or, quite bluntly, on strength. We have made ethical decisions at best *for* and not *with* the weak, the sick, the disenfranchised. It is little wonder that most of our concerns in ethics have been directed towards the problems of what I have elsewhere called rich man's ethics the ethical questions we, who are lucky enough to have good access to medical care, trouble ourselves about (Loewy, 1996).

In this chapter (and although that is not its main topic) I shall briefly describe various possibilities of donation. After all, the shortage of transplantable organs is the very reason for troubling oneself about thorny questions of allocation. While organs will (until they can be grown artificially) always be in short supply, increasing the supply of organs for transplantation would greatly ameliorate problems of allocation. For that reason, I shall suggest another possibility that could both increase the supply and decrease the (legitimate) demand for organs. Beyond this I hope to show that the particular instruments of donation prevalent in a given society both reflect the world-view towards community which such a society has and affect the way in which a public dialogue about such issues can come about. Following this introduction I will address the question of who should decide by examining the way communities are conceived and maintained. Finally, and moving from the question of macro-allocation, I will speak about the various mechanisms of allocating organs to individual patients.

OBTAINING ORGANS

(Caplan & Coelho, Eds 1998)

Besides donation from living donors, there are three methods of obtaining organs from the newly dead: (1) routine harvest; (2) presumed refusal; and (3) presumed consent.

Routine harvest – a situation in which all organs suitable for transplantation would be harvested from all suitable newly dead patients – would certainly increase the supply of organs. It would, on the other hand, conflict with some deeply held societal feelings about individual liberty as well as conflicting with the beliefs and practices of some cultures. Enticing as it may be, it is not a procedure that in a setting giving a high value to individual choice and personal liberty recommends itself or one that could be readily translated into practice.

Presumed refusal means that the organs of suitable donors will be harvested only if special consent has been given. This consent can be given either by the donor prior to the event (donor cards are an example) or by the next of kin after the death has occurred. It requires persons, in a sense, to do something out of the ordinary. The general assumption is that most persons will refuse. Psychologically this places relatives in a position of doing something extraordinary and something that is, therefore, supererogatory. It is the method of obtaining organs in most of the States within the United States.

Presumed consent, on the other hand, presumes that most persons would be willing to donate organs they can no longer use themselves to others who need them badly. Prospective donors would have to state in a type of negative donor card that they do not wish to donate and relatives (absent any such instrument) would have to go out of their way to refuse. This method of harvesting organs is practised in a number of states of the European Community and is debated in some of the states of the United States.

In some areas a practice known as stimulated request occurs. Laws state that physicians are compelled to request organ donation from the relatives of suitable donors and, if donation is refused, to document the reason for such refusal. Such regulations, it was hoped, would increase the supply of transplantable organs. In practice it does not appear to have been very effective.

Persons who unexpectedly lose another who had been close to them are psychologically in a very negative state of mind. They are apt to go along with the prevalent habits in a society whatever these habits may be. The kinds of instruments of donation a society chooses reflects the way in which societies understand obligations of their members to one another. In societies with a strong ethos of mutual help and with strong solidarity helping another in need becomes a matter of course: such societies are apt to choose presumed consent. In societies in which the urge to help one another is less strong or virtually absent, refusal is more apt to be presumed.

Donor cards are frequently used. In many states they are a part of drivers licenses. Persons may specify that they wish to donate their organs and when such a gift is duly witnessed the donor card has legal standing. Unfortunately (at least in my view) the donor card is widely ignored when any member of the family objects. This state of affairs has caused the loss of a number of transplantable organs. Not honoring the wishes of the person whose organs these were is quite similar to setting aside (without good and sufficient cause) a duly executed advance directive – for a legally executed donor card is just that. Ethically not honoring such a request is a form of promise breaking; legally it may be (albeit that to date it has not been) challenged. The reason why hospitals hesitate to honor such cards is crassly pragmatic: they are afraid of being sued and are quite aware that the dead person cannot, in fact, bring suit. Nevertheless (and even on that argument) a next of kin might readily bring suit for violating what amounts to an advance directive.

There may be a way of making organ donations a more compelling issue. One of the reasons why organs so often fail to be donated is that the question of donation is raised at a psychologically most unfortunate time. Most suitable donors die unexpectedly. When persons are confronted with an unanticipated tragedy their reaction is very negative. They are likely to refuse a request which, under less terrible conditions, they might readily agree to. Elsewhere I have suggested that one might consider a very simple proposition: while persons maintain their right to donate or not those who refuse donation would forfeit their future right to a donated organ. Who should receive rides piggyback on the question of donation and those unwilling to donate should, perhaps, be precluded from receiving organs. One could conceive having everyone deciding by a particular age to donate or not. That decision would be entered into a computer. Persons unwilling to donate (this could likewise apply to blood which, after all, is an organ) would be precluded from becoming recipients (Loewy, 1996).

Living donors have been employed for some time. They offer ethical problems which are worthy of a chapter in itself and they will, therefore, be only briefly discussed. The first renal transplants were, in fact, from one to another identical twin and, until much more was learned about immunological processes and suppression closely related donors were the donors of choice for renal transplantation. There is a host of problems with living donors.

First of all, when we speak of living donors we are mainly speaking of kidneys, bone marrow and, recently, of segments of liver. Until recently only blood relatives and spouses were considered to be acceptable donors in the United States – under the interesting (but false) presumption that persons who give organs to strangers must be mentally unstable.

When patients are in need of bone marrow, kidney or segments of liver the entire family is examined in the hope that an excellent match may be found. Not all relatives are, however, anxious or willing to give an organ. Some are reluctant to admit this and frequently will request the physician to say that they were not good matches. Physicians must remember who their patient is – this is the reason why the transplant surgeon and the person evaluating the donor ought to be quite separate persons. Secondly, physicians like the rest of us, have a prima facie obligation not to lie – especially not to the patient or family. Problems of confidentiality – what the propsective donor has confided to the physician – can be very real. Physicians in such cases are well advised to offer their help in explaining the donor's refusal to the patient but should refrain from lying. They can say that they have been asked by the prospective donor not to discuss their status – but that lets the cat out of the bag. There is no really good answer to this problem other than to urge mutual openness and honesty upon all concerned.

Parents who have another child expressly so that it might serve as a bone marrow donor and save the life of its siblings are another problem. First of all, there is the problem of using a young child – unable to give its consent – for the sake of another; secondly there is the problem of "creating" such a child expressly for that purpose. Kantians will often object that creating a child for this purpose is using another as a means. The answer to this, of course, is that such an objection omits the word "merely" . . . Kant does not say not to use others as means but not merely as means. Parents who love both of their children arguably are not using the donor as merely but also as a means – and in this case as a means towards rescuing the life of a sibling. The donor may grow up to bless the day when he or she had that privilege.

Do we have an obligation to donate organs to another while alive? The answer to this depends upon the way we see community, relationships and obligation. I would argue that relationships are in part defined by the obligations one has to one another and that the obligation to donate to someone with whom one has a close relationship (and not necessarily a family member) depends upon our understanding of such a relationship. While I would argue that such an obligation exists, libertarians would deny this. There is, furthermore, a vast distance between having an ethical and having a legal obligation. Even if an argument sketching such a duty can be made one would be, I think, ill advised to translate this into a legal stricture. Translating ethical precepts into laws is a bit like two porcupines making love – it is something which ought to be done most carefully! When we translate ethical principles into law two conditions must be met: first of all there must be wide consensus (not unanimity but wide consensus) that a given thing is ethically unacceptable. Secondly not having such a law would have to "threaten the king's peace" . . . that is, to cause problems within the community which threatened peaceful coexistence. This is why lying to one's spouse is not illegal and murder is.

We have never used the permanently vegetative as organ donors but have insisted on the criterion of whole brain death. The use of the permanently vegetative or permanently comatose has been suggested. It rests on the rather reasonable (but unproven and in the current state of our knowledge unprovable) assumption that such people while they are alive do not have a life – that is they are not knowing subjects of their life. Here we again need to ask not "what shall we do" but "who is to decide what should be done". Ultimately the way we deal with death or the vegetative state, what we consider the state to be, is a philosophical decision informed by biological "facts" which depends upon the world-view of the community making such a decision. Only once the decision of what death is is made, can criteria for it be set and can decisions as to what to do with such people be made.

WHO SHALL DECIDE – THE ROLE of COMMUNITY: IDENTIFIED vs. UNIDENTIFIED LIVES

Before we can decide how organs should be allocated (whether allocation involves micro- or macro-allocation) we need to be clear about who legitimately should decide. It is not obvious that such decisions are made best by experts. Certainly transplant physicians must be involved. But transplant physicians by themselves (or even the transplant team) are hardly legitimate decision makers. After all and quite legitimately, transplant physicians and their program have their own vested interests. Transplantation is a complex enterprise involving many areas of expertise. Among others transplantation involves transplant physicians, economists, psychologists, social scientists, social workers and many others each of which have some corner on a specific and essential piece of knowledge. One could conceive of constituting committees of such persons and allowing them to formulate criteria which in turn would serve as a basis for discussion. Such criteria would then be publicly discussed and through elected representative become law. There might be a committee that deals with the question of how donated organs shall be made available nationally – in other words a committee that would make macro-allocation suggestions, suggestions about procedure. Such a committee would be a committee dealing with unidentified or statistical lives. Another committee would be charged with making specific decisions about specific cases i.e. micro-allocation decisions. It would be a committee dealing with identified lives. Such committees, however, must derive their authority from another body. Such bodies must be connected to the community for which they purport to speak in a significant and meaningful way.

Allocation has been done locally, regionally and nationally. There is no ethically compelling reason why our considerations of community should stop at a given border be it local, regional or national. The first consideration (as always good ethics starts with good facts) is the viability of explanted specific organs and the ease with which such organs can be transported from one to another region. Viability differs among the various organs and likewise changes over time as better methods of preservation are developed, viability is lengthened. In the European Community a joint program for sharing organs among the various EU (and some non-EU) countries is in place. In the United States there has been and is a brisk discussion as to the priority to be given to local over regional over national needs. Under the current program stark inequities exist. A critically ill patient may not receive a vitally needed organ and in consequence may die while another less critically ill is transplanted a few scant miles away: a state or regional border happened to run between them. Internationally even starker inequities exist (Newspaper articles, 1999) (website).

Like many questions in health-care ethics, the question of organ allocation is a question that involves both micro-allocation and macro-allocation. Both of these questions, however, depend upon the way we conceive obligations to one another, to the community and in turn what we expect community to owe to us as individuals. Macro-allocation deals with the crafting of rules for what types of patients will be eligible to receive organs and how, once generically judged to have been eligible, they will be prioritized. Such patients are patients we do not know personally. They are what has been called unidentified or statistical lives. When it comes to micro-allocation we concern ourselves in allocating organs to individual patients, patients who are identified or easily identifiable.

Whichever is the case – our perception of obligation to one another has, among other things, much to do with three factors: (1) the way we conceive our relationship to specific others; (2) the way we perceive our relationship to the others within our community to whom we are not personally related; and (3) the way we integrate these sometimes conflicting obligations with each other. In a sense the first of these involves identified lives, the second statistical or unidentified lives and the third attempts to reconcile the first with the second.

We can view community as composed of a loose association of individuals. These can be seen as bound to one another by nothing more than an obligation of mutual non-harm as well as an obligation assumed by freely entering a contract. Such an obligation rests on a Hobbesian notion of social contract (Hobbes, 1962) and, in modern clothes is well expressed by the libertarian world view.(Nozick, 1974; Engelhardt, 1986, 1991) Such a view entails no obligations of beneficence or mutual assistance except where explicitly stipulated by contract. One is obliged not to directly harm but not obligated to come to the help of others. Such a point of view makes freedom into a near-absolute modified and modifiable only so as to assure the maximal liberty to all others. Such a view would consider help for the poor or giving health-care to the sick to be a matter of private charity. Organ donation would be supererogatory. In such a community the market might well serve to distribute organs. There would be no need to trouble oneself to evolve elaborate rules for organ allocation; those who could pay would receive (perhaps on the basis of an auction with the needed organ going to the highest bidder) and those not able to outbid their neighbor would not. This, in a nutshell, is capitalism in its crassest form.

One can adopt a different view. Community can be seen as an organic whole composed of individuals united by common goals and dedicated to common ends. Such a community, when driven to its extreme, could submerge all individual interests and instead drive merely for a common good. In such communities the poor would be helped to the point that helping them would serve the community and not beyond. Organs, likewise, would be given to those whose ongoing contributions to the community would be expected to be the greatest. In a nutshell such a community would be a crass form of communism.

Neither of these two communities seems viable. A viable community not about to shatter easily requires solidarity – solidarity which comes about because the individuals within the community see their private aims and interests as enabled within the embrace of community and difficult or impossible to be realized outside it. When individuals know that others will not harm them but also realize that others are unlikely to come to their aid, solidarity is weak and little cohesiveness exists. Persons are far too occupied struggling for their private good to realize that they could far more easily achieve their private aims and pursue their personal interests by altering the condition of association. A community in which individuals are related to one another only by obligations of mutual non-harm and where obligations of mutual help are given short shrift, will inevitably have a large and increasing body of poor, poorly educated and frustrated individuals exploited by the ever more powerful wealthy. Solidarity is not to be expected and revolution can easily occur. On the other hand, when individuals are neglected and relegated to a position in which they are seen as merely existing to serve the common good a similar situation exists: private lives are ignored and while persons may not be hungry or starving they are unfulfilled and frustrated. Solidarity will be absent and revolution may readily occur.

There are other ways of conceptualizing a community. Humans are social animals. Along with other higher animals, humans have certain natural inborn traits and capacities which underwrite the way they live and associate. Some of these are beneficial for personal as well as ultimately group survival; others may not be. Those which tend to help individuals survive and communities to thrive are likely to be perpetuated those that do not, are likely to be extinguished. Rousseau suggests that humans along with other higher animals are, among other traits, born with two: a sense of compassion and a sense of self-regard or self-worth. The former causes us to feel uncomfortable when confronted with the suffering of others; the latter is translated into the drive to self-preservation. Both self-regard (and its resultant drive to self-preservation) and compassion have positive survival value. Self-preservation prompts the individual to engage in activities which allow it to survive and breed; compassion causes solidarity within a group to increase and helps the particular group or species to survive. (Rousseau, 1965, 1993, 1996)

Both compassion and self-regard are prone to social conditioning: compassion can be fostered or crushed, self-regard can be exaggerated to self-love or, by training, be diminished to almost the point of extinction. These two traits often hold each other in balance: our sense of self-preservation may prevent us from acting on compassion in a suicidal manner; compassion may allow us to do some rather uncomfortable things to help others in distress.

Our sense of innate compassion with one another as well as our sense of self-preservation help shape our view of community. Compassion will motivate us to care for the weaker, self-regard will allow us to understand that our individual aims and desires require a viable community to support them. In both the "capitalist" and the "communist" community individuals who wish to pursue their interests and develop their talents see themselves in a dialectic with their community: individual needs compete with communal interests and resolution is only an armed truth. Rather than conceive community in a dialectic fashion, one might more fruitfully conceive of the interaction within a community and among its members to be a homeostatic process -- a process in which a myriad of individual interests balance one another in pursuit of a common goal. A homeostatic process aims to achieve a sufficient stability so that adaptations to changes in the external and internal milieu can occur. It allows organisms, species (and I have argued communities) to evolve, develop and thrive. In such a community individuals come to realize that their individual thriving is enabled by the community and the community accepts that supporting individual interests is necessary if the community is to thrive and prosper. (Loewy 1995) Such communities can thrive because, among other things, solidarity is brought about when individuals within it realize that their personal interest requires the general good. Supporting the weak, the ill, the unfortunate is no longer merely an act of compassion or charity but becomes a communal responsibility necessary to solidarity, communal survival and ultimately to individual prosperity. Such communities are apt to see that helping others serves one own interest. Persons, not knowing what their own future might hold, would wish to create a community in which the basic needs of all would be met. In (and consistent with a Rawlsian view) such communities allocation of critical resources would be apt to follow a code of fairness consistent with the prevalent culture, values and world-view. Since all persons might, in the future, be in need of a transplantable organ their own self-interest as well as their compassion for those in need would motivate them to readily donate their organs (Rawls, 1971).

The decision as to how organs are to be distributed (the question of macro-distribution) would logically seem to be the first order of business. Before we can allocate fairly to individuals in need of organs, we must first create a way of supplying organs to various transplant centers and regions. All of us would agree that such distribution must be fair and equitable – our disagreement stems from the definition of these terms. In order to establish a base of fairness it would seem an elemental requirement of justice that all those affected have a fair say in what, after all, may critically affect them. All of us are potential organ recipients and all of us, therefore, have a vested interest in seeing that the procedures established and the way they are implemented supports our conception of what is fair.

Justice is often seen as blind. Justice, in a formal sense, is impartial – the more partial, the less just. This is one reason why to avoid conflicts of interest we should disqualify ourselves from judging our friends in a competition. It is, among others, one of the very reasons why the transplant community should not be the sole judge of what fair allocation should be. Justice in a functional sense, however, is a much more complex thing than that. Relationships – defined precisely by obligations owed within that context – certainly count: flipping a coin to decide whom to rescue when your best friend and a stranger are drowning might strike us as formally just but hardly as functionally fair.

When making decisions about macro-allocation we are dealing with unidentified or statistical lives. We do not directly or even by proxy know the persons concerned and are, therefore, able to reason dispassionately. There are several problems here. First of all, I shall argue that unidentified lives are an artifact – that what we call unidentified lives are merely lives we happen not to have identified but which are most certainly (by virtue of being lives) enmeshed in a social nexus and, therefore, identified by someone else. Community consists of an association of lives all of whom are identified by some others in that community and are, therefore, in relationship with one another. Secondly, I shall argue that using reason alone (for the very reason that we are not in fact dealing with artificial but with very real and identifiable lives) is neither possible nor desirable. Thirdly I shall argue that deciding how we should decide is something in which all potentially concerned and willing to be potentially concerned should have a fair voice.

It is well, when dealing with statistical lives, to bring them closer to one and to begin to see them as flesh and blood instead as merely figures on a sheet of paper. This process requires curiosity and imagination: sufficient curiosity to wonder what it would be like to be in the other's shoes and sufficient imagination to carry one some steps in that direction. What, for example, it would be like to be denied an organ transplant or to be asked to donate the organs of a close relative who had just unexpectedly died. When we begin to identify such unidentified lives we begin to feel emotionally involved, our sense of compassion is aroused and we are ready to temper our reason with compassion – I have, elsewhere, spoken of this as "compassionate rationality".

On the other hand when we are asked to make decisions about lives we know and which have touched us, we are apt to have our emotions engaged early on. These may range from compassion or love to hatred and disdain – but they are emotions. In medical practice it is generally compassion that is aroused – we feel for and with the weak, the sick, the person with little hope left. So as to prevent ourselves from acting foolishly and unjustly we need to temper these emotions with reason – a process I have referred to as "rational compassion". Again curiosity and imagination play a role in sorting out the outcomes of various courses of action (Loewy, 1998).

Certain decisions need to be made if organ distribution is to accord to our vision of fairness. Decisions as to how much standing should be given to medical urgency and how much weight to the chances for a good outcome. Should, for example, a patient who is desperately ill but whose chances for long-term success are relatively poor be preferred over a patient not as ill but with a better prognosis? Such medical factors are critical and need to be prioritized. There are no set or "good" answers to those questions – there are, as is usually the case when ethical problems are discussed, only relatively better and relatively worse answers. What is relatively better or relatively worse depends in large measure upon prevalent communal values.

Such decisions should be ones that are made by all those potentially affected. They are not decisions that can be made by the transplant community but they are decisions in which the transplant community must play its proper and critically important advisory role. In a polis or small town such decisions can be made in town meetings; on a larger scale that is not possible and we are obliged to make such decisions in the way that a representative democracy usually does. This does not mean that decisions are left to the legislators – albeit that ultimately legislative action is needed. It means that an interactive public needs to be involved to guide the legislative process – something which has, for example, been done in Oregon or in the so-called Danish ethics councils. In such meetings, options are discussed and all are given a chance to express and debate their points of view.

Public participation is crucial if a method of distribution acceptable to most of those affected will come about. In societies that have a policy of routinely salvaging all useable organs all will feel themselves affected. Such a society, however, is probably not acceptable to our current western ethos. Societies in which consent is presumed, in which donation is the norm and in which refusal is seen as unusual would be societies in which most would have a vested interest in such a dialogue and those who chose to opt out would have little incentive to participate. On the other hand, when refusal becomes the norm and persons see the donation of organs as being an unusual thing to do, most will feel little interest in participating. The dialogue in such societies is apt to be sluggish with most caring little what particular method of distribution is adopted.

The transplant community plays an important role in such a dialogue. Good ethics starts with good facts. The members of the transplant community must supply such facts in a way that the public can readily understand. In my view, the transplant community must not make such decisions by themselves. First of all the transplant community has natural vested interest and that certainly interferes with their ability to make an even-handed judgment. Secondly, the interest of the transplant community is quite different from the interest of either transplant recipients or donors. Those who donate organs do so for a variety of reasons – most are altruistic and are concerned chiefly with the welfare of another person in need and not with the interest of any particular program. Those of us who may be recipients are not interested in the welfare of a particular program but are interested in having our needs fairly considered and adjudicated. Both donor and recipients, while critically concerned about the interests of transplant programs in general, are less or not at all concerned with the interests of any particular program. The interests of the public and of individual transplant programs not only often fail to coincide but also may conflict. Therefore, members of the transplant community while they must be involved all along the way cannot be allowed to dominate the discussion.

Currently in the United States the vested interest of diverse transplant programs has tried to keep distribution on as much of a local level as possible. Various proposals have been made, enacted, modified and re-modified generally with a great deal of pressure exerted by local programs eager to assert their own parochial interests. Great inequities have resulted. (Cleveland Plain, Dealer, 1997) Waiting times differ enormously from location to location. In some areas patients who are less critically ill or who have only a slim chance of a successful outcome are transplanted so as not to lose a transplant for a particular program. This has resulted in a number of social inequities. While we pay lip-service to the idea that lives must not be measured in terms of money, our health-care system and with it our transplant programs have shown the opposite to be the case. In the United States one gets what one can (out of pocket or by insurance) pay for – those without insurance lack fair access to basic health-care not to speak of access to transplantation. But even those fully insured do not fare equally: if one can afford to register with various transplant programs, one's chance of expeditiously receiving a transplant is greatly increased. Registering with several programs, travelling there and incurring all of the other out of pocket expenses associated with such a venture is a very expensive thing to do. It is not something an ordinary worker on an ordinary income can readily do. Until a public which has good cause to be interested in the way organs are distributed engages in a brisk dialogue and translates its will into legislative action by its representatives inequities stimulated by vested interests will continue to occur.

It remains to decide how to define a "community" in practical terms. Are we speaking of cities, towns, counties, states, nations or a world community? In part the answer to this is technically determined – it depends on organ viability and ready access to rapid and reliable means of communication and transportation. As the length of viability increases and as transportation becomes more reliable the affected community grows. We have, as a species, moved from polis to metropolis, from nation-state to economic community and will, if we endure and prosper, move to a community whose possibilities embrace the world. For now we are still within a national borders frame of reference – albeit that transnational arrangements are more and more the order of the day. In practical terms today I see decisions in the United States as being on a federal level and eventually extending to neighboring states. For now realizing that we are indeed a community within this nation and not a loose association divided by petty vested interests will be a step forward.

ALLOCATING TO INDIVIDUAL PATIENTS

Once a framework of rules and procedures for sharing organs on a macro-level are made, a system of deciding on a more micro-level who receives a particular organ needs to be in place. The micro and the macro level are not entirely separate or separable. Decisions of priority on the micro-level as profoundly affects macro-distribution as procedures on the macro-level affect what individual patients may receive.

Despite the presence of overt rules that are supposed to prevent inequities, inequities continue to exist. Many of these are produced by the lack of a coherent or equitable health-care system in the United States. Others are subtler and not as readily addressed. In a recent study, for example, it was found that African Americans when corrected for extraneous factors, and with the same medical indications, were given significantly fewer kidney transplants than was a matched group of white patients. It is true that African Americans also tend to donate less readily than whites (Ayanian et al., 1999; Levinsky, 1999). In part this hesitancy results from the entirely justifiable and empirically demonstrable fact that such patients are and continue to be disadvantaged and indeed often disenfranchised in our society.

The first question when it comes to allocating organs to specific patients is, once again, not what should be done but who is entitled to set the criteria and establish the procedures for what eventually will be done. On this level, although the public ought to have its say on the general rules of procedure, a good deal of reliance will have to be placed on the health-care professionals involved. Many of these decisions require medical experience and expertise; some do not.

There are several ways of distributing scarce resources. Chief among these are: (1) medical indications and medical necessity; (2) the market; (3) queuing or first come first served; (4) a lottery; and (5) social value judgements.

Medical Indications

I shall assume and not argue for the proposition that transplanted organs first of all need to be well matched – that is that the danger of rejection must be minimized. To do other would be to waste organs. Care, however, must be taken to be certain that the various criteria used are truly proven to be related to graft survival and not merely used as a handy and sub rosa lottery.

At first blush, medical necessity would appear to be an exclusively "medical" decision. And yet many things can be subsumed under that heading. Physicians must determine diagnosis, prognosis, possible forms of therapy and various possibilities of outcome. These are mainly judgements which lay people cannot make. The decision whether to give preference to those at greatest risk or those with the best chance of long-term benefit is, however, not a decision which "experts" can make more readily than members of the general public. Here – and especially since what is being allocated is not renewable – societal values are at stake. No clear decision, I believe, will be possible and a trade-off which satisfies neither school of thinking but which is acceptable (even if grudgingly) to both will probably result.

Take a decision made in heart transplantation. Two candidates both of whom would be acceptable recipients for one donor heart are available. One is a person who without a transplant will die imminently but whose chance of survival is about 5%. The other is a person who is quite ill, badly disabled, not as imminently threatened as the other but with a chance for long term survival well in excess of 50%. In addition one must realize the fact that the general condition of patients who are not transplanted will inevitably deteriorate and their prognosis will inevitably worsen. Such decisions are not merely medical – they are based on communal values and worldviews. Their framework needs to be one set with the help of all those potentially affected and not only by those with technical or other expertise in transplantation.

Medical indications, then, fall into two separate albeit not entirely separable groups: the first is technical. It involves questions of matching donor and recipient, judgements which entail the effect other diagnoses may have on the feasibility of transplanting a particular organ into a particular recipient and so forth. These are judgements mainly made by "experts" in the field. The second is medical in a different sense: members of the transplant team must be guided by societal values in deciding which risk is worth taking, how to balance chance for success with gravity of need and so forth.

The Market

There have been repeated suggestions that the market be used to allocate organs. Although the market controls an overwhelming number of aspects of our daily lives we stop short of allowing whether one lives or dies to be controlled by market forces – at least we claim that we do. In fact this is not the case. We have, among other social ills, millions without access to health-care, a fourth of our children (and a third of our African American children) hungry at some time during a given year, a minimum wage which fails to lift many people above the poverty level. These are all factors materially controlling who lives and who dies. Nevertheless, we shrink back from overtly selling organs to the highest bidder. While we claim that while we are quite willing to allow market forces to control what the content of life shall be (undoubtedly the content for a grindingly poor person is quite different from that of an affluent!), we simultaneously claim that we do not allow financial considerations to dictate who shall live and who shall die.

If one were to be honest, one would indeed have to acknowledge that the market in the United States plays an important role – a role which most of us dedicated to the proposition that life is precious and ought not be measured in monetary terms would love to deny. Nevertheless: transplantation is expensive and unless health-care institutions are reimbursed adequately transplantation stops being a viable option. De facto persons who lack insurance, other coverage or who are not independently wealthy would have difficulty being accepted into a transplant program. Even those who are insured will fare better if they are well to do: they can register with several programs, stand, as it were, in several queues and reap the benefits of such multiple registration. The uninsured and disenfranchised have far greater worry than access to transplantable organs: they lack basic health-care. The health-care system in the United States as it exists today is, in my view, a national shame and the role that the market plays in organ transplantation is one of its more minor ills. Beyond this there are absurdities introduced by the decision to fund patients with end-stage kidney disease while they are receiving dialysis while not funding persons with other end stage diseases. Further, patients with end stage renal disease – once they have been transplanted – lose their medical benefits and unless insured may be unable to afford the long-term and expensive aftercare needed to maintain their graft.

Those who tout the market as a method of distribution cling to a libertarian worldview in which we are connected merely by obligations of mutual non-harm to one another. We have no obligation to help those who are worse off than ourselves. Illness, poverty or disability (insofar as they were not directly caused by the actions of another) may be unfortunate but they are not unjust or unfair – and we, in such a view, have only an obligation to those we have directly injured and none to those who happened to be the victims of bad luck (Engelhardt, 1981).

In our culture, selling and buying organs is not permitted. This prohibition is grounded both on a worldview that looks askance at placing a monetary price on life as well as on very negative experience with the buying and selling of blood. Lately there have been some suggestions (and indeed there have been some programs initiated) which offer the family of donors certain monetary benefits. Such offers (the benefits are not large and are given to all families who donate) would tend to disadvantage the poor – a poor family who is disinclined to donate organs may be far more easily coerced into agreeing than would a family which is well off.

The market has been used by wealthy people in need of organs by purchasing such organs abroad. In some third world country poor and often starving persons will sell one of their kidneys to support a family or perhaps to open the door for a better life to one of their children. In other cultures organs are taken from executed "criminals" with the date of the execution often matched to the convenience of transplant surgeons. A proposal to use organs of executed criminals in this country was made some time ago by none other than Dr. Kevorkian (Kevorkian, 1985, 1985, 1992).

Queuing

First come first served or queuing would give the person registered earlier a better chance to obtain an organ than one registered later. This, of course, tends to advantage the insured, the more affluent and the better educated. Those who are insured will be diagnosed earlier. Further, affluent and well-educated persons invariably tend to insist on earlier diagnosis and treatment than do the poor or ignorant. It is difficult to see how this can be avoided. To exclude the time a particular patient has been on a waiting list as one of the factors when considering who is to receive the next available organ seems hardly fair.

Queuing, if it is fair, has to be guided by definite criteria as to who can be placed on the waiting list. If earlier placement offers an advantage to patients, then physicians may very well be tempted to place patients on the waiting list quite early and, at times, even before it is clear that organ transplantation will be necessary. Therefore an independent mechanism for evaluating patients to be placed on the waiting list and criteria for in – and exclusion have to be carefully set, universally agreed to and stringently enforced.

A national uniform policy is desirable. If different centers are allowed to have different criteria so that patients and their physicians can pick and choose then a gross inequity controlled again by a patients ability to afford going to distant centers is introduced.

The Lottery

To the best of my knowledge, no one has ever overtly used a lottery as a method of allocating organs. Nevertheless, there have been some claims that extensive HLA-typing beyond the point where it makes a significant difference in outcome has been used to this purpose. A lottery indicates either that there are no relevant differences or that the problem is so trivial that one does not wish to take one's time to make a decision. No relevant differences would have to mean that two or more patients are of the same age, have the same disease at the same stage of development, be in identical physical condition, etc. Such a state of affairs is not apt to exist. The problem of who should live and who should die (or who should continue to be burdened with dialysis and who free of it) cannot be considered to be "so trivial" that one need not trouble oneself to make a decision. In many respects the use of a lottery (unless two patients are truly identical) is a moral cop-out.

Social Value Judgements

The question of using social value criteria comes in many guises. In a sense all the judgements we make – even those we call "scientific" – have a social component. The decision to accept a given set of data and call them statistically valid is a judgment that, like all others, is made "socially". That is not what I have in mind. I distinguish between judgements socially made (as all judgements are) and "social value judgements" which are judgements made about the value others have for and within society.

Social value judgements have in fact been made and undoubtedly explicitly or more frequently tacitly continue to be made. When dialysis was first introduced and dialysis machines were few and far between there was an attempt to have such decisions made by committees which soon (and deservedly) were nicknamed God committees. The result was a disaster acknowledged by all as unfair (Annas, 1985).

Using age as a criterion is, in many respects, a social value judgment. Using age is based on two assumptions, one overt, the other more hidden. The first is that older persons have first of all had a far greater (or at least longer) opportunity to experience life in its various manifestations and that secondly and in the natural order of things they will live a shorter time after the graft has been successfully placed. The second and less often overtly stated assumption is that the future contributions to society of an older person will be smaller than will those of a younger. These assumptions are difficult to defend when it comes to deciding for individual patients. Even if one were to grant that having a larger or smaller number of positive or negative life experiences should count (which I for one would not be readily willing to do) the fact that a person has lived longer does not mean that they have necessarily either had more positive experiences than one who has lived for a shorter time or that they have had the opportunity to have such positive experiences. The statistical observation, furthermore, that in the natural order of things persons of forty will have a longer time to live than will persons who are seventy does not hold in an individual case. As to the future contributions which a person can be expected to make – here indeed is a social value judgement par excellence! If we allow the possibility of future contributions to enter into the equation we do two things: first of all we claim that it is possible to place a value on one as opposed to another contribution, that, for example, writing a novel is a greater contribution than inventing a new recipe for chocolate cake. I would deny such a claim. Secondly we claim that – even if we could distinguish the value of one vis-à-vis the value of another contribution – the contribution one were able or expected to make should be seriously factored into the equation. This claim I likewise deny. Acknowledging such a claim could open the door to all sorts of mischief – experience with early "God committees" to admit or not admit patients to the few available opportunities for dialysis were less than encouraging. I do not deny that age may legitimately enter into allocation decisions – if it can be shown that patients past a certain age fare less well with transplantation, reject an organ more readily or recover poorly – an argument that can be made based on at least some technical information. But unfortunately many of these assumptions are just that – assumptions which may be testable but which, in fact, have not been tested.

I have used age as an example of hidden as well as overt social value judgements. We claim that we do not allow financial considerations to determine who shall live or die – but in the final analysis this statement proves to be false. Likewise we often wish to pretend that social value judgements are judgements we ought not and in fact do not make – and in the final analysis this is probably neither true nor even fair.

Consider the question of providing transplants to felons convicted of having committed a terrible crime – perhaps several times over. Would we, for example, rest easy knowing that a person like Mr. Barbie (the butcher of Lyons who sent thousands of children to their death in Auschwitz) might receive a heart-transplant and that, therefore, Monsieur Bouchard the baker next door could not? But such a judgement would, beyond doubt, be one of social value. This is not a theoretical matter – some felons need heart or liver transplants if they are to live or kidney transplants if they are to be relieved from dialysis. As has been pointed out, organs are not renewable resources: one cannot simply buy more.

Such judgements once again are judgements that need to be socially and democratically made. As matters stand they are often made and made differently by individual transplant programs. When the state imprisons a person certain things are taken away and others are promised. Prisoners are removed from society and deprived of liberty. In return they are promised that their basic necessities as well as medical care will be provided. Such a promise – tacit though it may be – is not limited. This problem is, I think, once again a procedural one. All of us are potential organ recipients just as we are potential felons. We as a society, after sufficient communal discussion and through our elected representatives may well decide that the promise made to persons convicted of certain crimes will be limited: they will be given medical care but will not be eligible to receive organs. Such a process is one in which social values most certainly play a role but it is a process in which all potentially affected have had a chance to have their fair say.

Using the criteria

In practice most of the ways of selecting patients discussed in the preceding pages are in use. Most certainly medical criteria are the necessary condition for all else: it would be clearly unacceptable to transplant an organ into a recipient bound to reject it or into a patient bound to die shortly from another disease. There is no doubt that market criteria indirectly and directly influence transplant decisions. That they do so is discordant with our expressed societal values and norms – we can see this when a child is refused a transplant and an enormous effort to collect the needed money is made. Leaving such decisions up to capricious value judgements is patently unfair – a well dressed, well spoken and weeping grandmother is apt to get support whereas a poorly dressed, poorly spoken and not as overtly desperate grandmother may not. Such a situation does not accord with the sense of fairness most would wish to claim as their own. Personally and for reasons stated I would accept a lottery only as a last ditch measure and then only in cases in which no relevant medical or social differences are evident. These different approaches to distributing organs will inevitably be used together – it becomes a question of how much weight and what priority is to be given to each. The answer to that question, I have argued, is less important than is the process of going about finding such an answer. In my view answers must be developed by dialogue among those potentially affected and implemented in a democratic representative way. (Habermas, 1992) As ways and answers are developed, these are used as experiments on the way to improvement – things we learn from and ultimately develop further and not things which we enshrine for all time.

BRINGING IT TOGETHER

In this chapter I have tried to show the relationship among our approaches to organ donation, allocation on a macro-level to various programs or regions and ultimately to individual patients awaiting transplantation. I have shown how our conception of communal structure and, therefore, of mutual obligation, can critically influence our approach to all of these questions. Our willingness to donate our organs after they no longer are of use to us in part is a function of how we view our relationship to others and to the community. When we feel obligated to refrain from directly injuring others but feel no strong obligation to help we are far more apt to accept implied refusal as the norm; when we feel more obligated to help others we are more apt to opt for implied consent. Communities in which individuals have a strong sense of being obligated to help one another are communities which have a stronger sense of solidarity and shared commitment. Such communities are apt to think more in terms of the larger community than in terms of individual vested interests and are more likely to develop national criteria and national procedures for equitable organ distribution. In such communities regional differences in waiting times as well as regional differences in the criteria for being accepted into a transplant program will tend to disappear or at the very least be ameliorated. Moreover, communities with a strong sense of communal solidarity will be more apt to make such decisions in a democratic way allowing all those potentially affected rather than only "experts" to participate in creating the framework within which experts then will have to make the ultimate individual decisions.

Let me be clear. I personally favor: (1) implied consent as the instrument of donation; (2) a system in which those unwilling to donate would be excluded as recipients; (3) a national and equitable mode of distributing organs so that regional differences would tend to disappear; and (4) distribution to individual patients which operates within a framework of agreed upon, democratically determined and evolving criteria. But above all I have argued for more communal participation guided but not controlled by experts. Such a process assumes a viable democracy something which, if we wish to have an equitable society in which an equitable system of organ distribution can thrive, we are obligated to help create and maintain. For a nation lacking personal, economic and educational democracy is (as John Dewey said long ago) ill equipped to maintain a meaningful and viable political democracy (Dewey, 1991).

REFERENCES

Annas, G. J. (1985). The prostitute, the playboy and the poet: rationing schemes for organ transplantation. *American Journal Public Health*, *75*(2), 187–189.

Ayanian, J. Z. et al. (1999). The effect of patient preference on racial differences in access to renal transplantation. *New England Journal of Medicine*, *341*(22), 1691–1692.

Caplan, A. L., & Coelho, D. H. (Eds) (1998). *The Ethics of Organ Transplantation*. Amherst, NY: Prometheus Books.

Cleveland Plain Dealer February 2–6, 1997. Transplanting Life: the triumphs, the traps, the tragedies.

Dewey, J. (1991). Creative Democracy: the work before us. In: J. A. Boydston & A. Sharpe (Eds), *John Dewey: the later works 1939–1941*. Carbondale, IL: Southern Illinois University Press.

Engelhardt, H. T. (1991). *Bioethics and Secular Humanism: the search for a common morality* Philadelphia, PA: The Trinity Press.

Engelhardt, H. T. (1981). Health-care allocations: responses to the unjust, the unfortunate and the undesirable. In: E. E. Shelp (Ed.), *Justice and Health Care* (pp. 121–138). Dordrecht, Netherlands: D. Reidel.

Engelhardt, H. T. (1994). *The Foundations of Bioethics* (2nd ed.). New York, NY: Oxford Publishers.

Engelhardt, H. T. (1991). *Bioethics and Secular Humanism: the search for a common morality* Philadelphia, PA: The Trinity Press.

http://www.hrsa.gov/osp/dot/chron.html

Habermas, J. (1992). *Moralbewusstsein und kommunikatives Handeln*. Frankfurt a/M: Suhrkamp.

Helderman, J. H. (1999). Allocation of cadaveric kidneys. *New England Journal of Medicine*, *341*(19), 1468–1469.

Hobbes, T. (1962). *Leviathan*. New York, NY: Collier Books.

Kevorkian, J. (1985). A brief history of experimentation on condemned and executed humans. *Journal National medical Association*, *77*(3), 215–226.

Kevorkian, J. (1992). A controlled auction market is a practical solution to the shortage of transplantable organs. *Medicine and Law*, *11*(2), 47–55.

Kevorkian, J. (1985). Opinions on capital punishment, executions and medical science. *Medicine and Law*, *4*(6), 515–533.

Levinsky, N. G. (1999). Quality and Equity in Dialysis and renal transplantation. *New England Journal of Medicine*, *341*(22), 1661–1669.

Loewy, E. H. (1987). Drunks, livers and values: should social value judgements enter into transplant decisions? *Journal Clinical Gastroenterology*, *9*(4), 436–441.

Loewy, E. H. (1996). *Textbook of Health Care Ethics*. Albany, NY: State University of New York Press.

Loewy, E. H. (1996). Of community, organs and transplantation: routine salvage with a twist. *Theoretical Medicine*, *17*, 61–74

Loewy, E. H. (1995). *Freedom and Community: the ethics of interdependence*. Albany, NY. SUNY Publishers.

Loewy, E. H. (1998). Curiosity, imagination, compassion, science and ethics: do curiosity and imagination serve a central function? *Health Care Analysis*, *6*, 286–294.

New York Times (1999). Misguided chauvinism on Organs. March 12.

New York Times (1999). Fight over organs shifts to states from Washington (S. G. Stolberg) March 11.

Nozick, R. (1974). *Anarchy, State and Utopia*. New York, NY: Basic Books.

Rousseau, J. J. (1965). Siscours sur l'origine et les Fondements de l'Inequalité parmis les Hommes Paris, France: Gallimard.

Rousseau, J. J. (1993). (by G. D. Cole, tr). In J. J. Rousseau, *The Social Contract and the Discourses*. New York, NY: Everyman's Library.

Rousseau, J. J. (1965). Siscours sur l'origine et les Fondements de l'Inequalité parmis les Hommes Paris, France: Gallimard.

Ubel, P. A., & Caplan, A. L. (1999). Geographical favoritism in liver transplantation: unfortunate or unfair? *New England Journal of Medicine*, *339*(18), 1322–1325.

6. THE ETHICS OF ORGAN RETRIEVAL

David C. Thomasma

INTRODUCTION

The ethical issues in transplant technology have always covered a broad range of clinical and social policy concerns. These can be addressed on their own, or within the context of psychological, social, and religious concerns arising from families and the organ procurement specialists involved in obtaining organs. I take the latter approach in this essay focusing on the ethics of organ retrieval. This ethics has been further complicated by new Federal Government rules and corresponding new duties and powers for retrieval specialists working for regional organ banks and sharing networks. At the same time, the deaths of prominent figures due to liver disease, such as Mickey Mantle and later, Walter Payton (Page, 1999), vividly demonstrated to the public how the shortage of organs affects all citizens (Anonymous, 1999a).[1]

After an introduction about the current situation, and the new HHS initiatives, I will briefly assess standard proposals to increase the organ supply as a background for the specific issues I will identify that arise under the new mechanisms for retrieving organs from donors and families. The focus then shifts to the moral problems encountered by caregivers of a potential donor, and by the organ retrieval specialists.

BACKGROUND

Despite world-wide and national widespread official acceptance of transplant technology as a last-ditch effort to save human lives while also redeeming the

The Ethics of Organ Transplantation, Volume 7, pages 149–165.
2001 by Elsevier Science Ltd.
ISBN: 0-7623-0764-1

tragic circumstances of dying and death, the number of individual patients on waiting lists for viable matching organs has grown far beyond the numbers of organs donated. This holds true for every organ. As of the end of 1999, for example, 66,000 people are awaiting organ donations. About 5,500 organ donations were made last year, yet in that same year, 4,300 people died while waiting for a transplant (Page, 1999).[2]

The shortage of organs arises from two facts: first, the surgical skills and technology for retrieval and transport of organs has continued to progress, as has the surgical and medical post-operative care (including immunosuppression and anti-rejection therapy), with the effect that the envelope of suitable transplant candidates is constantly expanding for each organ as well. A good example was the successful heart transplantation of a 79-year-old Canadian man (Associated Press, 2000). Not long ago the age cut-off was 55.

The success of organ transplantation is a remarkable achievement of our time. It has progressed from a very experimental activity in the 1980s with only a dismal outcome, to a major method of prolonging human life today (Starzomski, 1997). For example the five-year survival rate for kidney and liver transplants is over 75%. As organ transplant technology continues to improve, then, the increasing shortage of organs becomes more and more tragic. This dilemma will continue to bedevil the medical enterprise until it can grow a person's own organs in the laboratory and successfully transplant them. In the meanwhile, transplantation in this country and many others must continue to rely on altruism or other proposed methods of retrieval from live donors (when appropriate) or the families of the dying and newly dead.

This reliance leads to a second fact contributing to shortage of organs. The number of organs donated has remained relatively steady over time despite constant efforts to encourage donation. The data is discouraging. Voluntary donation has not met the need for increasing the number of donors (Hauptman & O'Connor, 1997). In 1988 the number of cadaveric donors in the U.S. was 4,080, while a decade later, that number grew only modestly to 4,300. During the same period, the number of living donors increased only modestly as well, from 1,825 to 2,902. No one wants to sniff at these increases, but recall that more than 50,000 people were listed, waiting for transplants in 1998.

Sometimes advertising has been effective. Illinois, for example, remains one of the highest states for obtaining organ donations due in large part to commitments by transplant centers to stress organ retrieval and to the vigorous campaign of the Secretary of State's office under now-governor Ryan. Still Illinois lags far behind Minnesota. The constant theme of groups working to improve organ donation is expressed well by the Gift of Life Foundation, a voluntary association of donor families, recipients, health care professionals, and business executives: "As we enter the year 2000 the most immediate problem in transplantation remains an inadequate organ supply. More donors are needed" (Koch, forthcoming).

HHS INITIATIVE

Ironically, pockets of greater or lesser success like those just mentioned around the country created an inequity among regions in the allocation of organs. Regional organ bank cooperatives that labored in more successful venues than others, allocated the organs within their region first, and then only to other regions if a suitable candidate could not be found. A similar strategy was used by the United Network of Organ Sharing (UNOS). The principle underlying this method of allocation is called the "neighbor effect," whereby retrieval is improved by knowing about local figures who donate or receive organs. An often-articulated principle, too, was the idea that organ donation cuts both ways: those centers and regions having higher than average donations, due to their efforts, deserve to have greater numbers available for donation compared to regions that do not have the same success rate. Hence UNOS devised a regionally-weighted allocation system that emphasized local over national distribution (McGulgan, 2000).

The resulting regionalized maldistribution also meant that more successful programs competed with one another within a context of density while other programs languished in parts of the country with lesser success at donation. Chicago, for example, had five liver transplant programs performing almost one-third of all liver transplants in the country (UNOS, 1998). The upshot of this success was that the waiting lists in Chicago were longer by average than in other sections of the country. That is why Chicagoan Walter Payton initially went to Minnesota for a work-up of his liver disease to be evaluated for a liver transplant, since that state has an excellent organ retrieval record and a shorter waiting list due to fewer competing programs.

Several other sequella due to competition and density occurred. The first was that the rules for placing one's patients on the waiting list were sometimes bent. Cheating appears to have occurred in order to boost one surgical center over another in competition for organs (Thomasma et al., 1999). Second, patients learned how to manipulate the system by finding out on the Internet where the best centers were (Thomasma et al., 1999), and for some organs, entering themselves on multiple waiting lists. Third, and most importantly for the analysis to follow, the sickest person in the country, due to the aforementioned regionalization of allocation, did not get first chance at the matched organ that might have saved his or her life. This is considered a violation of justice, since by law transplantable human organs are considered a national resource, and one's needs are assessed within the context of a national community (Davis, 1999).

This fact was brought home to Donna Shalala, Clinton's Secretary of HHS, when a close friend needing a liver transplant died. She then issued a directive that regional cooperative sharing banks should allocate organs on the basis of the sickest person first, no matter what the region.

The government was officially critical of UNOS policies, since, as noted, the United Network of Organ Sharing had developed the more regional policies that kept some livers from the sickest person in the country in favor of the sickest person in a region. UNOS defended itself. HHS rebuked UNOS (U.S. Congress, House Committee on Energy and Commerce, 1990). Congress became involved. Nonetheless, in the government-issued new guidelines for allocating organs, starting with livers, an appeal was made to the general principle that livers were a "scarce national resource." The language comes from earlier legislation. If this designation is accurate, then the government could begin to establish guidelines for allocation that might override those of previous voluntary associations like UNOS, just as it had to ration and allocate gasoline and meat during the Second World War.

Subsequently, Congress temporarily suspended the new rules in October 1999, since they seemed to involve government too much in the free and voluntary association of sharing organs through UNOS. Predictably, groups such as the American Society of Transplant Surgeons expressed concern that the HHS secretary should not be making medical decisions. According to the transplant surgeons, in the final ruling regarding the Organ Procurement and Transplantation Network (OPTN), the health secretary continued to insist on having the final word in how organs are allocated. Critics of the ruling assert that Congress intended such decisions to be made by the medical community, and not by a government agency (Anonymous 1999b). Further discussion and political maneuvering is anticipated. At the time of this writing, the rules are still suspended (Anonymous, 1999c; Neikirk, 1999).

POSSIBLE STRATEGIES TO INCREASE RETRIEVAL

How can we balance all the interests in organ transplantation? Before considering the pathway taken under the temporarily-suspended HHS rules, let us briefly examine other possibilities for retrieving organs. These can be distinguished into general strategies, and specific proposals.

General Strategies

By now it is commonplace to outline general categories for organ retrieval into buying/selling, required donation, gifting, donating.

The first category, buying and selling, is outlawed in the United States. Although philosophers and others have proposed that buying and selling, relying on the free market, is the most equitable way to obtain organs, there is still widespread mistrust of market forces intruding for what most consider to be an altruistic act. It is tempting to discuss the pros and cons of the free market proposal, but certainly now, and possibly in the foreseeable future, buying and selling organs will not be legalized in this country, so the question is somewhat moot. At the very least, it would add to an already-competitive environment, an incentive to obtain prisoners' organs (as China is accused of doing) (Dorning, 1999), or to prey on the poor and disenfranchised (Thomasma, 1997). Another concern is that the human body and its parts will be officially commodified. In support of this worry, a fashion photographer put pictures of eight models who sell their eggs on the web, opening bids at $15,000 to $150,000 per egg. Although there was widespread disgust over this entrepreneurism, the photographer Ron Harris had early-on received a serious bid for $42,000 (Loewy, 1998; Anonymous, 1999d, e). Later, buyers have offered $100,000 for the healthy eggs of a college athlete, and on eBay a human kidney was up for bid for $100,000, to be picked up in Zurich (Associated Press, 1999).

Yet, donation rates in Spain are three times that in the U.S., 30 per million compared to about 10 per million citizens. Thus, despite almost heroic public efforts to increase donations, the rate has remained rather steady. Because of this fact, many in the U.S. are open to considering other strategies.

Required donation is one of the alternate strategies. It is a form of default mode. According to this proposal, the U.S. would adopt the policy of other nations, in determining that organs as a scarce national resource should be presumed to be donated by all citizens, unless they opt out for religious or other reasons. Such individuals might carry a card like an organ donor card that expressed their wishes not to be a donor. Surely this strategy would increase the supply of organs. Further one could add to it certain disincentives. A good one might be that in the presence of refusal to donate, one would automatically be ineligible to receive organs.

The biggest problem facing this strategy is that it would seem to require an Amendment to the U.S. Constitution regarding the public rights to private bodies, and violates a sense of autonomy that is ingrained in the American culture (Reuters, 2000). Early on, the government did adopt "required request" rules, namely, that each potential donor's family would be approached about donation. Even this modest effort met with great resistance because, although a separate transplant team made the request, there was a perception that such requests from total strangers seemed to intrude upon the natural grieving process. This is a problem with the new guidelines as well.

In this context one should consider the discussion by Spital and others (Spital, 1997; Rhodes, 1994; Wear & Logue, 1995) about "mandated choice." According to this idea, generally all citizens would be required to choose whether or not to donate and execute an irrevocable will that the family could not supersede later upon the individual's death. This may remove concerns about intruding on the grief of families at death.

One other perception about current practices led to new rules about organ retrieval to be examined later. This perception was that unskilled individuals were making requests and failing to obtain potentially life-saving organs due to their ineptitude. As a result, only trained individuals will be authorized to discuss with families the possibility of donation.

Gifting is another promising strategy that avoids the pitfalls of an organ free market or of requiring donations. Gifting is also different from pure, altruistic donation. Gifting recognizes that, despite the presence of altruism, individuals and families who donate organs do "receive" something, even if that something is an honorable standing in the community. In the case of live-donation, the individual may enhance his or her recognition in the family as the one who "saved" her uncle's life. Apparently in India, where widespread organ selling occurred, the process was more comparable to gifting than selling. There was at the time no organ bank, so those in higher castes who had money, sought the "gift" of an organ. Those in lower castes were happy to help and volunteered to do so. A kidney was provided.

In the culture, however, there was an expectation of an outpouring of gratitude from the recipients of this largess, and that gratitude was expressed through an appreciation gift, usually in the form of money (Thomasma, 1997). Like an elaborate tip. Indeed, even the practice of using prisoners' organs is one in which, in exchange for the organs, the criminal under the death penalty removes shame from his family's good name. There is that recompense (and unfortunately, coercion) of families.

Recognizing tradeoffs like these has led to a series of proposals for an exchange involving organs and, perhaps, some financial reimbursements, like payment for the funeral. Even those who might oppose direct buying and selling may support this notion (Marshall et al., 1996). At academic medical centers, there are proposals to provide a free education to family members, and the like. Of all other general strategies, gifting carries the best chance of augmenting the standard donation policy. But for now, altruistic organ donation remains the standard general strategy for retrieving organs. It is time to consider specific initiatives under that strategy.

Specific Initiatives

1. Continue to use cessation of total brain function as the event that triggers the possibility of requesting donor organs. By coupling this with required request guidelines, all real and potential patient's families are to be approached about the possibility of transplant. Increased efforts at public education was thought to help the pool of potential donors grow. Despite all efforts thus far, however, this approach has not kept pace with the growing success of organ transplant technology. As noted, the level of organ donation has not substantially changed, while the need has sometimes quadrupled due to greater knowledge and techniques. Something more is needed.

2. Change the definition of death to cessation of higher brain function (Lawlor, 1999). The problem with establishing this criterion is that loss of higher brain function is not as easily measurable, objectively, as the loss of all brain function. Persons in a PVS or a permanent coma might then qualify as potential donors, depending upon the kinds of tests developed (Sorenson, 1988; Cohen, et al., 1988). These patients would be declared "dead" (which is a social definition) (Schaffner & Starzl, 1998), and their organs used to help others. Anencephalics would also be eligible for a declaration of death. We can assume that there would be widespread public abhorrence of taking the organs of living, vulnerable people without their current consent. This is because there would be no social consensus about what counts as "death." The current brain death criterion required a great deal of public discussion and legislative deliberation. One could only imagine how difficult it would be to broaden the definition of death in this way, although awareness about the inadequacy of the current brain death criteria is growing (Thomasma, 1997).

3. Permit individuals through advance directives to donate their organs upon attaining what, for them, would be unacceptable forms of living, including, but not limited to, neurological conditions like the aforementioned PVS, end-stage Alzheimer's, or a permanent coma. The problems mentioned in 2, above, would only be amplified in this strategy, since taking the organs, even if permitted, would create the physiological death. Furthermore, individuals might find living in chronic states unacceptable. Reportedly, this strategy was the guiding commitment of Kevorkian (Quill, 1999), who was only convicted of murder in the assisted suicide of his last "patient," who requested that his kidneys be donated. Kevorkian offered those organs upon the suicide of his patient, but he was convicted of causing the death in this way (Anonymous, 1999e).

4. Establish a legally-valid required donation national health policy. Under this policy, individuals would be presumed donors unless they opted out by signing a card that refused to donate for whatever reason. Since this effort would violate an Amendment to the U.S. Constitution, the chances of following this policy, or the less-restrictive one widely established in other countries, are virtually non-existent.

5. Establish a right to temporarily sustain organs in a brain-dead person until survivors could consent or not to retrieving organs (Youngner et al., 1999). This would violate the principle of personal and bodily integrity, but from one point of view, the person no longer "exists" because of the loss of total brain function. Controversy over test proposals and protocols like this still swirls around the variations in a pluralistic society regarding the integrity of a human person and the role of the union of body and spirit (Childress, 1996).

The Regional Organ Bank of Illinois (ROBI) supported a protocol for obtaining kidneys that fell into this category. The research was to prove that one could obtain viable kidneys from cadavers by perfusing kidneys to keep them at an ideal temperature while they were still in the body, prior to transplant. Animal models suggested the feasibility of this method. Yet, in order to be successful, the interventions had to occur right away, at the moment of death. Since most of the potential donors would be accident victims, this intervention would have to take place prior to notification of the family that their loved one had expired.

This protocol was tested at my own institution, Loyola University Chicago Medical Center, after due approval by the IRB. Although the research on human subjects under this protocol proved that the technique was very successful, it was only done with prior family approval. In order to help reduce the shortage of kidneys nationwide, of course, this procedure would have to be used without that prior family's consent in many cases. This violates the right to privacy, and would seem to be illegal at the present time since there would be an "assault" on one's body without prior consent.

6. Use the Pittsburgh Non Heart Beating Donor Cadavers (NHBDC) protocol (Fox & Swazey, 1992) or a variant of the same (Arnold & Youngner, 1993). Under this protocol, only individuals who raise the desire to donate their organs qualify. Shortly before their death, as their heart fibrillates during the dying process, their organs are taken in surgery. So far, very few organs have resulted from this initiative, and great controversy has resulted even over the mere discussion of the possibility using it in other centers. Although this protocol is based on the way death was defined before the brain-death criterion, it is now seen as a form of bringing about the death of the individual donating the organs by harvesting them while the individual is still legally alive (Agich,

1999; Koughan & Bogdanich, 1999). The essential ethical issues surround the distinction between physiological death and the medical and social determinations of death. Either one must argue for a broader concept of death than just the cessation of total brain function, or as Arnold and Youngner argue, one should expand the dead-donor rule itself to cover those that might still be perceived as "living" (Arnold & Youngner, 1993). They are judged to be "dead" for the purposes of retrieving their organs after two minutes of irregular or diminishing heart rhythms. Thus, not only are they not resuscitated, in the view of some, they are actually killed by the organ retrieval operations themselves. It should be noted that these patients are facing immanent death, are already DNR, and they or their proxy had already asked to remove life-support before asking to donate.

7. Continue to create artificial organs to substitute, most often temporarily, for the missing functions of biological organs until the latter become available. The new artificial liver device is a good current example of this technology, but it can only help for a maximum of 48 hours, and at great expense (Potts, 1997). It does not represent a long-term solution to the problem of organ shortage. It functions as a temporary bridge until transplant is possible. A recent success has occurred at the University of Chicago where the liver assist device saved a young woman's life until a liver became available. She has now gone home (Luh, 2000). Eventually new organs will be grown in the laboratory. Already there is a report, for example, of growing human heart valves in a test tube (Anonymous, 1999f), and of finding the genetic switch to make eyes (Cooke, 1995).[3]

8. Continue to promote live organ donation as an alternative to cadaveric organs. This can work for kidneys and livers, but one can raise the question of the degree of risk another person through altruism should be allowed to assume. Live liver donation, in which the liver is divided, is more risky than kidney donation at present.

Absent any serious national efforts to redefine the moment of death or to foster the cause of using organs from living beings as currently legally defined to benefit others, it is clear that the focus of new strategies must lie on improvement in the altruistic donation system now in place.

NEW RETRIEVAL STRATEGY

We may now turn to a discussion in more detail of the increased professionalization of organ donation request under the HHS initiative. The proposed rules in effect gave unprecedented powers to organ retrieval specialists (most of whom are nurses) working for regional organ banks, and greater and more intrusive powers to those organ bank associations over the doctor-patient, and institutional relationship taking place during the dying process and immediately after death.

These new powers arose from the worry that unskilled efforts by the managing physician, nurses, and other care givers to obtain organ donor permission either from the patient, or more often from the family, may have led to the loss of many potential organs and the subsequent loss of many lives that might have been saved by those organs.

To ensure against that probability, the new guidelines require the physician and other care givers to step aside at the point of first discussion about donating organs and call for a retrieval nurse from the regional organ bank, now renamed a "family care specialist," who is intensively trained and experienced in obtaining organ donations. Such training means it will be less likely that organs might be lost due to bungling, misstatements, or other causes. This rule is so important, that institutions are to notify the organ bank when patients are dying and might be good candidates for organ donation.

Nonetheless the health professionals most closely involved with the patient and family must now turn over an intimate part of the care at the end of life to a total stranger, one who is also subject to staff resentment for the intrusion and implication that the latter cannot do as good a job as the organ specialist. Further, after death has occurred the eye bank and other agencies that coordinate parts of the body that can survive a short time after death must be notified. They in turn contact the family about donation of these parts after the body is on the way or has arrived at the funeral parlor. Imagine the grieving family being petitioned in this way by additional strangers, or the possible anger at learning that one's loved one's death was reported behind one's back!

Instead of modifying for the better, these newer actions serve to reinforce more long-standing resistance factors that I will now briefly examine with respect to the ethical issues facing the new breed of organ procurers, the family care specialists.

NEW MORAL CONCERNS

The trained organ retrieval specialists, the "family care specialists" from the organ bank, have a double burden. First, as strangers they must approach patients and families involved in a profound and grief-filled relationship of dying. This problem has existed for some time. In the effort to ensure in the family's mind that the caregivers of the patient did not have a conflict of interest, a separate hospital team or a "procurement nurse" was dispatched to make the arrangements. Nonetheless, this person was a member of the hospital staff itself, not an institutional outsider. Family care specialists from the organ procurement agency are seen as outsiders by fellow nurses in hospital, something that was not anticipated. They are sometimes resented.

Part of that perception lies in the implicit judgment that authorizes only outside specialists to discuss organ transplantation. If a doctor does so with the family, he or she is violating the law, and the organ specialist may be required to report that doctor and create further ill-will with the hospital. Many physicians and their institutions are proud of their records of obtaining organs, and find it difficult to release their successes into the hands of strangers. Insisting on their rights, the organ specialists risk keeping the regional organ bank in good standing with the hospital, and risk contributing to the shortage of organs by creating additional obstacles to obtaining them. They are left with trying to do "damage control" in the aftermath of the previous discussion with the family.

There are some other ethical problems facing the family care specialists under this first burden. If the NHBDC protocol is in place in a hospital, as it is in several in the Chicago area, how much time should the specialist insist be given to saying final farewells, and moving the patient to the operating room? This is a very delicate matter, since most families do not want to be absent when the patient actually dies. It takes extraordinary sensitivity, especially if that person had not known the family or patient at all.

A second burden arises from the degree of persuasion to be used. Under this burden are some major difficulties identified by family care specialists themselves (Questions? 1998–1999):

(1) Is it wrong to tell the families that if they do not donate, their refusal will lead to other people dying?
(2) Is it ethical to persuade a family toward donation if the specialist already knows that the patient had not registered as a donor in the donor registry? Suppose the patient had refused, but the family does want to donate anyway. In this case is there a violation of patient rights by accepting her organs? As is widely recognized, the individual upon death, does not "own" his or her body. The family does (the legal next of kin makes decisions about donation and burial). So it sometimes seems appropriate to approach them no matter what the patient had said about donating.
(3) Does the end of the work, saving the lives of others, justify the means, turning up the intensity of trying to obtain organs and intruding ever further on the grieving process to the point of contacting the family while the body is on the way to the funeral parlor for eyes and other tissues?

(4) Is it appropriate to educate families of patients about their religion's acceptance or rejection of organ donation, if one is informed that the patient did not practice that religion? Suppose a patient belonged to a religion that would prohibit donation, and was alienated from the family, should efforts be used to persuade them anyway?
(5) Is it alright to accept consent for organ donation from someone who was involved in the potential donor's death? This moral quandary arises less in family brutality cases than in accidents, when a spouse was driving and survives the victim.
(6) Is it ethical for a prospective donor family or the donor him- or herself to limit the people who would be eligible to receive an organ? An example might be an advance directive indicating that "I wish to donate my organs only to someone of the Islamic faith."
(7) What about the failure of the family care specialist to obtain suitable organs? Is she or he to be held morally responsible for the failure to save, potentially say, seven other lives with the organs and tissues that might have been donated if she were successful.

These are only a few of the detailed moral problems facing the people trained to approach families about donating. Their heightened duties and responsibilities are accompanied by a moral sense that may overburden them, given that so many of them are nurses by training and are committed to saving lives. Placing them in highly emotional contexts as strangers with a duty to excel at what they do may create more ethical problems than ever anticipated.

MORE GENERAL CONCERNS

The ideals of organ transplantation continue to face a series of more general resistance factors that mitigate the compassionate idealism forming the desire to donate. These mitigating counter-forces are emotional, medical, social-cultural, and religious.

Many of the organs being transplanted today carry with them emotional content. The heart is an organ, especially, with deep cultural linkages to love and to life. Thus a transplant of a heart is accompanied by similar feelings and cultural concerns that in earlier times were present in ritual consumption of an enemy warrior's heart, or of the eating of a buffalo heart by an Indian hunter. The incorporation of another person's organ into one's own body and resultant medicalized body-image is a profound experience, the depths of which we may only still imagine (Rollins, 1999). Transplantation is still a relatively youthful technology.

However, medical technology usually views these organs as interchangeable, almost like buying a new toaster for one's kitchen. Patients report that this attitude on the part of transplant specialists is dangerous. There are also deep problems with interspecies transplants, as well as multiple re-transplantation. In particular, is there a cutoff on the number of organs to be used to save any one individual life?

Inconsistencies in both the retrieval and donation system create additional problems for both the donor families and the family care specialists. A policy of opting out of donation rather than opting in would respond to these challenges, but create problems of its own.

There are enormous social consequences of changing the system of organ transplantation now in place. In the U.S. we cannot require donations, and there is resistance to discussing these issues at the bedside of newly brain-dead patients (the problem addressed by requiring only certified organ bank specialists to make requests). Many argue that we simply must get better at "promoting" organ donation.

I have suggested that other options for obtaining organs should be explored. I oppose buying and selling organs (because of the potential for abuse), but think that other kinds of incentives might be appropriate, for example, providing more direct access to high-technology care for individual families who donate, donor families being placed higher on recipient lists than others, all other things being equal, if their own organ failure occurs, and so on.

All of these reasons need to be examined in light of fears individuals possess about donation, making the body an object, disputes about brain death, and concerns about the need for organs creating a kind of elasticity about the guidelines for determining the moment of death. The future of genetic developments is also a factor.

It may be possible, either by way of interspecies transplants or by immunological means, to harvest organs from animals that will not meet the body's normal reactions to foreign tissue, thus enhancing both availability and the success rate. At present a breed of pigs with a human immunological system has been patented for just this purpose. If this approach works out as planned many of the resistance factors will be bypassed, and many lives will be saved that are now lost on waiting lists for human organs. Among the major problems to this approach, however, is the growing conviction that animal life is owed the same or equivalent dignity as human life (Singer, 1998).

As long as the shortage of organs continues, I suggest that we might owe one another our organs when we cannot any longer use them, not so much because they are a scarce national resource, but for humanitarian and religious reasons of justice. If the new guidelines for organ bank specialist training of procurement nurses do not result in an anticipated increase in donor organs, then other government efforts may be justified. The problems arising from increased professionalization and concomitant increased bureaucratization of the retrieval process may be ameliorated by developments now that point to a rosier future for transplantation technology.

CONCLUSION

Too much power has shifted, pendulum-like, to the government and the patient specialists (organ retrieval organizations), especially as some organs like livers are now being viewed by the government as a "scarce resource" to be allocated under government control. Responding to continued shortages of organs, John Harris, an English philosopher, has lately argued that at death, our bodies ought to be seen as the property of the state so that the government may take organs as needed to preserve the lives of others (Harris, 1985).

Undeniably, the scarcity of organs has reached a critical stage, but so has the scarcity of many other medical services as both government and private insurers shrink-wrap medical care under diminished reimbursement schemes. The irony develops that, with respect to organs, the government may control retrieval and allocation mechanisms, but with respect to ordinary medical care, it can do little or nothing to allocate fairly.

Even more critically from a moral point of view, I have argued in this essay that the individuals identified and trained to obtain organs from donors and donor-families, are placed in a compromised position. They "intrude" into a private relationship between the care givers and the patient and family. Finally, family care specialists are placed under enormous moral burdens to be successful, and potentially save the lives of a number of dying people based upon this success. Yet they enter the rooms and relationships as strangers. They themselves need a great deal of moral and emotional support.

NOTES

1. Nonetheless, both died of liver cancer, Mantle after receiving a controversial transplant, and Payton after first being listed as a candidate, although once the bile duct cancer was identified in February, 1999, he was removed from any consideration, since the immunosuppressants needed for the transplant would make it likely the cancer would return.

2. The Regional Organ Bank of Illinois said that, while organ donations had been down in the previous year, 1999 had been a banner year nationally, with an increase of 5%, they attribute to Payton's case and advocacy. Even when he knew (but the public

did not) that he was not to be put on a waiting list, he went on TV in favor of organ transplants.

3. These have been grown and tested in animals, working as nature intended.

REFERENCES

Agich, G. J. (1999). From Pittsburgh to Cleveland: NHBD (non-heart-breathing-donor) controversies and bioethics. *Cambridge Quarterly of Healthcare Ethics*, *8*(3), 269–274.

Anonymous (1988). HHS pushes new organ distribution. *Chicago Tribune*, June 3, 16.

Anonymous (1999a). Payton's biggest triumph: football hero's big heart in facing illness has renewed interest in organ donations. *Chicago Sun-Times*, Nov. 7, 39A.

Anonymous (1999b). HHS pushes new organ distribution. *Chicago Tribune*, June 3, 16.

Anonymous (1999c). HHS secretary shouldn't make medical decisions. *Medical Ethics Advisor*, *16*(12), 146–147.

Anonymous (1999d). Photographer stirs controversy with human egg auction. *Chicago Tribune*, Oct. 25, 10.

Anonymous (1999e). Kevorkian gets 10 to 25 years for murder. *Chicago Tribune*, April 14.

Anonymous (1999f). Researcher reports producing human heart valves in a test tube. *Chicago Tribune*, Nov. 8, 10.

Arnold, R. M., & Youngner, S. J. (1993). Special Issue: Ethical, psycho social, and public policy: Implications of procuring organs from non-heart-beating cadavers. *Kennedy Institute of Ethics Journal*, *3*(2).

Associated Press (1999). To critics, auction of models' eggs an ugly moment in field of fertility. *Chicago Tribune*, Oct. 26, 9.

Associated Press (2000). Heart transplant to 79-year-old sets off ethics debate in Canada. *Chicago Tribune*, Jan. 8, 16.

Childress, J. F. (1996). The gift of life: ethical issues in organ transplantation. *Bulletin of the American College of Surgeons*, *81*(3), 8–22.

Cohen et al. (1988). Making treatment decisions for permanently unconscious patients. In: J. Monagle & D. C. Thomasma (Eds), *Medical Ethics*. Rockville, MD: Aspen Publishers.

Cooke. R. (1995). Science finds genetic switch to make eyes. *Chicago Sun-Times*, March 24, 4.

Davis, R. (1999). Site lists best places for transplants. *U.S.A Today*, Oct. 14, 1A.

Dorning, M. (1999). Delay likely on rules for transplants. *Chicago Tribune*, Oct. 12, 4.

Fox, R. C., & Swazey, J. P. (1992). *Spare Parts: Organ Replacement in American Society*. New York: Oxford University Press.

Harris, J. (1985). *The Value of Life: An Introduction to Medical Ethics*. London; Boston: Routledge & Kegan Paul.

Hauptman, P. J., & O'Connor, K. J. (1997). Medical progress: procurement and allocation of solid organs for transplantation. *New England Journal of Medicine*, *336*(6), 422–431.

Koch, T. (2000). They might as well be in Bolivia: race, ethnicity and the problem of solid organ donation. *Theoretical Medicine & Bioethics* forthcoming.

Koughan, F., & Bogdanich, W. (1999). *60 Minutes* sets the record straight. *Cambridge Quarterly of Healthcare Ethics*, *8*(4), 514–516.

Lawlor, E. F. (1999). The organ relationship revisited. *Chicago Tribune*, Nov. 28, 19.

Loewy, E. H. (1998). Waste not, want not: communities and presumed consent. In: J. Monagle & D. C. Thomasma (Eds), *Health Care Ethics: Critical Issues for the 21st Century* (pp. 342–350). Gaithersburg, MD: Aspen Publishers.

Luh, S. S. (2000). Liver machine keeps Joliet woman alive: time critical as she awaits transplant. *Chicago Sun-Times*, Jan. 7, 10.

Marshall, P. A. et al. (1996). Marketing human organs: the autonomy paradox. *Theoretical Medicine*, *17*(1), 1–18.

McGulgan, J. J. (2000). Message. *Gift of Life News*, Jan. 4(1), 1.

Neikirk, W. (1999). GOP leaders slow White House drive for organ transplant policy. *Chicago Tribune*, Nov. 19, 25.

Page, C. (1999). Another record: Payton put a face on organ crisis. *The Chicago Tribune*, Nov. 3, 29.

Potts, J. T. (1997). *Institutes of Medicine: Non-Heart-Beating Organ Transplantation: Medical and Ethical Issues in Procurement*. Washington, D.C.: National Academy Press.

Quill, T. E. (1999). Kevorkian: hero, villain, or somewhere in between? *Choices* (Newsletter of Choices in Dying), *8*(3), 1,4.

Reuters (2000). German Internet auction site stops bidding on human kidney. *Chicago Tribune*, Feb. 21, 9.

Rhodes, R. (1994). A review of ethical issues in transplantation. *Mount Sinai Journal of Medicine*, *61*(1), 77–82.

Roberts, E. J. D. (1999). Letter to the editor: selling models' eggs misses beauty of ethics. *U.S.A Today*, Oct 29, 17A.

Rollins, J. D. (1999). Medical chimera: the anniversary of an allograft. *Journal of Medical Humanities*, *30*(3), 177–190.

Schaffner, K. F., & Starzl, T. E. (Eds) (1998). Paradigm changes in organ transplantation. *Theoretical Medicine and Bioethics*, *19*(5).

Singer, P. (1998). *Ethics Into Action: Henry Spira and the Animal Rights Movement*. Lanham, MD: Rowman & Littlefield.

Sorenson, J. (1988). The determination of death: the need for a higher-brain death concept. In: J. Monagle & D. C. Thomasma (Eds), *Medical Ethics* (pp. 234–238). Rockville, MD: Aspen Publishers.

Spital, A. (1997). Ethical and policy issues in altruistic living and cadaveric organ donation. *Clinical Transplantation*, *11*(2), 77–87.

Starzomski, R. C. (1997). Dissertation: *Resource Allocation for Solid Organ Transplantation: Toward Public and Health Care Provider Dialogue*. Vancouver, Canada: The University of British Columbia.

Thomasma, D. C. (1997a). Bioethics and international human rights. *Journal of Law, Medicine, and Ethics*, *25*, 295–306.

Thomasma, D. C. (1997b). Tecnologia del trapianto: implicazione etsche e religiose. In: *La Questione dei Trapianti: Tra Etica Diritto, Economia*, tr. Christina Todeschini. Milano: Dott A. Giuffre Editore, 103–124.

Thomasma, B. C. et al. (1999). The ethics of competition among liver transplant programs. *Cambridge Quarterly of Healthcare Ethics*, *8*(3), 321–329.

UNOS (1998). UNOS analysis of proposed organ transplant regulations. UNOS.org/Newsroom/archives_other_regsanalysis_052798.httm.

U.S. Congress, House Committee on Energy and Commerce, Subcommittee on Health and the Environment (1990). *National Organ Transplantation Act: Hearing Before the Subcommittee on Health and the Environment of the Committee on Energy and Commerce, House of Representatives, One Hundred First Congress, second [sic] session, on H. R. 3968. . . April 20*. Washington D.C.: U.S., G.P.O.

Wear, S., & Logue, G. (1995). Informed consent for organ transplantation: mandating the participation of the family. *Law and Policy, 17*(2), 210–216.

Youngner, S. J. et al. (Eds) (1999). *The Definition of Death: Contemporary Controversies*. Baltimore, MD: Johns Hopkins University Press.

7. ETHICAL ISSUES IN NON-HEARTBEATING CADAVER DONORS

Shelly Ozark and Michael A. DeVita

INTRODUCTION

What is a Non-Heart-Beating Cadaver?

In non-heart-beating organ donation (NHBOD) the physician certifies death using traditional cardiac criteria; that is, the patient is considered dead after his or her heart has irreversibly ceased to beat. This may seem like a rather low-tech way of declaring death, and thus one less likely to provoke discussion than using the brain death criteria that historically has been at the center of many ethical discussions. However, the reintroduction of declaring death utilizing cardiac criteria and then procuring organs for transplantation sparked a fire-storm of questions and discussion about whether such practices were a morally acceptable means for procuring organs. That it is a reintroduction of criteria, rather than an introduction of new criteria has played no small part in the discussion. Originally, in the early days of transplantation, organs were removed from two sources: living donors, usually related to the recipient, and recently deceased donors who were declared dead when their hearts stopped beating. Death, in these circumstances, was declared based upon a cardiac-centered criteria rather than a brain-centered criteria because the concept of 'brain death' had not yet come into usage. After its introduction, the concept of brain death gradually grew to a point of wide acceptance, to the extent that it became the dominant standard used in organ procurement. Indeed, until

The Ethics of Organ Transplantation, Volume 7, pages 167–194.

ISBN: 0-7623-0764-1

recently it was a rather rare occurrence for transplant teams to procure organs from cadavers whose death had been determined using cardiac criteria. Severe organ shortages and patient or family demand to donate organs have forced the alteration of this trend.

The transplant waiting lists grew as both improved outcome and expanded indications for the procedure increased demand. Supply has always remained insufficient. Advocates for organ transplantation attempted to increase supply through a variety of interventions. Public education campaigns to increase public awareness of the shortage did increase public knowledge base, but did not lead to an expected rise in organs. Required request legislation required physicians or other caregivers to approach the families of all potential donors and request that they consider donation. Designated requestor regulation mandated that the requestors be trained in the most beneficial techniques in asking families to donate organs. These efforts, however, resulted in only a limited increase in actual donations. New sources needed to be found.

One possible solution seemed to lie in a previously largely ignored population: patients who were declared dead based upon cardiac criteria. Since more people have death determined using cardiac criteria than using neurologic (brain death) criteria, the potential donor pool may be greatly expanded. This potential pool of donors includes those patients with terminal conditions who are on heart-lung bypass machines, ventilators or blood pressure support and who rapidly progress to cardiac arrest when the support is withdrawn. For each of these patients, like for anyone whose heart stops beating, cessation of brain function is inevitable. Maintaining a distinction between patients declared dead based upon a brain criteria, that is patients who would commonly be considered prime candidates for donation, and patients declared dead based upon cardiac criteria, appeared to significantly limit the pool of potential donors. Allowing prompt recovery of organs from non-heart-beating donors, might be a reasonable means of expanding the donor pool and increasing organ supply.

It is important to note that there are two circumstances under which non-heart-beating donation may occur: controlled settings and uncontrolled settings. In controlled settings the death of the potential donor is predictable and can be manipulated. The potential donor is terminally ill, is dependent upon life support interventions, and a decision to remove life support has been made. Following that decision, consent for organ donation is obtained from either the donor or his or her surrogate. As it is foreseen that death will occur shortly after removal of life support, there is some latitude in when such support will be withdrawn, i.e. it will be withdrawn once the procurement team is ready and the family has gathered to say its good-byes. In contrast, uncontrolled NHBOD takes place randomly, yet occurs in a setting convenient to donation, such that after a patient suffers a fatal heart attack while in the emergency room. In uncontrolled NHBOD, more time may elapse between death and organ procurement because the potential donor's family must be contacted, informed about the death and consent for procurement obtained.

Some wonder, however, if the use of non-heart-beating donors is morally acceptable. Questions ranged from basic concerns about the overall moral acceptability of NHBD to ones which addressed more humanistic concerns which had developed. These questions included: Are non-heart-beating organ donors really dead? Is it permissible to manipulate a death so that organs can be procured? Is there a reasonable middle ground in the inherent conflict of interest between care of the donor and the recipient's need for functioning organs?

Within this chapter we will provide an overview and discuss the interplay of several of these issues. In turn, we will analyze how these issues have shifted over time. This chapter will also detail specific organ procurement protocols and discuss how organ procurement programs have responded to subsequent criticism. Finally, this chapter will discuss the consensus statement recently released by the Institute of Medicine about the use of and procedures surrounding NHBD and what impact such donation has actually had on organ procurement numbers in 1998, the first year following the legalization of NHBD.

DISCUSSION

Are Non-Heart-Beating Organ Donors Really Dead?

The determination of death prior to procurement is important. There is a concern that if surgeons removed a donor's organs before irreversibility was guaranteed, the procurement teams could be held morally culpable for their patient's deaths. While not resuscitating a patient would be seen as a letting die, a morally acceptable inaction, removing organs from a patient who could potentially self-resuscitate would be seen as a morally unacceptable action. The removal of organs from a patient who could be resuscitated by others, but upon whom no resuscitative efforts was initiated, is seen by some as equally morally unacceptable. As a result of this issue, a "rule" – the dead-donor rule – has emerged. It states that the procurement of organs can neither precede nor cause death of donors. Physicians who break this rule, in addition to the moral concerns run the risk of charges of homicide.

But what should the criteria for determining death be? Some wondered whether, despite its use in the early days of transplantation, the use of a cardiac standard is appropriate for use in the procurement of organs. Since NHBOD is frequently used in situations where, at least in theory, if the patient were treated, restoration of spontaneous circulation could occur, critics have questioned whether death is being declared prematurely. They argue that the waiting time between heart stoppage and the initiation of the organ removal process is insufficient to ensure that the donor's heart has irreversibly stopped and cannot ever be restarted. They argue that because the heart's function may be restored for a long time after cardiac arrest, the brain should be the sentinel organ for death determination. After all, irreversible cessation of brain function occurs in a shorter time frame, and has more "accepted" criteria for death determination. These questions seem to seek to define the very nature of death itself. This questioning illustrates the effect that the widespread adoption of a brain death criteria and the development of resuscitative technologies have had on perceptions of life and death. Perhaps such questions also indicate the discomfort that many feel at having multiple means for declaring a person dead.

After the heart stops beating, the organs including the brain cease to function. Although not currently functioning, these structures retain the ability to resume functioning if circulation is restored in a timely manner. Death, some argue, cannot be considered to have occurred until it is guaranteed that the brain loses this ability to resume functioning. Because of this, some clinicians and ethicists question whether we could truly consider a person dead based solely on the fact that their heart has ceased to beat. This is due in part to the fact that death of an individual extends beyond the physical changes of the body and into a changing of society's treatment of that individual and his or her corpse. "Yet the concept of death is not a purely biological one: death is not only a biological condition. It may be viewed as a cessation of experience, the departure of the soul from the body, or a passage into 'another mode of existence' " (Catherwood, 1992). Any criteria for determining death thus would have to carry not only strong clinical weight, but also be significant in its moral symbolism. This is because death alters the relationship between an individual and society, and shifts the line of what may be acceptable behavior and action upon that individual's body. "At the point of death their moral status changes. . . . With the change in moral status of the now dead human being, the duties of attending medical staff will change. It is for these reasons that we need a set of clear 'indicators', or criteria for death" (Catherwood, 1992).

Why Not Wait Longer Before Certifying Death?

There are clearly ramifications, both moral and legal, to misjudging when a person has died. So why not just wait a very long time and resolve all doubt as to the potential donor's death?

Warm ischemic time, the time between when oxygen supply to the tissue falls below oxygen demand until the organs are cooled, may make the difference between whether they function properly in the recipient. During warm ischemic time the organs are slowly dying. Cooling slows this process, and enables transport of organs across long distances to the awaiting recipients. The time during which the organ remains in the body after the heart has stopped is crucial for survival of the organ. A severely ischemic organ may not recover after transplant, and to transplant a failing organ that would further endanger the recipient's life, would be unethical. An absolute limit of warm ischemic is not known, but is approximately 45 minutes. Thus, minimizing the time between failed circulation and organ-removal is key, and waiting until complete absence of brain metabolism (just to 'make sure') is a luxury whose organ-deteriorating consequences cannot be afforded (Youngner & Arnold, 1993). While this may seem to be an issue of practicality and utility, it reflects a general belief that many ethicists and physicians have that the patient is dead when circulation stops, even though some cellular and biochemical functions may persist for a short period. However, to have a potential donor in a state of limbo in which not all members of the medical team agree that the patient is dead can only create confusion. "It is undesirable for there to be a protracted time during which it is not clear what the medical responsibilities are" (Cole, 1992).

The Importance of Irreversibility

Some have argued that if the heart can be restarted and the individual resume spontaneous circulation then life may be restored. Consequently, the questions about whether death is being declared prematurely and whether death, when it is declared by cardiac criteria, can really be said to be irreversible, are raised. But why should whether or not the death is an irreversible one be a concern?, claims Cole, "Most of these liberties which may be taken upon the death of a person have consequences which themselves are either irreversible or only reversible with great difficulty" (Cole, 1992). Indeed, for most it makes sense to think of death as irreversible – only in legends and religious teachings is the reversibility of death ever really challenged. Few outside of the imaginary world of soap operas have had to deal with a relative or former lover suddenly coming back from the dead.

> "Thus it is natural to view death as irreversible – otherwise, what would justify taking such irreversible actions involving the decedent's body and property? But irreversibility does not appear to be a characteristic of the ordinary concept of death . . . The underlying evidence for this is straightforward enough: if irreversibility were a component of the ordinary concept of death, then 'x was dead but was later brought back to life' would be clearly self-contradictory" (Cole, 1992).

Because of this, some argue that irreversibility should not be the central crux around which we make our ethical judgements about non-heart-beating organ donation.

To set at ease societal fears and to ensure that persons who could potentially become organs donors receive appropriate and adequate care, we employ ideological constructs and rules. "Two fundamental moral requirements have governed organ procurement. One is the dead donor rule – i.e. vital organs should only be taken from dead patients, and correlatively, living patients must not be killed by organ retrieval. In fact, our society quickly accepted brain death precisely because the new criterion facilitated effective organ procurement while maintaining the dead donor rule" (Youngner & Arnold, 1993). In other words we are willing to alter our views of what death constitutes when we believe that it is in society's best interest to do so. We hold this opinion as long as we feel that the alteration of the definition of death remains morally acceptable and when we create clear-cut rules by which determinations are made. Should then, irreversibility matter if a person pre-selects the criteria which they feel would indicate their death, even if that death might be temporarily staved off by resuscitative efforts? Some see this merely as an extension of the autonomous rights of the individual, and that to follow criteria for death other than what the person has already chosen or to intervene to prevent that person's death, is an affront to those rights. Tomlinson argues,

> An essential element of the present context is that the non-heart-beating donor under the Pittsburgh protocol[1] has volunteered to donate organs only after exercising his right to refuse any further life-prolonging treatments, including treatments aimed at resuscitation from cardiopulmonary arrest. To refuse to withdraw the life-prolonging respirator therapy or to institute other life-prolonging treatments would be a violation of the donor's wishes and of his rights, and so not ethically acceptable (Tomlinson, 1993).

An individual's right to self-determination and autonomous decision making, "trumps" other externally imposed requirements that society might wish to place on patient care (within certain limits), (Matter of Quinlan, 1976), but cannot be used to determine whether the patient is dead. Such a position is seen by some as nothing short of an unacceptably ghoulish means of cheating the ill and the dying for the sake of increasing the supply of transplantable organs. Weisbard claims about the Pittsburgh Protocol, "The protocol's encouragement, whether explicitly or merely tacit, of decisions to die earlier and differently, its willingness to conceptually gerrymander the criteria for determining death, and its unmistakably utilitarian approach to the reallocation of living organs, threatened far more than it promises – at least, unless and until we are prepared to rethink much of our existing conventional wisdom" (Weisbard, 1993).

Indeed, others see any attempt to define death beyond the common understanding that most have about it, as leading only to greater confusion, and from these artificial definitions could arise unacceptable and harmful consequences to the individual, the physician and society.

> [On the irreversibility clause] First, I wish to argue that these definitions form a significant departure from the ordinary concept of death, which is weaker. The medical definitions are not clarifications; a clarification would increase precision or would resolve ambiguity. . . . The introduction of irreversibility in medical definitions appears then to be a departure from the ordinary concepts of death. to start with, 'irreversible' suffers from ambiguity. 'irreversible' means 'cannot be reversed". Accordingly, a reasonable construal is that if something is irreversible then at no time present or future will anyone be able to reverse the condition (Cole, 1992).

Others though, see irreversible as meaning 'will not reverse on its own and without intervention', not that death could not be reversed through resuscitative efforts and that the question of irreversibility was merely a question of semantics (Lamb, 1992).

What is an Acceptable Waiting Period?

Within this discussion of irreversibility there arose a compromise, a waiting period past which the heart was not likely to auto-resuscitate. By waiting a short interval after heart stoppage to declare death, NHBOD proponents could address the fears of those who believed that death was being declared prematurely. But in place of the irreversibility argument, there arose another argument as to what was an appropriate interval to wait to determine death. If the interval is set to any time before two minutes after circulation has ceased, it is possible that the heart may restart on its own. However, after forty-five minutes the organs seem to lose all potential for future functionality and the question of death declaration prior to removing those organs for transplant becomes moot. Since during the entire range between these points in time, the heart could, in theory, be actively resuscitated, the question then is whether it is acceptable to use what some may see as a 'weaker' definition of death. It could be considered 'weaker' because it is a definition based not on a biological state of irreversibility, but instead on a choice not to resuscitate. This is because "the timing of practices that surround death, including the use of artificial ventilation add vagueness to the situation and blur the line between life and death" (Price, 1997).

Until now, time, specifically waiting time, has not been as significant an issue in the process of declaring death as there was adequate time to perform repeat exams to verify brain death. The organs of a brain dead potential donor could be sustained mechanically by artificial ventilation until it was convenient to remove them, at a point when the medical team and the family were ready. "Because the hearts of brain-dead patients could be kept beating for at least hours and usually days, there was less time pressure to declare death (by neurological criteria) and remove organs" (Youngner & Arnold, 1993). Little was lost in the way of usability if the medical team waited a while after the declaration of brain death to begin removal the organs. Given the extremely rigorous criteria the President's Commission had established for declaring brain death,[2] there was never any doubt that potential donors who were declared dead based upon the brain death standard had undeniably and irreversibly lost brain function. Indeed, the issue of irreversibility almost never actually entered the discussion. "Since the late 1960s . . . the requirement of irreversibility has been constant and uncontroversial in both philosophic discourse and public policy. . . . Since technology for restoring brain function in brain-dead patients did not exist then and does not exist today, reversibility was not an issue for the President's commission or its medical consultants" (Youngner & Arnold, 1993).

In its 1997 Consensus Statement,[3] The Institute of Medicine recognized the great variation in the practices transplant centers use to declare death and believed that such variation comes from confusion over how to define and declare irreversibility. "Great precision in the moment of death is rarely crucial in general practice from the custom of using simple and imprecise standards and technologies. A little more time can make the diagnosis obvious but in donors, may result in organs of poor or unusable quality." Thus, timing in donation situations is crucial from a viability standpoint, though it is also extremely important for allaying the public's fears that death is declared too hastily and merely for the sake of removing the organs. The Institute of Medicine concludes that a uniform standard of at least five minutes should be allowed to elapse between cardiac and circulatory stoppage and the declaration of death and organ removal. This window "could ensure that death has occurred, diminish the window of haste and reassure the public, and eliminate the uncomfortable situation whereby a donor could be defined as dead in one OPO region and still, however briefly, be defined as alive in another" while minimizing the potential impact that warm ischemia may have on the organs. Yet there is no data distinguishing two minutes from five minutes or longer on resuscitability of either the heart or the brain.

Does Irreversibility Really Matter?

Is thirty seconds an appropriate waiting time to declare death, as is usually the case for comfort-measures only patients who will not be donors? Are five and ten minutes too long to both ensure that the donor would not auto-resuscitate and to ensure that the medical team has sufficient time to carefully harvest the organs before they became hypoxic and unusable? Is two minutes a 'happy medium' that would satisfy the fearful and retain organ viability all at the same time? As the authors of the Pittsburgh Protocol explain, "It was considered important that it is common practice to pronounce death in 'comfort measures only' patients within 30 seconds of central arterial pulselessness when a progressive loss of vital signs was well documented" (DeVita & Snyder, 1993). If it was acceptable to declare non-donors dead after only thirty seconds after the heart ceased to beat, and the patient had decided they wanted no resuscitative efforts made, why would it not be considered acceptable to apply a similar standard to those who would donate their organs? Was the overall increased social utility of the donors' death, even in situations where the patient was basically guaranteed to die because he or she had refused resuscitative efforts, too ghoulish a concept to allow the same standard to be used?

> Imagine two physiologically identical patients who both request discontinuation of respirator support and refuse resuscitation. . . . Patient A is part of a controlled NHBD protocol. Patient C is simple DNR; nor is he donating organs. Following an arrest, Patient A must be observed for five minutes with invasive monitors before death is declared. Consistent with the practice of most deaths, however, Patient C is pronounced dead much earlier, at the moment when no heartbeat is heard or respiration observed (Youngner et al., 1999).

Thus there is a tension between trying to treat NHBOD like other comfort measures only patients (and have shorter observation times) and trying to ensure irreversible loss of brain function which requires over ten minutes. If the standard is that the heart must be irreversibly stopped even if resuscitation is attempted, the tension is even greater. If the act of organ removal itself precedes the stated wait, it would be considered prematurely ending the donor's life, despite whatever waiting period may have occurred.

Is NHBOD Killing the Patient by Prematurely Removing His or Her Organs?

[The answer to the question as to whether removal of organs through NHBOD is morally permissible] may turn in part on issues of the relation of killing to letting die" (Cole, 1992). The question of whether a physician becomes responsible for a donor's death because he or she has removed the donor's organs is even further muddied by asking whether the physician has a duty to attempt to resuscitate the donor rather than begin organ retrieval. The morality or immorality of an action must be separated from the morality or immorality of inaction, when we attempt to define the parameters of what should be considered ethically acceptable medical practice. We must also separate the ethical issues of organ removal from the ethical issues that surround allowing the patient to die [or in some opinions, to remain dead].

First, let us deal with the issues surrounding the patient's death.

Respecting Patient Autonomy

Patients who have consented to be organ donors after their death (perhaps by way of an indication on their driver's license) but who have not requested that resuscitative efforts be withheld should be resuscitated. The duty a physician has to attempt to restart such a patient's heart trumps any duty that the physician may feel to remove the patient's organs stemming from the patient's consent.

Similarly in situations in which the patient is 'comfort-measures only' but either does not wish to or is medically unable to donate their organs, we find no harm in the inaction of a physician who does not attempt to resuscitate that patient. We would find it disagreeable and disturbing to go against the terminal patient's wishes that any efforts to restore and sustain his or her life be made. For patients who have declared their treatment wishes in advance through an advance directive, or for those whom a surrogate decision-maker has spoken as to what he or she believes the patient's wishes are, the decision may be clear. If the patient has asked that no resuscitative efforts be made so as to ensure that a minimal amount of time will elapse before his or her organs are removed, the physician, accordingly, has no duty to resuscitate the patient. To do so would violate the patient rights. "the failure to restore cardiac function will result not from lack of present means, but from a deliberate decision not to use them" (Youngner & Arnold, 1993). Again, respect for patient autonomy may be used to justify in action on the part of the physician. Thus, while the physician may not be held morally culpable for the patient's death due to his or her lack of efforts to resuscitate the patient, whether or not the actions of removing the organs actually caused (or perhaps guaranteed) the patient's permanent demise may still be within question.

Conflicts of Interest

Do the medical staff involved in declaring death and procuring the organs have inherent conflicts of interest? What types of conflicts of interest occur within the transplant setting, and how should they best be addressed? How do fears about conflicts of interest affect societal trust and perceptions? These questions arise from a possible perception that transplant programs might have too much incentive to declare someone dead. In this case the incentive is to give these organs to recipients for whom the transplant team has responsibility and for whom the team is an advocate. As a consequence, there could be concern that patients might be declared dead or organs procured prematurely in order to improve donations and patient survival statistics. There is a consensus that there needs to be clear separations of staff, such that physicians associated with declaring death are not involved in the procurement of the organs or their transplant into the recipient. Furthermore, as the separation between organ procurement organizations (OPO) and individual hospitals narrows, it may be impossible to avoid situations in which the team caring for a dying patient is also familiar with the potential recipient. In these situations, efforts must be made to ensure at least the separation of the duties of declaring death and organ procurement.

In addition to concerns that non-heart-beating donors weren't dead, and consequent criticism that physicians who removed donor organs might be killing those donors in the process, there have also been concerns that there may be prohibitive conflicts of interest within the transplantation system. Some examples of possible conflicts of interests included: conflicts between a physician's duties to the dying patient and duties to the potential recipients of the donated organs; and conflicts for the institution regarding its duties to the potential donor and the financial incentive for a transplant center to do as many transplants per year as possible.

Does the Medical Staff Involved in Declaring Death and Removing the Organs have Inherent Conflicts of Interest?

Yes. "Under ideal circumstances, the potential donor patient would be cared for by people whose sole desire is to maximize the potential for quality of life and minimize the potential for suffering among such gravely ill patients without regard to potential transplant recipients" (Shaw, 1993). However, such ideal circumstances aren't always possible. For example, physicians may feel a duty to the potential recipients to procure the donated organs in as good a condition as possible, that is, as oxygenated as possible. Likewise, one would expect that the potential donors probably want to donate organs which function as well as possible. Under circumstances where it may seem clear to the physician that the donor is going to die anyway and that the viability of the organs rests upon how long the dying process will take, the physician may be tempted to 'hurry the process up a bit' for the sake of the recipients whose lives may hinge on the rapidity of the donor's death. Given the extensive preparations that must be made for organ removal to take place (the surgical suite must be prepared and trained personnel must be on hand and ready for the event) there may be pressure to ensure that everything goes as planned. If the patient does not die on "schedule" and the organs cannot be removed, consequences that at the very least may be uncomfortable to the physician may ensue. "What is the plan for informing the family of the patient of the events? Whose responsibility will it be to tell them the doctors were, after all wrong. . . the loved one didn't die? These questions underscore the tremendous pressure that the responsible physician will feel to make the whole planned event come off smoothly" (Shaw, 1993).

What other Types of Conflicts of Interest are Important to Avoid Within the Transplant Setting?

Frader has pointed out that, "the hospitals with major transplantation centers may also have major economic and academic interests that may be hurt by organ shortages" (Frader, 1993). This could influence the center to perhaps be more of less selective (depending upon the numbers) in their donor acceptance criteria. Thus, organs of marginal or even less than perfect quality might be rejected for transplantation in fear that those organs would be more likely to fail and bring the rate of success for that center down, or conversely, used to increase volume and revenue.

How Can Conflicts of Interest be Avoided?

Dealing with inevitable conflicts of interest is important. Faced with the perception of such large and seemingly unavoidable conflicts of interest, it is of little wonder that some members of the public are wary of any type of organ donation. People have decided that they will never sign an organ donor card out of fear that they will not receive appropriate care once the medical team finds out that they are organ donors (Arnold & Siminoff, 1996). Overcoming these fears requires trust: "Three important principles provide the moral framework for organ procurement in America . . . the dead donor rule . . . prohibition against active euthanasia . . . the primacy of consent . . . These rules serve to reassure people that when they enter hospitals they will not be killed or mistreated so that their organs can be taken" (Fox, 1993). So too there are means of preventing the above mentioned conflicts of interest from occurring. In general, there are three techniques for addressing conflicts of interest: (1) separations in time or space of individuals, tasks, or decisions, (2) attempting to maintain practice that is as close to "normal" as is possible; and (3) providing internal and external accountability and oversight.

Transplantation protocols and regulations require, where possible, a separation of the medical team involved in the determination of death, and the team performing the procurement and doing the transplant. This is meant to prevent situations in which the physician who is responsible for obtaining consent to remove treatment and then declaring death, could be biased by the awaiting recipient who may be his patient. The physician who declares death must have as objective a view as possible, and this is not possible, it is believed, if he or she is the care-giver of the potential recipient and thus has a stake (basically his patient's survival) in the donor's death. Having separate teams for declaring death and transplanting the removed organs resolves this conflict in most cases.

The best way to prevent the appearance of coercion on the part of the healthcare team is to not allow them to approach families regarding organ donation. Thus only families who wanted donation would be able to have discussions. However, this would preclude families who want to donate, but who do not raise the issue on their own. Therefore, some centers allow OPO professionals to approach families. However, the potential for inappropriately influencing withdrawal of life support and consent to organ donation, can be mitigated by only approaching the patient or surrogate for consent after the decision to forgo life-sustaining treatment has been made. The purpose of this priority and separation is to allow for a decision to terminate life support that is independent of a decision to donate organs. Put another way, the decision to forgo life-sustaining treatment must be made on its own merit. Another method of addressing those conflicts is to deliver care for the potential donor as similar as possible to that provided to any other dying ICU patient. To the extent that care differs, the conflict becomes more palpable.

Finally, watchfulness through the use of an internal ethics committee and an external community oversight group may be one way of preventing or resolving such conflicts. Shaw suggests, "Conflicts of interest problems associated with separation of transplant staff are resolvable through the use of arbitrators who will monitor the proceedings" (Shaw, 1993). These arbitrators will be informed, though objective third parties who have neither a stake in the donor's survival nor a stake in the recipient's receipt of a transplant (except at of course the very most basic empathetic sense that would be difficult to avoid in any situation). In the best case scenario, the arbitrator will also have no stake in improving or sustaining the hospital's image as a transplant center, in order that he or she may objectively screen for decisions that are deliberately biased in favor of the hospital. "The arbitrators must be able to examine each potential case, sort out the biases – real or potential – of the individuals involved, and monitor each step and decision for any harm that might occur from the unavoidable conflicts of interest" (Shaw, 1993). Thus, there are solutions for resolving conflicts of interest that may arise in the transplantation setting, though it may be noted that to some extent we may be deluding ourselves if we believe that these methods will ensure that all that can possibly be done for a patient will be done, "We live with an unfortunate medical myth. Many continue to assert that individual physicians have medical and moral obligations to seek all beneficial care for each patient. This has never been possible, at least in the literal sense, and the injunction now makes little sense, given the technology that one could, in theory, employ" (Frader, 1993).

Are there Pressures to Consent?

Families and the patients themselves may face pressure, either real or perceived, to make the decision whether or not to donate. Before the decision to donate should be the decision whether or not to consent to treatments that could, in theory, save or prolong the donor's life. These treatments could include aggressive and invasive interventions including resuscitative efforts. Treatments that prolong a dying patient's life obviously prevent them from becoming an organ donor. The treatments may not only fail to save the potential donor's life, but they may decrease the number of organs that may be viable for removal. This creates an incentive to forgo treatment sooner. "Non-heart beating organ donation puts pressure on patients and families to forgo potentially lifesaving treatments to provide organs to save others" (Frader, 1993). A family that is inadequately informed (and consequently has a skewed and pessimistic view of the odds of their loved one's survival) may feel pressure to forsake treatment of the patient in hopes that the good of saving the lives of others may come of the death of the patient.

In such instances it may seem that the dying patient is seen as being more valuable to society when divided into transplantable parts than when he or she is "left whole". In such situations it seems reasonable to question whether a potential donor would receive adequate care and treatment (palliative or restorative). Joel Frader questions whether a utility-based approach may come to be employed, "might potential organ donors not receive all reasonable care because their parts can be seen to have greater value than their whole being? . . . If such a patient can serve as a donor of several organs rather than a recipient of one – a new heart – who should make that choice and on what grounds?" (Frader, 1993). In our opinion, this is a decision that only the patient should make.

Comfort Care for the Patient and Attention to Family Needs

Many critics of the NHBOD process are concerned that amid the efforts to maximize organ removal the patient's needs may get lost in the shuffle. These needs could include those for comfort care measures like ensuring pain relief and providing a caring, warm environment which permits the family members at the bedside. Indeed the role and needs of the family at the time of their loved one's death has been seen to be nearly as important as the needs of the patient, and this has been the basis for much discussion. What are the most appropriate ways to provide comfort measures to the dying patient? How should these comfort measures be considered and adjusted in the face of the need to maximize the viability of the donated organs?

What are Comfort Measures?

Simply put, comfort measures are any interventions – medical, environmental and emotional – that make a patient's condition and in this case, their death, more peaceful and unencumbered. Comfort measures may be as obvious and traditional as the administration of pain-relieving medications, or they may be as not so obvious as ensuring that the environmental conditions of the patient's room are not disturbing or distracting. This may include making sure that the room temperature is not uncomfortably cold and providing blankets when the room temperature cannot be adjusted. It may also include attempts to filter out and reduce routine hospital and hallway noises that may be distracting. Comfort measures for both patients and family should include permitting the family to remain at the patient's bedside for as long as desired including past the moment of death if necessary and offering the family pastoral care.

What are "Appropriate" Comfort Measures?

It seems reasonable to speak of the above comfort measures for patients who are still conscious or who may become conscious, but are there comfort measures for patients who are not conscious and who perhaps have no realistic hope of ever regaining consciousness? Comfort measures in these situations also serve a role, though perhaps more of a role of reassurance for the family and even the medical staff than for the patient. "In the case of an unconscious patient who demonstrates no signs of distress, comfort strategies may have a greater symbolic value than a concrete one. These symbolic strategies provide comfort and satisfaction to the attendant family, and in many ways to the care-giving staff, and cannot be discounted" (Campbell & Weber, 1995).

Yet there are claims that the protocols for NHBOD address comfort care issues inadequately and risk patient and family pain, discomfort and suffering.

Some view the potential donor's passing as a peaceless, utilitarian death. "A significant number of [critical care physicians] were concerned that patients might receive excessive sedation in order to hasten death or, equally concerning, inadequate sedation which could result in unnecessary patient suffering, solely to avoid the appearance of hastening death" (DeVita & Snyder, 1993). Excessive sedation could, of course, cross the line between killing and letting die. Active euthanasia, or intention to kill would make the whole process morally unacceptable. Not giving adequate attention to a patient's needs for comfort care measures, though, might lead to severe, unnecessary pain and a less dignified death for the patient. Similarly family members would go through the additional psychological pain of watching their loved one die under less than optimal circumstances.

Is it Ethical to Pre-medicate for the Prevention of Pain?

On the issue of when pain medication should be given to prevent or alleviate suffering, many believe that it is better to "err" on the side of being humane and maximally reducing the patient's suffering by preventing it from ever occurring. For them, to wait for signals of distress and discomfort is to act in a manner which is not humane to the patient. "Some physicians believe that all pain must be avoided rather than merely treated after the fact, and that using distress as an indicator requires that some patients will feel some pain in order to receive medication" (DeVita, Vukmir et al., 1995).

Treating pain and discomfort requires an amount of medication that may also hasten the patient's death. The principle of double effect comes into play and we find that it is morally permissible to administer a dose of medication sufficient to potentially kill the patient if the patient's pain necessitates it. Youngner and Arnold remind us, "We may not intentionally kill a patient but are permitted, with patient or surrogate consent, to withdraw therapy or provide pain relief, even at the risk of hastening death, so long as comfort is the goal" (Youngner & Arnold, 1993).

Others believe, that relying on the Principle of Double Effect may lead to situations in which more than treatment would be refused. For example, Childress believes that current NHBOD protocols do not adequately address these situations and also raise further questions. "Would patients have the right to choose to forgo not only life-sustaining treatments but also certain comfort measures in order to increase the possibility of successful organ donation (if such a conflict could technically arise? Should their choices be restricted in this regard? The protocol does not adequately address these issues" (Childress, 1993).

"Erring" on the side of patient comfort

Some clinicians choose to "err" on the side of patient comfort by, pre-medicating to prevent pain and discomfort. Others argue though, that pre-medication is unnecessary, and potentially risky as society could view such pre-medication as a means of hurrying death for the sake of organ extraction. "If there is no evidence of patient distress, we suggest that there is no indication for pre-medication and that its administration could be interpreted as a means of ensuring that the patient's dying is not protracted, thereby avoiding warm ischemia and the loss of organ viability" (Campbell & Weber, 1995). Campbell and Weber argue that NHBOD protocols violate some modern standards of comfort care. "At least four aspects of the care of patients whose organs are to be procured following the pronouncement of death by cardiac criterias appear to be at odds with the evolving standards of comfort care for other patients (non-organ donors) during the withdrawal of life-sustaining ventilation: (1) the patient may be a 'full code' patient prior to organ procurement; (2) sedation/analgesia may be routinely provided without indication of patient need; (3) comfort strategies other than pharmacological may not be adequately addressed; and (4) family needs may not be adequately addressed" (Campbell & Weber, 1995).

Others however see the decisions about the employment of comfort care measures as less blanket in nature. For them, comfort care is about considering all the factors at hand. Clinicians and ethicists connected with the Pittsburgh protocol see comfort measures as requiring a five element calculus, one that would tailor the measures employed to the needs of the individual situation. "It is generally agreed that: (1) ensuring informed decision making, (2) supporting patient autonomy, (3) minimizing or eliminating discomfort (using the standards that Campbell and Weber suggest), (4) maximizing Human dignity (including support of the family and loved ones) and (5) maintaining accountability are important components of this process" (DeVita, Vukmir et al., 1995).

Within this, protocol they feel that contrary to popular belief there is no "standard" comfort care. Instead, the appropriateness of various measures are best left to the judgement or at least the guidance of the *patient's* wishes, whether directly stated or indicated by his or her surrogate. This is because "If a specific protocol were utilized, it is likely that some patients would receive care they do not wish and others would not receive care that they do wish" (DeVita, Vukmir et al., 1995). Additionally, by believing that the patient has adequately understood and consented to various interventions (including resuscitation or the use of chemical agents) that were geared towards promoting the viability of their organs for donation, to follow a patient's wishes by engaging in these interventions is merely following the guidelines of patient autonomy, and promoting the patient's dignity.

Is it Appropriate for Potential NHBODS to have a Full-Code Status?
Campbell and Weber and others who took offense with the NHBOD protocols on the basis of their treatment (or perceived lack thereof) of comfort care frequently included within their arguments the apparent dichotomy that was established between patients who would become donors and those who would not make efforts to donate their organs. In particular, they argued that organ removal was being used as an excuse, both for not providing adequate comfort care, and for declaring that a patient who would otherwise be designated 'comfort measures only' to be in need of resuscitation if heart stoppage occurred before the transplant team was ready. Say Campbell and Weber, "It is only the fact that the patient is scheduled for organ procurement that leads to full code decisions [in which all efforts are made to resuscitate the patient]. In other words, the patient is treated contrary to standard comfort-care protocol because of the decision to remove the organs" (Campbell & Weber, 1995).

For them, a decision to resuscitate the patient in the event of a cardiac arrest for the sake of the death being convenient is the ultimate insult to the patient's dignity. "The decision to place a patient on 'full code' status means that every effort will be made to restore a dying patient to life, simply so that she can die a little later, when everyone is ready for her organs. This kind of indignity is clearly not compatible with the ordinary understanding of comfort care" (Campbell & Weber, 1995). Campbell and Weber argue that comfort care includes more than just the alleviation of pain. They argue it also includes efforts to preserve and promote patient comfort on all levels, including psychological, emotional, and dignitary. Given the risk of harm to the patient by requiring resuscitation, they argue, it is even more important to respect an individual's right to decide for him or herself and not to have decision about their care, life, and death made for them. The decision to remove a patient from full code status is, in Campbell and Weber's words "one which patients alone should be permitted to consent to" (Campbell & Weber, 1995).

Thus, while they recognize the potential harm involved in allowing NHBOD, they do concede that if we fully respect a patient's autonomy, then we must allow such means of obtaining organs to take place. This recognition however, is not without the admonition that we must strive to remain cognizant of the potential harm that may occur and attempt to prevent them from occurring lest the patient's interests become supplanted in the process. "In the case of [NHBOD]s, the dying of a patient is so closely connected with the procedure to remove organs that focus on the patient's dying can easily be subordinated to the transplant procedure" (Campbell & Weber, 1995).

The Needs and Role of the Family

In addition to the patient's needs and comfort, the needs of the patient's family, some argue, should be paramount to the organ removal process. "The goal of procuring more organs for transplant should not interfere with optimal care of dying patients and concern for their families" (Campbell & Weber, 1993). Concern for the patient's family may be as simple as keeping them well informed of the patient's status and reassuring them that their loved one is being kept comfortable. Or, it may involve allowing the family to be at the patient's bedside up to the time of death. Allowing the family to remain with the patient is difficult. In the case of controlled NHBOD, it is possible to time death such that it occurs in the surgical suite when the medical team is ready to begin removal, a time and place that helps to reduce warm ischemia time. In some instances, families may feel forced to choose between donating their loved one's organs or spending the last few moments of life with that person. This could be a wrenching decision for many families, and understandably so, that when given such options they choose not to donate.

Having the family present in the room where the organs will be removed seems for some, at the least, logistically difficult (due to the need to maintain sterile conditions). Difficult however, does not equate to impossible, but merely to the requirement that extra effort be expended. "Although it is not customary, it is certainly possible to maintain the sterility of the surgical suite while permitting the family to stay with the patient until death is pronounced; doing so, however, requires both creativity and a commitment to the objectives of comfort/dignity care" (Campbell & Weber, 1995). Some protocols have dealt with this by allowing the family and patient to go to a room near the operating room, and then rapidly move the patient after death to the operating room.

Some NHBOD protocols have addressed and resolved this issue while others have not. "The UPMC protocol unlike the ROBI, [Regional Organ Bank of Illinois] procedure, requires that explicit consent be obtained before any intrusion upon the patient and that the timing of the removal of support takes the family's needs into account" (DeVita, Snyder et al., 1993). As we live in an age where families no longer all live in the same town as one another (sometimes not even in the same country), the needs of the family may include time – time to travel from far and near to say final good-byes before the patient is removed from life support. "At times, the withdrawal may be delayed for as much as a day to allow family members to arrive from out of town" (DeVita, Vukmir et al., 1995).

Unfortunately not all transplant centers have given adequate attention to these ways of meeting the family's needs. Until all transplant centers develop protocols for allowing the family to remain at the patient's bedside until his or her death, families may be forced to make an unnecessary choice. "As non-heart beating donation will, for now, require transfer of the patient to the operating room prior to death, the family members will have to choose between donation and physical contact with the child at time of death" (Frader, 1993).

How can the Viability of Organs Removed through Non-Heart-beating Conditions be Maximized? Are Interventions that are Directed at Improving Organ Viability Ethical?

As not all NHBOD occurs under controlled circumstances where the patient is expected to die, families are not always prepared to simultaneously hear that their loved one has died and make a decision whether to donate his or her organs. There is an empiric limit to the amount of warm ischmia that an organ can tolerate. Variably estimated between thirty and sixty minutes, the time is not long. It may seem prudent to artificially maintain organ viability after death through cooling and the ante-mortem use of anticoagulants and other drugs which do not benefit the donor. However, it might not be considered ethical.

As discussed earlier, there is a certain degree of utilitarian thinking that enters into the discussion of the morality of Non-Heart-beating Organ Donation. Indeed, state Arnold and Youngner, "For the most part, their judgements about non-heart-beating cadaver donor protocols rest on whether they would increase the number of transplantable organs without violating existing ethical norms" (Arnold & Youngner, 1993). Given the short period of warm ischemic time that is tolerable before the organs lose viability, methods have been sought to expand this vital window of time. Several techniques for use both before death and after death has been declared, have been explored. In this section we will discuss these methods and the controversy surrounding their use and their timing. Organ procurement organizations have heretofore lacked any agreement over the employment of such methods to increase organ viability. Recently, the Institute of Medicine issued a report recommending means of bridging these disputes.

In controlled NHBOD, death is expected and occurs after the patient is removed from life support. "These patients are either competent with intolerable quality of life or incompetent, but not brain dead, because of severe, generally neurological, illness or injury with an extremely poor prognosis as to survival or any meaningful functional status" (Herdman & Potts, IOM, 1997). Since the removal of life support can be scheduled, it can occur when transplant staff is available to harvest the cadaver's organs and when other resources are available to help minimize warm ischemia. "[Controlling death circumstances as] an alternate method for reducing warm ischemia allows patients and families the option of donating organs after they have decided to forgo life-sustaining treatment.1) there is time for discussion, reflection and adequate consent prior to initiating an invasive procedure. Second, the time and place of death are controlled to minimize warm ischemia time" (Youngner & Arnold, 1993). This is perhaps the simplest and least invasive means of increasing organ viability. It is not without controversy, however, as some argue that maintaining the potential donor on life support any longer than necessary, solely for the purpose of maintaining organ quality in preparation for removal is wrong. "In October 1994 the health department of England and Wales issued guidelines stating that [ventilation] for transplantation purposes constituted an unlawful battery – being non-therapeutic and not done in the best interests of the individual" (Price, 1997). In the U.S., it has been argued that organ donation is a desired outcome for the donor (or his family). Therefore, with consent, provision of continued support is morally acceptable because it is acceptable to the impacted individuals.

Is the Use of Cold Perfusion and Medications Ethical?

Additional and more invasive means of expanding the window of organ viability include the use of cold perfusion and medications either before or after death is declared. Cold perfusion involves the insertion of perfusion cannulae into the femoral arteries. The insertion may occur before life support is removed and death declared, (occasionally even while the potential donor is still conscious and capable of feeling pain) or it may be done immediately after death is declared. While cannulation itself does not accelerate death, "perfusion, since it usually involves solutions that will stop heart action immediately, must always await the declaration of death" (Herdman & Potts, IOM, 1997). Upon the placement of cannulae and the death of the potential donor, rapid cooling of the body to slow deterioration of the organs is undertaken by perfusing the body with cold fluids. Additionally, some organ procurement programs infuse cold fluids into the cadaver's abdomen as well in order to maximize the benefits that reduced temperatures have on organ viability (Herdman & Potts, 1997).

Medications including anticoagulants (e.g. Heparin) and vasodilators (e.g. phenotolamine or Regitine) may be injected into the potential donor to reduce clotting in the organs to be removed. Unlike the fluids used in perfusion, these are less likely to cause a patient's death. Generally the use of such drugs to promote later organ viability would have little discernable effect on the patient's outcome; there are however, exceptions to this. "In the occasional NHBD with ongoing intracranial bleeding or deficiencies in blood volume, the administration of anticoagulants or vasodilators such as heparin or [Regitine] is not indicated because it could actively cause death" (Herdman & Potts, IOM, 1997). Others believe that in the time frame in question – usually a few minutes before death – no harm can occur. For example, a patient who receives heparin is extremely unlikely to have a lethal bleeding event after a single dose while hypotensive, during the last 10 minutes or so of life. Phenotolamine, a blood pressure reducing medicine, is also argued to have an immeasurably small risk of causing death given the dose and time frame involved. In some transplant centers that have used such pre-mortem medication, the principle of double effect has been used to justify the potential life shortening consequences that may occur, though there is little consensus as to whether the Principle of Double Effect could hold up to close scrutiny in these situations. Still other transplant centers instead inject these medications after death has been declared in order to avoid any semblance of moral impropriety, and rely upon chest compressions and flushes to adequately circulate the drugs through the cadaver's system.

The use of medications such as Regitine (phentolamine) and heparin to promote later organ viability while the patient is still alive is considered ethically permissible under most circumstances. However, given the small percentage of cases in which these drugs may actually hasten the donor's death, "a blanket policy cannot be recommended because of possible untoward effects in some donor patients" (Herdman & Potts, IOM, 1997). Instead, the decision as to when to use these drugs, since their use is no longer in question, is up to the medical judgement of the physician. The decision of when to inject anticoagulant and vasodilator medications, the IOM recommends, should take place in consultation with the transplant staff. Every effort should be made to inform the donor's family about the use of the medications and permit them to request that the medications not be used until after death is declared. Additionally, the Institute recommends that efforts be taken to avoid conflicts of interest within the hospital and the transplant team, though it also recognizes that all organ procurement organizations currently have such safeguards in place.

Are Interventions Without Consent (in Order to Promote Choice) Ethical?

As the title of this subsection paradoxically suggests, viability-promoting interventions may also serve as means of ensuring free decision making by the donor's family. These interventions allow greater time for the family to decide whether or not to donate the patient's organs. Emergent post-mortem placement of cold perfusion catheters without consent occurs largely in uncontrolled death situations where the family may not be present at the hospital or even able to be located at the time of the patient's death. Organ donation for these patients would normally be impossible because warm ischemia would destroy the organs before consent was obtained. Furthermore, without the implementation of cold perfusion, the family may have only a few minutes to simultaneously attempt to cope with their loved one's death and decide whether to donate the organs. This time frame is expanded as far as a few hours once cold perfusion, vasodilatation and anticoagulants are implemented. Because patients and families may donate if given sufficient time to process the barrages of events and questions surrounding death, some OPOs feel compelled to insert cannulae, begin cold perfusion and to inject medications immediately following cardiac arrest. These interventions increase the odds that the organs will be usable if consent is achieved, allow families the time they need, and perhaps increase the odds that consent will be obtained. If consent for organ donation is achieved via an organ donor card, it would seem that cold perfusion would be an acceptable step in organ preservation, one that would not require additional consent from the donor's family.

However, donor consent to organ donation is not always so explicit and such interventions, without consent, are controversial. Some argue that intervening without consent amounts to battery of the corpse, while others see it as acceptable because it grants the family the opportunity to make a decision of which time might otherwise rob them. In that sense, it promotes choice rather than prevents it. "[Regarding perfusion and consent] One center, the Regional Organ Bank of Illinois, after being refused permission in 35 consecutive cases decided to infuse preservation fluid prior to requesting family consent. Proponents of this practice have responded to obvious ethical objections by arguing that these interventions are essentially 'non-deforming' and 'non-mutilating' procedures that do not require family consent. Moreover, this procedure gives families the option to donate" (Youngner & Arnold, 1993).

Obviously, some would argue that given that the cadaver is already dead, there is little chance of harm being done by introducing chemicals into the patient's body in order to potentially benefit others. However, such an stance would be met with argument as well since, "If the controversy about practising intubation on dead patients is any indication, there is little consensus about the moral acceptability of performing invasive procedures on dead patients to benefit others" (Youngner & Arnold, 1993).

Is the impact of NHBOD "worth the 'trouble' "?

If there is so much dispute surrounding NHBOD, even down to how and when the removal of organs is performed, why should we use NHBOD as a source of organs for transplant? Will the number of organs obtained from NHBOD be significant enough to warrant procuring organs through such a hotly debated means? Some worry that even if NHBOD became widely accepted, and was seen as morally defensible that it would have little impact on the actual number of useable organs removed, and that working out the answers to the moral ambiguities currently present in NHBOD would have little practical use. On this matter, DeVita et al. argue, "First, other countries – notably Japan and Holland – have demonstrated that NHBOD can be a major, or even the sole, source of donor organs. In Japan, where brain death was not recognized until recently, non-heart-beating cadavers are the sole source of cadaveric organs, and in Holland, one-third of cadaveric organs come from NHBOD" (DeVita, Vukmir et al., 1995). Thus, NHBOD can account for significant numbers of organs, even the totality of all organs transplanted under some systems internationally where determining death by neurological criteria was not accepted. In the U.S., the current numbers of organs that are being obtained by NHBOD indicate the potential for a significant impact. The number of organs procured through these methods at a single transplant center can be indicative of this. "UPMC [University of Pittsburgh Medical Center] has had two NHBODs per year from this protocol, a small number to be sure, but it constitutes 10% of the total annual procurements. Extrapolating that 10% to the national experience indicates an increase of 500 donors per year, with a potential yield of 1000 kidneys and 500 livers and pancreas" (DeVita, Vukmir et al., 1993).

Despite such promising numbers, some worry that the adoption of NHBOD protocols may actually reduce the number of organs procured as clinicians may become too impatient to wait for brain death to occur in patients for whom such a diagnosis may be a foreseeable clinical course. "Fewer organs would be utilized if a severely brain damaged, but not yet brain dead donor was moved prematurely through the [NHBOD] process rather than waiting for 'brain death' to develop. Because successful preservation and transplantation of [NHBOD] organs have occurred mainly with kidneys, transplant programs may be reluctant to use other organs from this source. Therefore choosing to take organs from [NHBOD] might yield only kidneys while waiting for brain death might allow the retrieval of multiple extra-renal organs" (Burdick, 1993).

It is important to note that the IOM finds that it is appropriate to allow the placement of cannulas for cold perfusion to take place after death is officially declared. However, they do not prohibit the placement of cannulae in the time between heart stoppage and the declaration of death. With explicit consent from the patient or his or her family and the use of proper comfort measures, especially local anesthetic, cannulae may be placed before the patient's heart stops, though perfusion is not permitted until death is declared. The IOM is still largely undecided on the issue of anti-mortem cannulization, however, and states that "a decision based upon deference to what the public is prepared to accept may be the wisest policy at the moment" (Herdman & Potts, 1997). They do however, recognize that organ donor cards can be seen as clear and legal indicators of the consent to organ removal, and therefore because cannulization can be seen as a routine aspect of this process, it is permissible.

CONCLUSION: THE IMPACT OF NON-HEART-BEATING ORGAN DONATION

It is still too early to say whether NHBOD will actually live up to the hopes that some have held for its ability to increase the supply of transplantable organs significantly. Given that the Institute of Medicine's 1997 Consensus statement casts NHBOD in a favorable ethical light, it is likely that that those transplant centers that have shied away from attempts to procure organs through non-heart-beating protocols will slowly embrace NHBOD as a source of organs that is morally justifiable and worthy of pursuit. In the not yet released 1999 Consensus Statement, the IOM recognizes that most centers are not actually engaging in organ procurement from non-heart beating cadavers and that they should be encouraged to not only adopt but also utilize NHBOD as a source of transplantable organs. In 1997 alone, kidneys removed from non-heart-beating cadaveric donors comprised roughly one percent of all cadaveric-source kidney transplants that took place in the United States. As hospitals begin to more widely adopt the use of organ viability enhancing medications in cadavers who are seen to be potential donors, it is possible that families will give greater consideration and more frequent consent to organ donation when given a longer time frame in which to consider donation. Given the endorsement granted by the IOM statement for hospitals to more aggressively pursue the development of non-heart-beating organ donation, it is hoped that obtaining organs through such sources will no longer be discouraged for fear of public outcry. Should public objection and disapproval occur out of fear and misconception, it is also hoped that means of educating the public to allay such fears will be properly implemented.

NOTES

1. The 'Pittsburgh Protocol' is considered to be a landmark in transplantation policy. Indeed it was one of the first major attempts by a transplantation center to establish a position on death certification and a process for the management of dying patients and removal of organs from non-heart-beating donors. This protocol, which has been greatly debated and which has since evolved through many incarnations, requires that the decision to forgo life-sustaining treatments must be made independent of the decision to donate. It requires that two minutes must elapse between when the heart stops and when death is certified. Organ removal processes commence after death.

2. To determine an individual is dead based upon brain-death criteria, several steps must be taken. The individual must be completely unresponsive to stimuli and must register a completely 'flat-line' electroencephalogram. Some protocols require that a second electroencephalogram must be performed twenty-four hours later and exhibit no change from the first, that is, it must produce a second 'flat line'. While it may seem self-contradictory to require a second EEG, the requirement of a second test is for the purpose of insuring that human or mechanical errors during the initial testing process (including the possibility that the EEG may be flat from other causes, such as drug use) do not result in a person who has brain activity being prematurely and incorrectly declared dead.

3. In response to concerns expressed by the Department of Health and Human Services, the Institute of Medicine examined organ procurement protocols from the various organ procurement organizations (OPOs) and individual transplant centers across the country. In 1997 they issued the Non-Heart-beating Organ Transplantation: Medical and Ethical Issues in Transplantation Report, more commonly referred to as the consensus statement. This is the most detailed and thorough medical and ethical analysis of the issues that surround non-heart-beating donation, and as such, it holds great weight in terms of how NHBOD will be perceived. While much of the consensus statement speaks along the lines of strong recommendations rather than strict policy, it is the closest in format and stature to a national policy in this area that we have to outright legislation on these issues. Though there isn't space to include a thorough analysis of the conclusions presented in the statement, a brief summary of its major points is in order, as they indicate future trends and practices that may occur, as well as what is more commonly seen as ethically justifiable conduct.

REFERENCES

Arnold et al. (1996). Ethical Issues in Organ Procurement: a Review for Intensivists. *Critical Care Clinics*, *12*(1), 29–48.

Arnold et al. (1993). Back to the Future: Obtaining Organs from Non-Heart-Beating Cadavers? *Kennedy Institute of Ethics Journal*, *3*(2), 103–111.

Arnold et al. (1993). The Dead Donor Rule: Should We Stretch It, Bend It, or Abandon It? *Kennedy Institute of Ethics Journal*, *3*(2), 263–278.

Burdick, J. F. (1993). Potential Conflicts of Interest Generated by the Use of Non-Heart-Beating Cadavers. *Kennedy Institute of Ethics Journal*, *3*(2), 199–202.

Campbell et al. (1995). Procuring Organs From a Non-Heart-Beating Cadaver: Commentary on a Case-Report. *Kennedy Institute of Ethics Journal*, *5*(1), 35–42.

Caplan, A. L. (1993). The Telltale Heart: Public Policy and the Utilization of Non-Heart-Beating Donors. *Kennedy Institute of Ethics Journal*, *3*(2), 251–262.

Catherwood, J. (1992). Rosencrantz and Guildenstern are 'dead'? *Journal of Medical Ethics*, *18*, 34–39.

Childress, J. F. (1993). Non-Heart-Beating Donors of Organs: Are the Distinctions Between Direct and Indirect Effects and Between Killing and Letting Die Relevant and Helpful? *Kennedy Institute of Ethics Journal*, *3*(2), 203–216.

Cole, D. J. (1992). The Reversibility of Death. *Journal of Medical Ethics*, *18*, 26–30.

Cole, D. J. (1993). Statutory Definitions of Death and the Management of Terminally Ill Patients Who May Become Organ Donors after Death. *Kennedy Institute of Ethics Journal*, *3*(2), 145–155.

DeVita, M. A., & Snyder, J. V. (1993). Development of the University of Pittsburgh Medical Center Policy for the Care of Terminally Ill Patients Who May Become Organ Donors after Death Following the Removal of Life Support. *Kennedy Institute of Ethics Journal*, *3*(2), 131–143.

DeVita, M. A. et al. (1993). History of Organ Donation by Patients with Cardiac Death. *Kennedy Institute of Ethics Journal*, *3*(2), 113–129.

DeVita, M. A. et al. (1995). Non-Heart-Beating Organ Donation: A Reply to Campbell and Weber. *Kennedy Institute for Ethics Journal*, *5*(1), 43–49.

Dombrowiak, D. T. (1997). Ethical Issues Concerning Non-Heart Beating Cadaver Organ Procurement and the UPMC Protocol. *St. Francis Journal of Medicine*, *3*(3).

Fox, R. C. (1993). An Ignoble Form of Cannibalism: Reflections on the Pittsburgh Protocol for Procuring Organs from Non-Heart-Beating Cadavers. *Kennedy Institute of Ethics Journal*, *3*(2), 231–239.

Fox, R. C., & Christakis, N. A. (1995). Perish and Publish: Non-Heart-Beating Organ Donation and Unduly Iterative Ethical Review. *Kennedy Institute for Ethics Journal*, *5*(4), 335–342.

Frader, J. (1993). Non-Heart-Beating Organ Donation: Personal and Institutional Conflicts of Interest. *Kennedy Institute of Ethics Journal*, *3*(2), 189–198.

Herdman, R., & Potts, J. T. (Eds) (1997) (Institute of Medicine). *Non-Heart-Beating Organ Transplantation*. Washington D.C.: National Academy Press.

Kushner, T. (1992). When Do Organs Become "Spare Parts"? *Cambridge Quarterly of Healthcare Ethics*, *4*, 349–353.

Lamb, D. (1992). Reversibility and Death: a Reply to David J. Cole. *Journal of Medical Ethics*, *18*, 31–33.

Lynn, J. (1993). Are Patients Who Become Organ Donors under the Pittsburgh Protocol for "Non-Heart-Beating Donors" Really Dead? *Kennedy Institute of Ethics Journal*, *3*(2), 167–178.

Matter of Quinlan 70 N.J. 10 (1976). Supreme Court of New Jersey.

Orr et al. (1997). Reanimation: overcoming objections and obstacles to organ retrieval from non-heart-beating cadaver donors. *Journal of Medical Ethics*, 7–11.

Price, D. T. (1997). Organ Transplant Initiatives: the twilight zone. *Journal of Medical Ethics*, 170–175.

Robertson, J. A. (1993). Policy Issues in a Non-Heart-Beating Donor Protocol. *Kennedy Institute of Ethics Journal*, *3*(2), 241–250.

Shaw, B. W. Jr. (1993). Conflict of Interest in the Procurement of Organs from Cadavers Following Withdrawal of Life Support. *Kennedy Institute of Ethics Journal*, *3*(2), 179–187.

Spielman, B., & Simmons McCarthy, C. (1995). Beyond Pittsburgh: Protocols for Controlled Non-Heart-Beating Cadaver Organ Recovery. *Kennedy Institute of Ethics Journal*, *5*(4), 323–333.

Thomasma, D. C. (1992). Ethical Issues and Transplantation Technology. *Cambridge Quarterly of Healthcare Ethics*, *4*, 333–343.

Tomlinson, T. (1993). The Irreversibility of Death: Reply to Cole. *Kennedy Institute of Ethics Journal*, *3*(2), 157–165.

Weisbard, A. J. (1993). A polemic on Principles: Reflections on the Pittsburgh Protocol. *Kennedy Institute of Ethics Journal*, *3*(2), 217–230.

Younger, S. J., & Arnold, R. M. (1993). Ethical, Psychosocial, and Public Policy Implications of Procuring Organs From Non-Heart-Beating Cadaver Donors. *JAMA*, June 2, 1993. 2769–2774.

Youngner et al. (1999). When is Dead? *Hastings Center Report*. Nov-Dec 1999. 2–8.

8. THE ETHICS OF XENOTRANSPLANTATION

Richard A. Demme

INTRODUCTION

Organ Transplantation: A Growing Demand

The field of organ transplantation has proven a practical testing ground for ethical issues in medicine. During the early years of transplantation, common issues were those of "lifeboat ethics" – the ethics of scarcity. How should we allocate scarce lifesaving resources? Who decides who lives or dies? Who should be selected or excluded from being pulled out of the water; who should receive an organ?

Radical egalitarians might argue that none should be saved if all cannot be, or that all should be pulled onto the boat, giving everyone an equal risk of being saved – or of drowning. In medicine, we are not comfortable with that analogy; if some real individuals *can* be saved by judicious use of a scarce therapy, we *ought* to attempt to save them. We have been reluctant to let all die when some might be saved. And, in saving them, we ought not significantly imperil others.

When chronic hemodialysis first became available for people with failing kidneys, "Life and Death" committees had to choose which one out of fifty persons would be allowed to receive it. Patient selection committees, as described by Shana Alexander in her landmark article in *Life* magazine (Alexander), were criticized for the subjective criteria that were often used in making their selections, such as whether a person was married, had children, or

The Ethics of Organ Transplantation, Volume 7, pages 195–229.
2001 by Elsevier Science Ltd.
ISBN: 0-7623-0764-1

went to church. In the late 1960s dialysis patients were largely Caucasian, married, male high school graduates, between twenty-five and forty-five; and over forty percent were employed (Beauchamp & Childress, 1989). This demographic clearly did not represent the cross section of the population with kidney failure, which was, and still remains overrepresented in African American, Hispanic and Native American minorities. In the United States, this scarcity was "alleviated" by building more dialysis machines, building large dialysis units, training nurses, technicians and nephrologists, and, since 1972, paying for much of dialysis costs through Medicare funds obtained by taxation of the general population. The goal was to eliminate shortage of the life-extending resource, rather than to limit its application to the "best" recipients. At the present time, a large proportion of dialysis patients are over 60, and are retired or unemployed. Only a small percentage of the people who receive hemodialysis now would have been eligible for hemodialysis according to the early selection criteria.

Organ transplantation continues to serve as the paradigm for allocation of scarce medical resources. In America, when scarcity of medical treatments cannot be overcome by manufacturing more units, the selection criteria for who will receive treatment has primarily focused on medical need and the probability of success, and has shied away from subjective or social criteria. When the medical need is comparable among potential recipients, the probability of success is weighted to a greater extent. For example, medical need is roughly equivalent among most persons with kidney failure due to the availability of dialysis, so kidney transplant candidates receive more points and a greater chance of receiving an organ if they are a closer antigenic match, as there is a lesser risk of rejection and a greater possibility of long term success.

More weight is given to the urgency of medical need for those awaiting liver transplantation, as there is no artificial liver therapy comparable to dialysis available yet. We also give some priority to those who have been on the waiting list longer following the principle of allocation on a first come, first served basis, or queuing. And in general, those under the age of 18 years receive more points, and a greater chance to receive an organ; they have the greatest likelihood of benefiting for the longest time.

Organ transplantation has been successful in extending a number of lives, and success rates for transplants continue to improve each decade. From 1988 to 1996, the one year survival rates for kidney transplant from living donors increased from 88.8 to 93.9%, and the survival rate for cadaveric kidney transplants increased from 75.7 to 87.7 %. During that time period, the half-life for kidneys from living donors increased from 12.7 to 21.6 years, while cadaveric grafts increased from 7.9 to 13.8 years (Hariharan et al., 2000).

Yet it is, in part, the growing success of transplantation that has generated its own growing problem – the demand for transplantable organs has far outstripped the usual supply. Advances in transplantation science and immunosuppression have led to increased application of the technology. Whereas once transplantation was reserved for either the most desperately ill, or situations where it was most likely to be successful, such as in identical twins, it is now offered as a possible therapy for numerous conditions. Older, and more medically complex candidates are listed. The internet website for United Network for Organ Sharing (UNOS) currently displays in large print "Every 14 minutes a new name is added to the national organ transplant waiting list" (http://www.unos.org). As of August 2000, over 71,000 patients are now waiting for organs; more than 46,000 are wait-listed for kidneys, and over 16,000 are waiting for livers. The number of hepatitis C infections could increase the demand for liver transplants by several times in the next decade. Others are waiting for pancreatic tissue, intestines, hearts, and lungs to become available.

As the waiting lists for organs continue to grow at a rapid pace, the average time waiting for an organ also increases. Because people wait longer for organs, a number of them die before an organ becomes available. A person might be sustained on dialysis and wait 2 to 4 years or more for a cadaveric kidney to become available; the median wait for a heart is over 200 days. One source suggests that in 1998, 50,000 Americans "needed a new heart", while only 7,683 were "lucky" to land on the national transplant list and only 2,340 received "new" hearts (Fox, 1999). In 1999, 6,448 people in the United States died while waiting for an organ transplant (Levinsky, 2000). In May, 2000, a U.S. Department of Health and Human Services (HHS) Fact Sheet reported that approximately 13 die each day while awaiting a transplant (HHS). The number of people who might benefit from an organ transplant is likely much greater than the number of people who are actually evaluated and listed by transplant centers due to lack of access and other factors.

Expanding the Donor Pool

Our current organ matching system is cumbersome. We would prefer not to have to select among patients, or to have them wait fruitlessly. The well-publicized death of people on transplant waiting lists has fueled a search to expand the organ donor pool. As we are not comfortable enforcing limitations as to who can receive an organ, one solution would be to increase the organ supply so that all who might achieve a benefit have the opportunity to do so.

Several plans have been proposed to meet the demand for organs. However, expansion of the organ pool using new sources risks decrease in the number of organ donations from conventional sources if such strategies do not meet public approval.

Approaches to expand the organ donor pool have included suggestions for obtaining an increased number of cadaver donors, living human donors, non-human donors or development of biomechanical devices. For instance, we might increase the number of cadaver donors if we adopted a presumed consent model, as in some European countries, where the law encourages recovery of organs from those who have died unless the deceased had previously expressly forbidden it. (As it is, in the U.S., we still only retrieve organs from about 50% of "conventional" brain dead cadavers, due to lack of consent from family members.) Or, the use of living donors might increase, as it has in India, by allowing the sale of organs. The sale of human organs for transplantation is illegal in most countries. Over the past few years, there has been a growing acceptance and use of genetically unrelated but "emotionally-related" kidney donors, such as spouses, with good technical success. Obviously, one cannot obtain a heart from a living donor, so such a strategy still limits the supply. Biomechanical devices are undergoing research and development such as the renal tubule assist device (Humes). Left-ventricular assist devices are commonly used as "bridge" therapy for those awaiting cardiac transplants, and the Oxford Heart Centre and the Texas Heart Institute have been recently testing the Jarvik 2000, a new mechanical pump which may be inserted into failing hearts (Rogers, August 2000). *Xenotransplantation* has come to the forefront as a possible means of providing a virtually unlimited supply of organs.

Xenotransplantation – What is it?

Xenotransplantation is derived from the Greek root *xenos*, meaning foreign, or strange. In simple terms, it generally refers to the transfer or transplantation of animal tissues or organs into humans. The U.S. Public Health Service (PHS) recently defined xenotransplantation "to include any procedure that involves transplantation, implantation, or infusion into a human recipient of either: (a) live cells, tissues, or organs from a non-human animal source or (b) human body fluids, cells, tissues or organs that have had *ex vivo* contact with live non-human animal cells, tissues, or organs. Furthermore, xenotransplantation products have been defined to include live cells, tissues or organs used in xenotransplantation" (PHS).

The choice of which animal organs might be placed into humans and still function is limited, because our bodies have natural defense mechanisms that identify foreign tissue as foreign, and attempt to reject it. Although some might poetically wish for the heart of a lion or the kidneys of a camel, such transplants are unlikely to come about. We are genetically closest to other primates, and therefore less likely to reject their tissues, which most resemble ours genetically, anatomically, and chemically. These animals, closer in genetic kinship, have been termed *concordant. Discordant* species include animals that arc more distant on the evolutionary tree, having a more distant genetic relationship. Baboons have been proposed as a concordant source, and pigs as a discordant source of organs for transplantation into humans.

This use of animals to further human ends has led to considerable ethical debate. Many animal rights activists see xenotransplantation as an unfair exploitation and improper use of living creatures; others see the use of these animals as legitimate, acceptable and their use in saving of human lives as a high moral achievement. In this chapter, we will identify the ethical questions that the use of such animal organs in transplantation provokes.

Slippery Slopes in Transplantation

A "slippery slope" in ethics can be envisioned as follows: Some practices are morally acceptable, they can be imagined at the top of a slope. Some practices are clearly immoral, and they are at the bottom of the slope. However, there are a number of practices that lie between what is clearly acceptable and what is unacceptable. This is where most ethical dilemmas lie. A slippery slope argument suggests that as soon as we allow practices that are not clearly acceptable, we will have a tendency over time to accept practices which are even less acceptable and so on, until we have rapidly reached the bottom; propelled unimpeded into unacceptable behavior, as if sliding down a slippery slope (Fig. 1).

The slippery slope argument implies that at some point along the slope, we lose our moral discernment, and can no longer distinguish which are truly unacceptable activities, nor reverse our trajectory. If we can no longer discern right from wrong, nor take corrective action, it implies we are no longer moral creatures, and can no longer exercise choice. I envision more of a two-way moral stairway, rather than a slippery slope (Fig. 2).

I believe that there are discrete steps we may take, and remain in the range of acceptable behavior, and still be able to stop and say we should go no further, or we may even reverse our course. For instance, some experiments

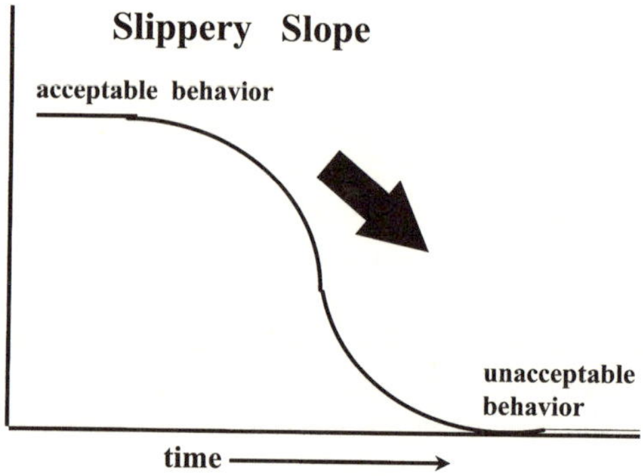

Fig. 1. Slippery Slope.

performed by Nazi physicians were immoral and unacceptable, but the ensuing Nuremberg Code and Declaration of Helsinki have led to steps upward in medical experimentation, particularly in emphasizing the need for informed consent of subjects. Still, considering the slippery slope analogy is a useful technique, and demands that we ask whether there are actions that put us beyond the point of no return.

Each strategy to expand the donor pool has raised ethical concerns in at least one of the following broad categories:

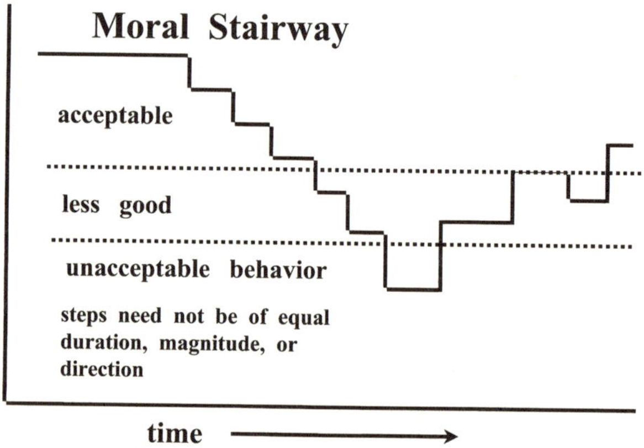

Fig. 2. Moral Stairway.

Categories of Ethical Concern

- WILLINGNESS
- QUALITY OF ORGAN
- COMMERCIALISM
- RISK TO DONOR
- RISK TO RECIPIENT.

Each strategy suggested to expand the organ donor pool must be examined with regard to each of these ethical concerns. For it is certainly true that public support for transplantation would wane if organs of *poor quality* were retrieved *at significant risk* from *unwilling donors*, *sold* to the highest bidder, and *transmitted other illness*.

Such an unacceptable practice would represent the very bottom of a frankly frightening slope.

The goal of this chapter is to examine each of these categories of ethical concern as it relates to xenotransplantation. In this manner, we may identify the ethical challenges of xenotransplantation, and be better able to compare this strategy with other proposed strategies to expand the organ pool.

WILLINGNESS

Willingness refers to a donor's desire or motivation to give up an organ or body part. Willingness is grounded in *autonomy*, or self-rule. Our current system of organ donation is based on altruism, or voluntary gifting. Some authors suggest that all people should be considered as potential organ donors, and that such donation is a communal obligation (see Nelson's chapter).

For the most part, the donation of a body part from a living being has been considered supererogatory; it is a noble and generous act, but beyond what is usually an ordinary obligation. People who are newly dead are unable to voice a desire or objection to organ donation at that critical time, but they can indicate such a desire beforehand by signing an organ donor card, or their families may use a substituted judgment to allow for donation.

Although current policy allows for directed donation, where family members are allowed to donate organs from their dead relative to a specific person or locale, this is not widely publicized (as there is usually the possibility of a better match or a chance to get an organ for someone who has been waiting longer if the organ is donated to the general larger "pool"). However, a living person may willingly choose to donate a kidney while still alive, and usually donates to a family member or a friend.

While many parents would be willing to donate an organ to their child, they might be less willing to have one of their organs removed for a stranger, or a stranger's child. A spouse may choose to donate a kidney to their own spouse, if their blood types are compatible, but there is a possibility of coercion in this instance. A wife may be the one providing transportation for a husband to and from hemodialysis sessions three times a week, or a husband may carry the supplies and set up an "automated cycler" machine for daily peritoneal dialysis for his wife. These examples are commonplace. The divorce rate in this country is still near 50% of all marriages, and it is foolish to think that the rate is any lower among those with chronic illness. The majority of spousal donations have been from wives to husbands. Although wives may be sensitized to more antigens through pregnancy, and may sometimes not be able to receive a kidney from a husband, one still has to question whether this is the only factor accounting for the disparity. A spouse might be pressured into donating a kidney, and then live to regret it.

However, who else might benefit *as much* from donating a kidney? Improving a spouse's health and quality of life may represent a great gift of love, and could certainly improve one's own stress level and quality of life on a daily basis. Premenopausal kidney transplant recipients sometimes become fertile again, and may pursue raising a family, which might not have been possible while receiving dialysis. This discussion is not meant to discourage spousal donation, but merely to point out the potential for subtle or not so subtle pressures that influence willingness. Likewise, a sibling may feel pressured to donate a kidney to a sibling, because they find they are the closest match after blood testing. Again, this is not to discourage organ donation among siblings, but to point out that there are degrees of influence that may occur in organ donation. A person may feel some reluctance about undergoing a major operation, but still decide it is the right thing for them to do. It is *undue* coercion that is unacceptable. The decision to donate should be a voluntary choice, but it frequently goes without saying that the person most likely to ask you to donate an organ to them is a person who has great emotional influence on you – one may feel that there is no real choice.

It is clearly wrong to obtain an organ from an unwilling or involuntary donor. Transplant centers allow for private meetings of potential donors with members of the transplant team. If unwillingness or suspicion of undue coercion is detected, the team will not proceed to remove an organ from that person.

Willingness is at the heart of altruism, and autonomy, choosing one's own path is at the center of the western medical morality. If one has no choice in one's actions, then one cannot choose to do a right or wrong thing. If a man cannot distinguish right from wrong, then he is not acting as a moral agent.

It is highly unlikely that animals would be willing to sacrifice their lives to serve as donors of organs for humans. In fact, one surgeon who assisted in the harvesting of the baboon livers at Pittsburgh for transplantation into humans noted that the baboons were not willing participants (Bronsther). This leads to two broad moral questions; first, are animals moral agents, i.e.; can they make moral choices? Secondly, does it matter? Even if animals are not moral agents or members of the moral community, and even if *they* have no choice, what about *our* choice? How ought we to treat animals? Do animals have "rights"? If they have different rights than humans, does it matter if we treat them well or use them for our own purposes?

The main reason we are exploring xenotransplantation as an option is that *we can* coerce animals with limited risk of reprisal, while it's generally accepted that *we shouldn't* coerce other humans to obtain their organs. This demonstrates a broad acceptance of the Kantian view, as described further below.

Philosophers and scientists have offered differing opinions on the nature of animals throughout the ages. Aristotle noted "[O]f all animals man alone is capable of deliberation (Aristotle, Berlin No.488b).

About choice, he states . . . [W]e must next discuss choice; for it is thought to be most closely bound up with virtue and to discriminate characters better than actions do. Choice, then, seems to be voluntary, but not the same thing as the voluntary; the latter extends more widely. For both children and the lower animals share in voluntary action, but not in choice, and acts done on the spur of the moment we describe as voluntary, but not as chosen" (Aristotle, Berlin No. 1111b).

In Nichomachean Ethics, Aristotle writes "We have good reason therefore for not speaking of an ox or horse or any other animal as being happy, because none of these is able to participate in noble activities" (Aristotle, Berlin No. 1099b).

For Aristotle, man was the only rational animal, and his ability to deliberate and choose a course of action was intricately linked to virtue and morality. He did not think animals (or even children) had this ability. Animals therefore could not be moral agents.

Rene Descartes, the French philosopher and scientist who wrote in the early 1600s, derived his entire philosophy from the precept *cogito ergo sum* – "I think, therefore I am". Rationality was the centerpiece of his philosophy; the ability to think and reason was the core of being human. But he believed that animals are "devoid of reason." He believed that the "the rules of mechanics" were "the same as the rules of nature". He noted that even "imbeciles" could arrange a few different words together; and, because animals cannot speak, he thought that proved " not only that animals have less reason than men, but that they have none at all." He goes on to explain that he thinks animals function as mechanical automata, like machines:

> . . . rather it proves that they do not have a mind, and that it is nature which acts in them according to the disposition of their organs, as one sees that a clock, which is made up of only wheels and springs . . . (Descartes).

The Cartesian belief that animals don't feel pain, and therefore cannot suffer was, surprisingly, well accepted by many twentieth century scientists.

The modern medical bioethicist will often try to apply the influential philosophy of the Prussian Immanuel Kant to current moral problems. In this case, Kant's views were clear. He stated "Beings whose existence depends not on our will but on nature's, have nevertheless, if they are irrational beings, only a relative value as means, and are therefore called things; rational beings are called persons, because their very nature points them out as ends in themselves . . ." (Kant, 1952). Kant wrote that nature exists to serve human interests. It followed, for Kant, that since only humans are rational, only *persons* are of moral concern, and "Animals are not self-conscious, and are there merely as means to an end. That end is man" (Kant, 1975). Kant might have encouraged xenotransplantation.

For Aristotle, Descartes, and Kant, animals were not considered moral agents, and might serve as appropriate sources of organs for humans. There are always at least two sides to every argument, however, and such is the case here. David Hume, an English contemporary of Kant in the 1700s bluntly asserted "[N]o truth appears to me more evident than that beasts are endowed with thought and reason as well as men. The arguments are in this case so obvious, that they never escape the most stupid and ignorant" (Hume, 1920).

Charles Darwin introduced the revolutionary concept of evolution in the late 19th century. While he "freely admitted that no animal is self-conscious if by this term it is implied he reflects on such points as whence he comes or whither he will go, or what is life and death, and so forth," Darwin believed that despite the difference in degree of mental power between humans and apes, no fundamental difference exists in kind between humans and many forms of animal life (Darwin, 1872). If humans evolved from other primates, then we have an animal nature, and animals might be considered as our distant relatives.

One can follow this Darwinian thread further: perhaps animals that are closer to humans on the evolutionary tree, or those that have more human-like traits have a higher moral status than those more discordant. This is a reason why many feel it would be unsuitable to use chimpanzees or other primates as donors of organs for humans: they are closer genetic relatives, they look more like humans, and exhibit several human-like behaviors.

Following Aristotle's system of distributive justice, we ought to treat equals equally, and treat those that are not equals in proportion to their inequality. Pigs are genetically more distant from humans than primates, but Peter Singer notes "Of all the animals commonly eaten in the western world, the pig is without doubt the most intelligent . . . The high intelligence of pigs must be borne in mind when we consider whether the conditions in which they are reared are satisfactory". Singer argues that most humans are speciesists (an analogy to being racists or sexists). He maintains "If possessing a higher degree of intelligence does not entitle one human to use another for his own ends, how can it entitle humans to exploit non-humans for the same purpose?" He holds humans have no morally relevant characteristics not also possessed by non-humans, and that "to discriminate against beings solely on account of their species is a form of prejudice, immoral and indefensible in the same way that discrimination on the basis of race is immoral and indefensible." (Singer, 1975).

Many believe that biblical man was given dominion over animals. But *how* are we to dominate them? Rollin observes "Even if humans have been placed by God at the peak of the Great Chain of Being, or even in command of it, it does not follow that the creatures beneath them may be treated by them in any way they see fit." He further maintains that "if animals are objects of moral concern, then they have moral rights and correlatively, they must have legal rights" (Rollin, 1992).

An international animal rights organization, People for the Ethical Treatment of Animals, known by their acronym PETA, refute the need for use of animals for transplantation or most other research purposes.

However, most Americans are carnivores. I have recently seen an organization use the PETA acronym satirically, for them meaning People Eating Tasty Animals. Through the centuries, we have seen the human palate have an influence on our moral relationships with animals. Even Jeremy Bentham, a founder of the utilitarian / consequentialist school wrote "the day may come when the rest of the animal creation may acquire those rights which never could have been withholden from them but by the hand of tyranny. He stated "the question is not, Can they reason? Or Can they talk, but Can they suffer". But Bentham also wrote

> . . . there is a very good reason why we should be suffered to eat such of them as we like to eat; we are the better for it, and they are never the worse. They have none of those long-protracted anticipations of future misery which we have. The death they suffer in our hands commonly is, and always may be, a speedier, and by that means a less painful one, than that which would await them in the inevitable course of nature (Bentham, 1780).

Benjamin Franklin, the early American sage was a vegetarian as a youth. He says he considered the "taking of every fish as a kind of unprovoked murder, since none of them had done or could do us any injury that might justify this massacre." But, one day he noted that some of the fish his friends caught had eaten other fish. He concluded, "if you eat one another, I don't see why we may not eat you". He admitted that he reached this conclusion when the fish was in the frying pan, and had begun to smell "admirably well"; adding that " So convenient a thing it is to be a reasonable creature, since it enables one to find or make a reason for everything one has a mind to do" (Franklin, 1936).

It is unlikely that pigs or baboons will become willing or voluntary organ donors. The conflict between researchers and animal activists has been long, sometimes shrill, and is destined to continue. But if it is morally acceptable to kill animals to provide ourselves with food in the short term, it is illogical to argue that killing animals to provide organs for longer-term survival of some humans is immoral. So long as Americans continue to enjoy bacon for breakfast, and ham sandwiches for lunch, this moral concern will not likely inhibit the use of animals as xenotransplant organ donors if such practice can be shown to save human lives.

It is respect for persons and need for voluntary consent that has been the major difficulty in obtaining human organs for transplant. If we imagine organ donors on an ethical slope, willing donors are at the top. Somewhere along the slope, influence becomes pressure, which can develop into coercion; it is unacceptable to use unwilling donors at the bottom of the slope (Fig. 3). However, we have turned to use animals as organ donors because many feel their lack of willingness is morally and merely irrelevant.

Choosing Xenotransplant Donors

An optimal organ donor should be ready, willing, and available to donate. Even if unwilling, the availability of animals as donors must now be briefly explored. Chimpanzees are our closest non-human relatives, having 99% similarity to the human genome. In fact, several chimps were used as kidney donors in the mid-1960s, when organ transplantation was in the early stage of development. Importantly, chimps and many other primates are endangered or in very limited supply. (Of course, with a population approaching 6 billion, the only primates that are in superabundance are humans!) In the wild, only baboons exist in large enough numbers to serve as potential organ donors. However, baboons only grow to about 70 lbs. at the largest, which may restrict use of their organs to children or small adults. It might be possible to transplant a pair of kidneys from a single baboon into a larger human adult. On the positive side, liver

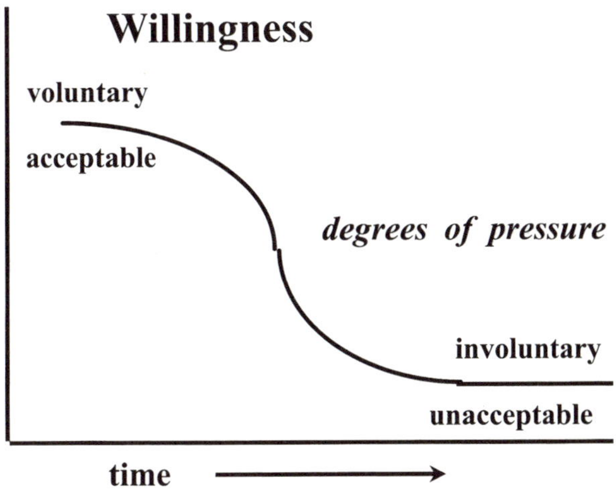

Fig. 3. Willingness.

tissue is the only tissue that regenerates well in humans. After partial liver transplantation from human donors, livers have been demonstrated to grow. The recipient of a baboon liver transplant in Pittsburgh was noted to have had extensive growth of the transplanted liver on his autopsy.

The use of baboons as organ donors causes moral concern for some people due to their status as primates, having some humanoid characteristics. Moreover, they are difficult to raise. They have extensive social groups, and need to be raised in colonies. They reproduce and mature slowly, having only one offspring at a time, and they raise few young. They are relatively dirty, and it is expensive to raise them in clean conditions. In addition, they harbor numerous viruses.

Pigs are further discordant from humans than baboons are. Pigs can be grown very large, have litters of several piglets at a time, and are easier to raise in captivity than primates. The miniature swine grows to about 350 pounds. Although their outward appearance does not resemble humans, the internal anatomy of pigs is similar to humans; it is common for biology students to dissect fetal pigs to learn anatomy. Humans have domesticated pigs for thousands of years, and well know how to breed them in captivity. Pigs are commonly slaughtered to provide food for humans, so there is less moral objection to their use in transplantation (compared to primates). For these reasons, the pig has been selected as the most likely source of organs for xenotransplantation into humans. However, as pigs are genetically distant from primates, they present a greater number of foreign antigens, and use of pig organs will likely require higher levels of immunosuppression in recipients to prevent organ rejection.

QUALITY OF ORGAN

The quality of the organs available is important for the probability of successful transplantation. Quality refers not only to the status of the organ before it is transplanted, but also to its likelihood of functioning well in its new host. It makes little sense to transplant organs of poor quality which fail in a short time. Such practice would be expensive, and would expose the recipient to multiple courses of high levels of immunosuppressive medicines, as well as greater risks of infections and surgical misadventure. The transplant community has long debated whether any transplant patients should be allowed a second organ while others on the waiting list still have not received a first. At the present time, a number of organs are used for repeat transplantation, and some kidney transplant recipients have received three, four, or even more transplant organs. The practice of xenotransplantation might make a great number of organs available, so repeat transplants would be of lesser ethical concern. Yet there is great concern about whether organs from animal sources will work well at all, and if pig or baboon organs cannot work well in humans, then our research efforts and resources should be directed elsewhere. This is an opportune juncture to briefly review the history of xenotransplantation, and to explore its "success" so far.

Xenotransplantion History

In 1906, M. Jaboulay carried out the first two recorded animal to human kidney transplants, using organs from a pig and a goat, but each kidney worked for only one hour (Hamilton, D). In 1963 and 1964, Keith Reemtsma, then at Tulane University, transplanted kidneys from chimpanzees into six patients, one who lived for 9 months. During the same years, Thomas Starzl, then at the University of Colorado transplanted six baboon kidneys into humans, and patients survived between 19 and 98 days. By 1974, about 20 persons had received primate kidneys. Most of the recipients died from graft rejection, or infection from the use of immunosuppressive drugs, and a voluntary moratorium on xenografting was established in the United States by the transplant community (Institute of Medicine). Xenotransplantation trials were reported to have continued in the 1980s in Sweden, China, and Hungary, but as these trials have not been well publicized, it is unlikely that they were successful.

In 1985, xenotranplantation was brought to public light again at Loma Linda, where Leonard Bailey implanted a baboon heart into Baby Fae, who had been born with an underdeveloped heart. Despite the availability of cyclosporine as an immunosuppressant at that time, she only survived for 20 days. There have been at least eight other attempts at cardiac xenotransplantation, although they have been less well publicized. In 1964, Hardy at the University of Mississippi attempted the first heart transplant from a chimp to a human, four years prior to Barnard's human to human heart transplant. Other attempts, also unsuccessful, have used hearts from baboons, pigs, and sheep. (Michler, 1996).

Thomas Starzl reexamined the promise of xenotransplantation in 1992 and 1993 when he transplanted baboon livers into two patients with advanced hepatitis B. The baboon is thought to be resistant to that virus. Both of these patients died, the first after 70 days, and the other after 26 days. Due to the outcome of these operations, Starzl again recommended a moratorium on xenotransplantation, observing "we are too far from being able to do anything [clinically]; we are tremendously interested but we think the research endeavors are going in the wrong direction"(Butler).

In 1995, Jeff Getty, a man with AIDS, underwent a baboon bone marrow transplant, in an attempt to provide him with a new immune system. He survived, but the marrow did not engraft.

Although the focus of this chapter has been on use of whole-organ transplants, trials of xenotransplantation of animal tissues and cells continue, including use of pancreatic tissue from pigs, cows, and rabbits to obtain islet cells for use in insulin-requiring diabetics. In addition, fetal pig cells have been recently injected into brains of stroke patients, and those with Parkinson's disease; and are being considered for use in spinal cord injuries, multiple sclerosis, and amyotrophic lateral sclerosis (ALS), Lou Gherig's disease.

Making It Work

The above instances demonstrate that to this point, xenotransplants have not been generally considered successful, and the organs used, although of good quality and function in animals, have not worked well or for long in humans. In fact, one anti-xenotransplantation group pointedly notes that xenotransplants have had a 100% failure rate.

There have been several recent major technological advances in the field, however. First, success with xenotransplantation into other animals has improved; one research group has kept pig hearts alive in baboons for as long as 99 days. (Stolberg, 1999).

Second, In March of 2000, PPL Therapeutics Plc. announced the successful cloning of pigs by nuclear transfer using adult cells, a similar process that was used in the cloning of Dolly, the celebrated sheep. The method successfully produced five female piglet clones. The successful development of a cloning process means that if a few pigs can be developed to which humans are tolerant, their body cells might be used to clone hundreds of genetically identical animals for use in transplantation. In addition, mice have recently been cloned through six generations, with no signs of premature aging, alleviating some concern that cloned animals might die prematurely (Associated Press, 2000).

Finally, there has been continued success in development of transgenic pigs. *Transgenic* means that the pig's genetic structure has been changed by the addition of a human gene or genes. For example, pig herds have been developed that express human complement regulatory proteins, such as CD55 (also known as decay accelerating factor, DAF), which may block a human recipient's response to reject the organ rapidly. Not only may genes be added, but work is progressing on developing gene deletion, inactivation, or "knockout" pigs for the gene encoding galactosyltransferase, which may be the main xeno-antigen that human immune systems recognize on porcine endothelial cells (Weiss). This is another strategy to decrease the risk of hyperacute (immediate) rejection of the xenotransplant organ.

Despite all these advances, it appears we may still be a considerable distance from our goal, the development of "stealth" organs, which remain undetectable to the human immune system, but continue to function.

We want organs of good quality for transplant. The shortage of organs has led doctors to take greater risks in accepting organs of lesser quality. Whereas only 2% of heart donors were over 50 years old in 1988, 10% of hearts were retrieved from donors over 50 in 1998 (Fox, 1999).

Organ banks are willing to routinely consider cadaveric donation of some organs and tissues up to the age of 70 or more, and some suggest using organs from people who are significantly obese, diabetic, or hypertensive. In fact, some centers now offer kidney transplants of mismatched blood types from living donors (Davis, 1999). We have moved to using organs of lesser quality over the past decade, but our immunosuppressive techniques appear to be better, so in general, transplanted organs are lasting longer. Still, organs have to be good enough to offer a reasonable probability of success. Xenotransplantation efforts so far have not yielded organs that will work for any reasonable length of time in humans. And, if they cannot work well, they should not be used. It seems trivial, but true to say that it would be unethical to transplant organs of poor quality into humans – although some latitude is given during experimental phases of transplantation. The possibility of the success of xenotransplantation is tantalizing, yet remains out of our grasp. And it may remain out of reach, because despite our advanced genetic matching techniques and immunosuppressive medications, rejection of *human* kidneys still occurs in over 20% of transplantations (although this can frequently be successfully treated with further immunosuppression. But organs that have episodes of rejection do not tend to last as long as those that never have rejection).

Further Questions

We can add selected human genes to the pig genome, but how many human genes can be added to a pig before the pig becomes "humanized"? If we change enough genes, is the pig still a pig? One is reminded of Orwell's Animal Farm, where pigs develop human characteristics: "The creatures outside looked from pig to man, and from man to pig, and from pig to man again; but already it was impossible to say which was which."

And we recall how Circe transformed men into swine in ancient Greek mythology. Does a "humanized" pig deserve any more rights than wild or domesticated swine? Will a human who has received multiple organs from animal donors be any less human?

What psychological effects will there be in recipients? Should we eat pork from pigs that have some human genes but are not used for transplant? Ideas such as these populate science fiction novels. These are important questions, but I will not expand on them here.

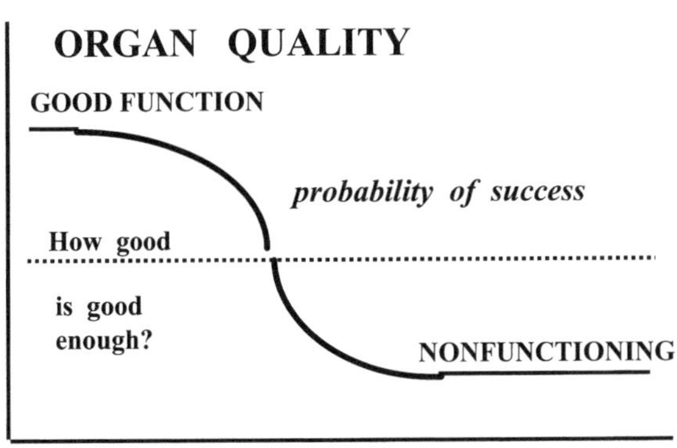

Fig. 4. Organ Quality.

COMMERCIALISM

Development of pig organs that will not be rejected by humans is an area of feverish activity by researchers, for if xentransplantation becomes widely available, it will likely become a very profitable industry.

While the sale of live humans into slavery is morally deplorable, the sale, trade or unauthorized use of human bodies or body parts has long been considered ghoulish and macabre. Frankenstein's monster was conceived by Mary Shelley during the era in England when "resurrectionists" were known to exhume bodies for sale to schools of anatomy. The trade was widespread and profitable. Sir Astley Cooper, President of the Royal College of Surgeons paid as much as seventy-two pounds for six cadavers, and in 1828 testified to a committee of Parliament "There is no person, let his station in life be what it may, who, if I were disposed to dissect, I could not obtain" (Newman, 1988).

Although this practice may have improved physicians understanding of anatomy, it did little to improve the reputation of medical morality.

The sale of organs for transplantation is forbidden in the United States, and most parts of the world. The National Organ Transplant Act (NOTA) from 1984 ruled "It shall be unlawful for any person to knowingly acquire, receive, or otherwise transfer any human organ for valuable consideration for use in human transplantation if the transfer affects interstate commerce." The Amended Uniform Anatomical Gift Act of 1987 states that "a person may not knowingly, for valuable consideration, purchase or sell a part for transplantation or therapy, if removal of the part is intended to occur after the death of the decedent".

As far back as 1971, the Transplant Society's Committee on Morals and Ethics declared that "the sale of organs by donors living or dead is indefensible under any circumstances" (Daar, 1972), and, in 1985, the Council of the Transplantation Society passed a special resolution that "no transplant surgeon/team shall be involved directly or indirectly in the buying or selling of organs/tissues or in any transplant activity aimed at commercial gain", at the risk of expulsion from the Society (Council of the Transplantation Society, 1985).

The sale of kidneys by living donors has been condemned by the World Health Organization. Despite wide condemnation of the practice, in the early 1990s it was estimated that more than 2000 kidneys from living donors were sold annually in India to wealthy recipients (Abouna, 1993), and in 1998, two Chinese nationals were arrested in New York for attempting to sell organs of executed Chinese prisoners; the price of a kidney was $20,000 (Gorman, 1998).

In May, 2000, Interpol began coordinating a worldwide hunt for a woman from Moldova who is alleged to have led a group of intermediaries who talked at least 100 young people from remote villages in the former Soviet republic into traveling to Istanbul. There, they each had a left kidney removed in return for L1800 *(pounds sterling).* The kidneys were given to patients who paid up to L15,000 pounds each (Franchetti, 2000).

Bernard Dickens sums up the objections against the sale of organs: "that paid donation is repugnant in itself, would unavoidably exploit the poor, would be counterproductive in deterring altruistic donation, would make donating patients fear that their life-sustaining care might be compromised, and that commodification sullies all donation and places a money value on the refusal to donate." On the other hand, he notes "it may be incongruous and hypocritical that, when hospitals make volumes of money from transplantation, physicians and associated health professionals advance careers and incomes, drug companies profiteer, and the medical-industrial complex is enriched, the original donor of tissues is supposed to be altruistic" (Dickens, 1990). Furthermore, in India and other developing countries, dialysis is only available to a small percentage of those who develop end stage renal disease, and the argument, because some *can* be kept alive through purchase of an organ, has been concisely stated "To buy or let die"(Daar, 1992).

In general, we have a visceral unease of the sale of human viscera. The current organ transplant system encourages altruistic donation in the manner of gift giving. This widely accepted policy can be envisioned at the top of an incline, with organ brokerage at the bottom, allowing middlemen to reap benefits by exploiting the poor and seeking out the highest bidders for human body parts (Fig. 4).

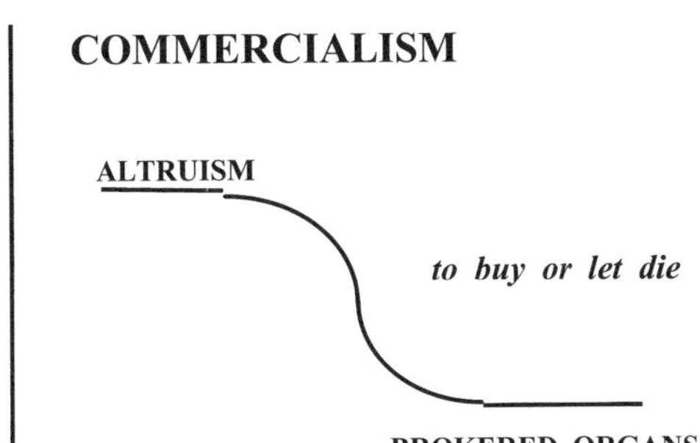

Fig. 5. Commercialism.

The introduction of exchange of money can cloud judgment, and increases the likelihood that arrangement of financially appealing deals may not be in a donor's best interests; along the lines of arguments against prostitution, but to a different degree. Somewhere along the slope can be placed "rewarded gifting", "remunerated donations" and "futures contracts", and other financial incentives discussed as enticements to increase organ "donation", but all of which, in some sense, transform the transaction into a sale. Is it less acceptable for a living donor to "voluntarily" give up their own kidney for compensation or for a family member to sell the organs of a relative who has died (who cannot give consent or refusal, nor can they use the organ any more)? Willingness is a necessary criterion for donating, but it is not sufficient alone.

Clearly, if it were very unsafe to perform living organ donation, then it should be forbidden in most instances. If we argue that kidney or partial liver donation is generally safe for selectively-screened living donors, our moral arguments must lie elsewhere.

With regards to commerce, the sale of animal organs or human transplantation poses less troubling moral questions in contemporary America. "Pork belly futures" are sold openly on the stock market. Animal organs are routinely "commodified"; most supermarkets in the country sell pork products as meat, and other animal parts are commonly sold as meat, clothing, and upholstery. The use of pig organs in xenotransplantation could greatly increase availability of organs, and allow most who are on the waiting list to be transplanted.

Because other organs would be available, xenotranplantation might decrease the likelihood of continued sale of human organs or execution of humans for the use of their organs. However, with pig organs available, donation of human organs for transplantation might decline.

Access to Health Care/Distributive Justice

Even if organs were available in sufficient quantity, it is not clear that all who might benefit from an organ replacement would receive one. Access to health care in the United States continues to be a vexing social problem; millions of persons have inadequate or no health insurance at all, and therefore avoid even routine medical care. Who would pay for all of these transplants, or would they only be available to the rich? General support for transplantation would likely wane if only the wealthy could afford them. The transplantation of an organ, a gift that keeps on giving, also continues to keep on costing. UNOS reminds patients that the cost of anti-rejection and other drugs may "easily exceed $8500 per year" (UNOS), even after the initial expense of the operation itself.

The use of newer immunosuppressant medications may increase that cost further.

In the mid-1960s, only about 800 people were receiving hemodialysis in the United States, at the cost of about $15,000 per patient per year. By 1972, the year that Congress authorized funding for dialysis through Medicare the cost was $229,000,000 to care for 11,000 people on dialysis. Later, much of the cost of kidney transplantation also became covered by Medicare. Over the past thirty years, the cost has escalated, and in the year 2000, the projected Medicare cost for those on dialysis or having a kidney transplant is $17,000,000,000.00 to benefit about 300,000 people, who would otherwise have died of kidney failure. (I have shown all the zeroes rather than writing out "billions", so it is easier to recognize the tremendous growth of these expenses.) Cardiac transplants may cost as much as $250,000 apiece to perform.

Can we afford to give an organ to anyone who might wish? Should we? Shouldn't our priority in allocation of health care dollars be the prevention of organ failure, rather than a fixation on expensive "rescue" technologies"? Is it right to focus our research energy, time, and dollars on developing a "spare parts industry" when we do not adequately disseminate basic health care to those who may benefit from already proven medications and therapies?

One response is that the funding need not be all or none. It is not necessarily true that by increasing funding for transplantation we must also decrease funding for preventative health care. We could increase or decrease funding in either or both areas if we wished; those are political decisions. We could build fewer tanks or roads; our budget is not fixed. Another response is that transplantation has clearly lengthened lives that would otherwise be lost. Some medical care, plastic surgery, for instance, does not typically provide that benefit. If goals of medicine are to extend life and increase quality of life, then organ transplantation may remain highly valued health care.

While the purpose of this chapter is not to solve the inequities in health care, it remains important and appropriate to ask how we will finance greatly expanded transplant care. In Britain, National Health Service patients waiting for transplants are being refused operations because of a lack of intensive care unit beds, while organs go to private paying patients from abroad (Rogers, 2000). The questions of access and fairness cannot be ignored. Neil Goldschmidt, then Governor of Oregon, signed a bill in 1987 to discontinue Medicaid organ transplant coverage for an estimated 34 recipients over two years at an estimated cost of 2.2 million dollars in order to provide basic health care for approximately 1500 low-income children and pregnant women. He stated "We all hate it, but we can't walk away from this issue any more. It goes way beyond transplants. How can we spend every nickel in support of a few people when thousands never see a doctor or eat a decent meal?" (Beauchamp & Childress, 1989).

RISK TO DONOR

"First, do no harm" is commonly accepted as a general rule of medical ethics, yet we in medicine cause harm on a daily basis with venipunctures, deep incisions and use of toxic chemotherapies. In fact, every drug that is used to alter normal physiologic process can cause multiple harms, which is why every book that lists drug "side effects" is likely to be very thick. But we choose to inject or operate for the chance of a greater benefit, and we use medications to achieve net improvement of our patients' welfare. For practical purposes, the ethical maxim might be better stated as "Do no harm without a reasonable chance of greater benefit".

Organ donation is unique in that the risk of physical harm is to the donor, while the benefit is to someone else, namely, the organ recipient. The donor, if living, or the dead donor's family may derive some psychological satisfaction from organ donation, and in that way may benefit.

The risks of donating an organ depend on which organ is donated, and whether the donor can be harmed. Obviously, a living person cannot serve as a heart donor. The first heart transplant in Japan resulted in charges of murder against the physician in charge for removal of the heart from the donor in 1968 (Lock, 1995). But the Japanese have been slow to accept the concept of brain death, and even in 1984, a group of Japanese doctors lodged a complaint of murder against the transplant surgeons who performed a combined kidney-pancreas transplant using organs procured from a brain dead donor (Amemiya et al., 1992).

In earlier years it was thought that a living person could not donate a liver, but partial liver donations from living donors are now being successfully carried out at several transplant centers. Although Dr. Starzl was one of the first to use living donation of kidneys, he discontinued this practice in 1972 after identifying two dozen living-related donor fatalities (although none were at his hands) (Gutkind, 1988). The operative risks to a living donor of a kidney are measurable; out of 10,000 living donors, three might die and as many as 1000 might have various complications from the surgery (Levinsky, 2000). A very small percentage of donors may go on to develop kidney failure themselves at a later time in life, but not at a significantly higher rate than the general population. Recently, advances in surgical techniques allow for laparoscopic donation of a kidney, an operation that allows for a smaller surgical incision and a shorter recovery time for the donor.

There is little risk of harm to a cadaver during the organ retrieval process. Most religions allow the donation of organs, *e.g.* Pope John Paul II, head of the Catholic Church recently praised organ donation as an "act of brotherly love" (CNN, 2000), but some people believe they require or desire bodily integrity for their afterlife, and will choose not to donate. A person who is "brain dead" risks loss of blood circulation, but in other respects has as little to lose as those with cardiorespiratory failure.

One proposed means to increase the number of potential organ donors is to change our definition of brain death from the current definition, which requires demonstrated lack of function of the whole brain and brainstem, to "merely" the lack of function of the higher brain. It is worth recollecting that early brain death definitions were formulated in part to facilitate organ donation. Why not use organs from those in persistent vegetative states? What part of brain function is still required for "personhood"? These debates are commonly given as an example of steps down an ethical slippery slope, and raise concern that the transplant community might lose respect for life, or use human donors as a means, rather than an end in themselves.

As one partial solution to the "organ shortage", more living donations have been encouraged and accepted. In 1988, only 4% of kidney transplants in the U.S. came from unrelated living donors. During the years 1993–1997, kidney donation from spousal and biologically unrelated donors increased annually by 37.5%, and by 1997, 15% of kidney transplants came from unrelated living donors. The total number of living donors doubled in the United States between 1988 and 1997 (USRDS).

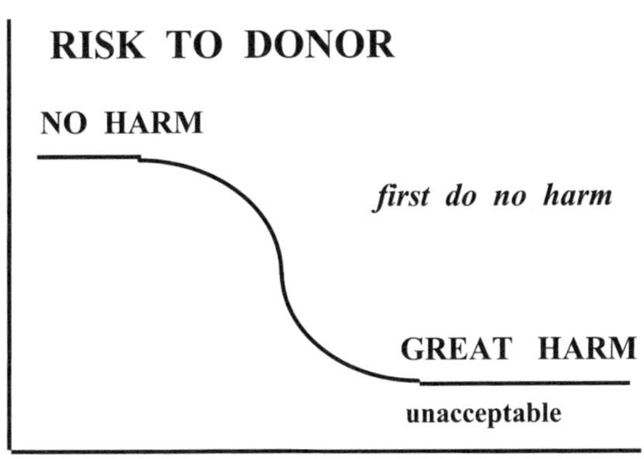

Fig. 6. Risk to Donor.

Using our slope analogy, we envision those donors who will be harmed least at the top of the slope, and those who can be greatly harmed at the bottom.

Living human donors are at greater risk than cadavers; and animal donors are difficult to compare. Humans who wish to donate but are not otherwise healthy may wish to take greater risks than surgeons may allow.

Animal donors will undergo great harm to themselves, (if they are considered *selves*), undergoing enforced upbringing in sterile environments, and sacrifice of multiple organs and life at the time and manner which suits humans. But, as noted in our concerns about willingness and commercialism, pigs are already sacrificed in such a manner to serve as a foodstuff for humans. To object to the use of animals as donors of organs to humans, we must object to our current practices in agribusiness. For those who do object, this is a slope of great moral concern.

RISK TO RECIPIENT

Considering risk to a transplant recipient comes almost as an afterthought, seemingly of less concern than risk to the organ donor. After all, it is presumed that transplant candidates willingly undergo some, even significant risk from organ transplant surgery and use of immunosuppressive medications. They accept these risks due to the potential great benefits of transplantation – the possibility of improved quality of life and even extension of their lives.

They are apprised of the more common risks prior to undergoing the operation, and must sign an informed consent document acknowledging the risks, benefits, possible complications, and alternative therapies, if any. In some cases, where patients await liver or heart transplants, comfort care or hospice care may be the only other reasonable available care. Some patients may be so ill from their disease, i.e., having encephalopathy from liver failure, that they may not fully appreciate the risks or be able to give informed consent for transplant themselves, so designated others may give consent. Some patients may truly not understand what they are choosing, or may be desperate, and willing to accept tremendous risks to themselves. Rapidly approaching death alters ones perceptions and priorities.

It is not the purpose here to discuss in detail the quality of informed consent obtained for organ transplantation from individuals, but recipients of xenotransplants must be made aware of the attendant risks. In general, risks to transplant recipients include operative risks, failed or non-functioning organs, rejection, infections, increased risks of malignancy, and recurrent disease, that is, the return of the same disease process which initially caused organ failure in their transplanted organ. Medications used to suppress the immune system to decrease the risk of rejection hamper the body's ability to fight infections and even to suppress some types of tumors. For instance, patients on immunosuppressive medications have a higher incidence of skin tumors. But again, it is presumed that transplant recipients assume these risks willingly, given the possibility of improving the quality or length of their lives.

Xenotransplantation increases the risks to recipients in very significant ways. The surgical risks remain; the risk of rejection is possibly higher than receiving a human organ due to the increased number of foreign antigens that the immune system might detect (despite "organ modification" that might occur from gene deletion or addition to the donor animal). The immunosuppressive regimen of medications is likely to be stronger to decrease the chance of organ rejection, and therefore more likely to increase the risk for life threatening infections. Not only will a patient who receives an animal organ be susceptible to infection from usual organisms in their environment, but they may also be exposed to xenozoonoses. A zoonosis is defined in the PHS Guideline on Infectious Disease Issues in Xenotransplantation as "[a] disease of animals that may be transmitted to humans under natural conditions (e.g. brucellosis, rabies)." (PHS, 2000).

Xenozoonoses are therefore animal infections that might be transplanted with the animal's organ or tissue and cause human illness.

Xenozoonoses: Risk to Other Humans

Because transplant patients are significantly immunosuppressed to prevent rejection, they are all susceptible to infections. We allow transplant patients to accept significant risks to themselves, as they are the individuals most likely to receive great benefit. We might allow xenotransplant recipients to subject themselves to the risk of xenozoonoses, if the risk is primarily to themselves. The most compelling argument against xenotransplantation is the risk that an animal infection might be transmitted to a human during a xenotransplantation procedure, and then be spread to other humans. Unlike other concerns in the field of transplantation, this fundamentally changes the nature of ethical debate; for in such an instance, the risk would be accepted by an individual, but the harm could extend to others who have not consented. If this possibility exists, then we must explore the following questions:

- Is there real risk to humans?
- How much risk is acceptable?
- Are there strategies to decrease risks?

To answer these questions, we must examine what is currently known about zoonoses, and whether such infections could be transmitted via transplantation.

First, experience with transplantation of human organs has shown that infectious agents can be transmitted from donors to recipients. HIV/AIDS, Creutzfeldt-Jakob disease (CJD), rabies, hepatitis B and C have all been transmitted between humans via transplantation (PHS).

Some of the non-viral zoonoses that swine have been known to harbor include brucella and erysipelothrix.

Baboons may carry toxoplasma and mycobacteria. In addition, each of these species may be infected with numerous viruses. Monkeys and apes harbor approximately 50 simian viruses (EID). Baboons may carry lymphocytic choriomeningitis virus, encephalomyocarditis virus, and herpes viruses including cytomegalovirus (CMV) and Epstein Barr virus. New simian viruses continue to be discovered; Kaposi's – sarcoma-associated herpes-like viruses (KSHV) have recently been detected in chimpanzees and gorillas (Lacoste et al., 2000).

Tissue from one of the Pittsburgh baboon-liver transplant recipients was recently discovered to be infected from CMV derived from the baboon.

It is important to discuss whether zoonoses can be harmful to humans, for even if such viruses are transmitted, they might remain dormant in humans. However, this cannot be assumed to be the case. In Germany, in 1967, the Marburg virus was transmitted from vervet monkeys to humans, infecting 31 persons and having a 23% case fatality rate. In 1976, a single person infected with the zoonotic virus Ebola in Zaire transmitted the disease to other humans; it spread to over 200 persons with an alarming case fatality rate of 88% (Institute of Medicine, 1996), and fueled the imagination of paperback writers. Other zoonoses that have spread to humans and resulted in high fatality rates include viruses causing Crimean Congo Hemorrhagic fever, and hantavirus.

More recently, we have examples of the H5N1 fatal flu in Hong Kong in 1997, which was spread from chickens to humans, and led to six deaths. There was no evidence of human to human spread. But Hong Kong is an island; all of the chickens were exterminated, thus halting the spread of disease. We are currently assessing the risk of the bird-borne West Nile virus in New York, which is transmitted by mosquitoes and has led to human deaths in the last two summers.

It is not too far past to recall the "mad-cow" disease scare in the United Kingdom where spongiform encephalopathy (SE) was transmitted to people who ate beef infected by the culprit prions. Ten cases of CJD occurred in the United Kingdom due to consumption of contaminated meat products. British beef herds were slaughtered to prevent spread of the disease. Again, fortuitously, Britain is an island nation – the disease was contained, but at great expense. How would spread of such infections be curtailed if they occurred in

Nebraska? People who spent an extended period of time in the United Kingdom during certain years are not allowed to donate blood products in America, due to the possibility of transmitting disease further.

The Nipah virus is a newly recognized virus transmitted from pigs to people. It was discovered in Malaysia in late 1998, infected 269 people, causing encephalitis and death in 117 people, and led to the slaughter of about one million pigs. (CRT).

It is possible that the flu epidemic of 1918, which killed over 20 million people, could have been a swine flu transmitted by pigs to humans. The list of other known xenozoonoses could go further, but the point that zoonoses can lead to significant human suffering and death has been adequately illustrated. Before concluding, however, it is important to mention that it is believed that HIV disease and AIDS are caused by a retrovirus derived from simian immunodificiency virus (SIV) from a chimpanzee species, which was introduced across species lines into humans, where it adapted, and was transmitted. Unlike Ebola, which causes rapid death of its new human hosts, some diseases like HIV may be tolerated by their new human hosts for years, being spread to other humans silently before they are discovered to cause serious illness. HIV disease may have infected over 40 million people at this time. When the horse (or in this instance, pig virus), is out of the barn, closing the door may be of little help.

Retroviruses

As noted above, HIV is a retrovirus, likely derived from a simian virus. Baboon endogenous retrovirus (BaEV) proviral DNA can be detected in tissues of all baboon species, and porcine endogenous retroviruses (PERVs) have been found in at least two different laboratories to infect human cells in vitro (Weiss, 1998). The implications of this finding are unclear, but suggest at least the possibility that a patient might receive an organ infected with a PERV, which could live on in the human. Because the transplant patient will be immunosuppressed, he may not make an adequate response to the virus, thus allowing it to live on, and perhaps adapt better to the human environment, and be transmitted in an altered form to other human contacts. Like HIV, this virus might be spread silently for years, and might contaminate the blood supply. A new study reveals mice who received experimental transplants of pig islet cells became infected with a pig virus (Associated Press, 2000).

It should be noted that all of the above episodes and epidemics of zoonoses occurred without the "assistance" of xenotransplantation as a vector, and other outbreaks of zoonoses will undoubtedly continue to occur, whether or not we proceed further with xenotransplantation. Important questions are "How much more likely are pathologic xenozoonoses to occur as a result of xenotransplantation?", and "How likely are they to spread to non-immunosuppressed people?" These questions are unanswerable at this time, in part because there may be other transmissible diseases that we do not even know of yet, and have therefore not developed means to detect, much less treat.

The discovery of PERV's ability to infect human cells in January 1998 led the Council of Europe Parliamentary Assembly to call for a moratorium on clinical xenotransplantation, until guidelines and regulations could be established. The prominent Harvard xenotransplant scientist Fritz Bach also called for a moratorium, noting that informed public debate was needed before embarking on clinical xenotransplantation (Bach & Fineberg, 1998). The public debate would have to include a discussion of how much risk from xenotransplantation is acceptable.

H. Vanderpool argues that the "worrisome risks identified two years ago have subsided", chiefly due to better understanding of PERVs and a commitment to improve testing and monitoring of such viruses (Vanderpool, 1999).

Limiting Risk

Humans and pigs have lived in close proximity for centuries. Pork insulin and heparin have been used for decades without evidence of disease transmission, and pig valves have been implanted into human hearts for decades, although they are rendered biologically inert first. Some argue that if pigs harbored serious zoonoses, man has already been exposed to them, and would not likely be harmed further by exposure through xenotransplantation. Others note that xenotransplantation eliminates many of our natural protections against disease, by breaching our skin or mucosal barriers, as well as blunting usual responses to infection with medication. These arguments do not prove or disprove whether xenotransplantion might allow for the spread of unusual infections.

There are risks involved in every medical manipulation of the human system. Given that there are increased risks to humans of xenozoonoses (particularly retroviruses) as a result of xenotransplantation, it is appropriate to ask how or whether these risks might be curtailed.

Strategies to control risk range from forbidding further xenotransplantation into humans, to a temporary stay on clinical trials while animal research continues, to advancing on to clinical trials and evaluating outcomes. In addition, they include prescreening measures of animal donors and post transplant surveillance of recipients.

The PHS guideline on Infectious Disease Issues in Xenotransplantation discusses in detail a number of safety techniques, including:

- procurement of tissues for transplantation only from animals bred in captivity, and that have a documented, well characterized health history and lineage
- raising the animals in facilities with adequate barriers to prevent the introduction or spread of infectious agents
- breeding programs utilizing caesarian derivation of animals to reduce risk of maternal-fetal transmission of infectious agents
- periodic surveillance of the herd or colony for exposure to known infectious agents
- quarantine of imported animals
- avoidance of importation of source animals from countries or regions where transmissible spongiform encephalopathies are known to be present
- availability of veterinarians with expertise in infectious diseases, and experts in research virology and microbiology to source animal facilities
- facility cleaning and disinfecting arrangements
- monitoring of feed components at such facilities
- maintaining medical records for source animals for 50 years beyond the date of xenotransplantation, as well as archiving biopsies of tissues or organs intended for use in xenotransplantation.

Recipients of xenotransplants would have to agree to *lifetime* monitoring for adverse clinical events potentially associated with xenogeneic infections, and possible periods of isolation or quarantine if they developed symptoms of illness. They would be counseled regarding behavioral modifications that diminish the likelihood of transmitting infectious agents. Recipients would be advised to educate family members and close contacts of the uncertainty regarding risks of xenogeneic infections, and recipients would be required to have a complete autopsy at their death. . In addition, they should defer from donating blood, blood products or other tissues or body parts. In the United Kingdom, organ recipients would have to sign contracts agreeing not to have children and never to have sex without barrier contraception.

There is no guarantee that any xenozoonotic illness would only be spread by intimate contact; "flu-type" viruses can be spread easily to limited contacts. Some xenozoonoses may be highly contagious and spread in respiratory fashion. Once a xenozoonotic virus began to spread, it might not be possible to check further transmission of the disease or even offer any effective therapy.

The PHS also recommends establishment of a National Xenotransplantation Database to allow tracking of adverse health events and notification of

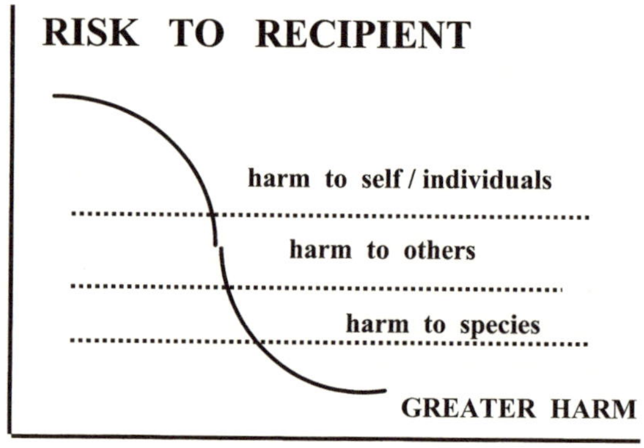

Fig. 7. Risk to Recipient.

individuals and clinical centers of epidemiologically significant adverse events related to xenotransplantation.

The development and implementation of such a system of precautions and maintenance of the database registry, archived tissues and records would be extremely expensive. Given the current state of transportation in our global village, where one (and any disease one carries) can be on the other side of the world in a matter of hours, the database would have to be available internationally.

Depending on circumstances, the records in such a database might have only limited confidentiality. Recording or monitoring of close contacts would strain confidentiality, and tracing contacts of these close contacts could be virtually impossible.

The nature of informed consent will have to be addressed prior to proceeding with xenotransplantation. How can single individuals give consent for a procedure that might benefit them, but put others at risk? How is it possible to obtain national or even international consensus to proceed with xenotransplantation, as risk is extended to the human species?

John Stuart Mill, the Utilitarian philosopher, declared "[T]he only purpose for which power can be rightfully exercised over any member of a civilized community, against his will, is to prevent harm to others . . . To justify that, the conduct from which it is desired to deter him must be calculated to produce evil to someone else" (Mill).

Perhaps the threat of xenozoonoses may be considered an evil to others. Informed consent will be changed in another sense, as well. Both the Nuremburg Code and the Declaration of Helsinki recommend that the subject of an experiment be able to withdraw permission for research to be continued and bring the experiment to an end. It would *not* be allowable for recipients of xenotransplants to withdraw from close monitoring once an animal organ had been placed within them. Society would be justified in enforced monitoring, along with diminished confidentiality, which would constitute significant departures from the usual informed consent process.

It is unlikely that countries with a high percentage of people of eastern religions would agree to use of animals for xenotransplantation. It is likely that countries where people are not adequately fed nor have access to basic medical care will find the concept of xenotransplantation as frivolous and wasteful, due to the tremendous expense and the limited number of people who may benefit.

On our slope of risk to recipient, xenotransplantation would be more risky to recipients than conventional human organ transplantation (Fig. 6), but we allow individuals great liberty with regard to taking risks that may delay their own death. It is the extension of risk of xenozoonoses to others who have not benefited from the transplant nor given consent to exposure to possible danger that is ethically troublesome.

SUMMARY AND CONCLUSIONS

Lewis Thomas describes organ transplantation as "halfway technology", representing treatment that must be "done after the fact, in efforts to compensate for the incapacitating effects of certain diseases whose course one is unable to do very much about". Thomas notes, "It is characteristic of this kind of technology that it costs an enormous amount of money and requires a continuing expansion of hospital facilities. There is no end to the need for new, highly trained people to run the enterprise." He concludes "the only thing that can move medicine away from this level of technology is new information, and the only imaginable source of this information is research" (Thomas, 1974).

Rather than "halfway", some see transplantation as double-edged, offering life extension and quality of life benefits, but in a costly fashion, fraught with the risks of immunosuppression, and leading to ethical dilemmas. The transplantation of an organ from one being into another may no longer be *uncommon*, but it should not be considered an *ordinary* procedure. In America, we have a fixation on "high-tech" solutions to our problems not shared by much of the world, which must still struggle to meet the basic needs of nutrition and sanitation.

Yet, while noting an increase in attention being paid to preventative care and health maintenance in the past few years, we remain concerned about the growing number of people on transplant lists, a number of whom will die without receiving an organ. We are frustrated by the concept of "rationing" care, and uncomfortable with the ethics of scarcity. Xenotransplantation has been proposed as a solution that could yield animal organs to anyone who might need a "spare part" to stay alive. However, xenotransplantation is not the *only* possible solution to the organ shortage. I have chosen to focus on the concerns of willingness, quality of organ, commercialism, risk to donor, and risk to recipient because these are the most common concerns posed by other proposed solutions to the organ shortage, to allow for comparison.

In summary: *Willingness* has been a critical issue in efforts to increase the number of human organ donations. Despite polls showing that many people are generally in favor of transplantation, this has not been demonstrated by a great increase in organ donation. Xenotransplantation offers a solution to this aspect of the organ "donation" problem. To many, it is not morally relevant if pigs are unwilling organ donors. Animal rights activists disagree.

The *quality of organ* that xenotransplants provide is critical—if xenotransplanted organs could be shown to work well in humans, I believe the other ethical issues would pale in comparison to the probability of success. Since xenotransplantation has not been adequately demonstrated to be effective treatments, this remains an area of great concern.

While there has been long debate about whether human organs should be sold or donors compensated, the ethical concern of selling pig parts is of much lesser concern, as that is a commonplace and widely accepted practice. More than 90 million pigs are slaughtered each year in the United States. And it's not likely anyone would recommend compensating a pig's relatives – who would likely also be organ donors or dinner fare. But in addressing the issues of *commercialism,* we tangentially must note that it is not clear whether we should or could possibly finance such a broad expansion of transplantation, when, as a nation, we have not been able to develop an adequate system to allow a large proportion of our citizens to have access to less costly therapy. Providing funding, access, and treatment for illness at earlier stages might prevent organ failure and the need for transplant, leaving us to consider whether concentrating our efforts and attention to advance transplant and high-tech science delays advancements in the less glamorous arena of preventative medicine. Research in other areas might provide a greater good to a greater number. We must examine our medical priorities and budgeting process.

It is certain that the informed consent process for xenotransplantation would differ from our usual practice, as animal organ recipients would not be allowed to withdraw from monitoring processes, would likely have only limited confidentiality, and might infringe upon the privacy of their intimate contacts who might also require monitoring.

On the positive side, xenotransplantation appears a potential solution to the organ shortage that in some manner avoids or diminishes ethical concerns about willingness of donors, sale of organs, and even *risk to donors*. And, we might not be concerned much about risk to recipients who choose organ transplantation over death, except that in this case, the *risk to recipients* may be extended to the human species. It is not clear whether individuals should be allowed to put other humans at risk of xenozoonoses.

As a nephrologist, I have seen the exuberant energy and miraculous transformation of those who have received a new lease on life through kidney transplantation, and will continue to advocate for placement of eligible patients on the waiting list. As an ethicist, I often pause to consider whether we might help more people by expanding access to basic care, better nutrition, and expanding research for prevention of end-stage organ failure rather than focusing our efforts on "rescue therapies". Yet preventing disease in future patients does little to help our current patients; we need to balance our efforts. In expanding the organ donor pool, we should strive for solutions that are the most likely to be successful, least risky, and most cost effective. At the present time, expanded use of human organs seems more likely to meet these three criteria than does xenotransplantation. It is of interest to note that Geron Biomed, which merged with Edinburgh's Roslin Institute where Dolly was cloned, recently announced a cut in funding and a halt in research in genetically modifying pig organs for transplant into humans, while at least three other research firms in Britain have drawn up proposals to begin xenotransplantation trials in humans next year.

A final sobering note is that there are over 5 billion people in the world. Before embarking on development of large-scale xenotransplant programs, we are compelled to search for acceptable means to increase the number of human organ donors. If we cannot significantly increase the number of human donors, we ought to explore whether the general public truly supports transplantation as a top health care priority. As Ben Franklin noted, it is convenient to be reasonable creatures, as we can find good reasons to justify whatever we wish to do.

ACKNOWLEDGMENTS

I am indebted to my parents for my interest in medical ethics: to my father, who taught me to try to do well; to my mother, who taught me to try to do good.

REFERENCES

Abouna, G. M. (1993). Negative Impact of Trading in Human Organs on the Development of Transplantation in the Middle East. *Transplantation Proc.*, *25*, 2310–2313.

Alexander, S. (1962).They Decide Who Lives, Who Dies. *Life Magazine*, Nov, 103f.

Amemiya et al. (1992). Special Issues Related to Transplantation in Japan. *Transplantation Proc.*, *24*, 2428–2429.

Aristotle. (1952). History of Animals, Book I. The Works of Aristotle, Volume II. Encyclopedia Brittannica, Inc. Berlin No. 488b.

Aristotle. (1952). Nichomachean Ethics, Book III. The Works of Aristotle, Vol II. Encyclopedia Brittanica, Inc. Berlin No. 1111b.

Associated Press. (17 Aug. 2000). Study raises concern over pig transplants. USAtoday. www.usatoday.com/life/health/transpla/lhtra39.htm.

Associated Press. (20 Sept. 2000). Cloned mice show no premature aging after several generations. www.cnn.com/2000/NATURE/09/20/mouse-clones.ap/index.html.

Bach, F. H., & Fineberg, H. V. (1998). Call for a moratorium on xenotransplants. *Nature*, *391*, 326.

Beauchamp, T. L., & Childress, J. F. (1989). *Principles of Biomedical Ethics* (3rd ed.), Oxford University Press. 289.

Bentham, J. (1780). Introduction to the Principles of Morals and Legislation. As cited in Singer, P. (1975) below.

Bronsther, O. Personal communication.

Butler, D. Briefing xenotransplantation. Last chance to stop and think on risks of xenotransplants. *Nature*, *391*, 320–324.

CNN.com. (29 Aug 2000). Pope condemns human embryo cloning. www.cnn.com/2000/WORLD/europe/08/29/pope.cloning/

Council of the Transplantation Society. (28 Sept. 1985). Commercialisation in Transplantation: The Problems and Some Guidelines for Practice. *Lancet*, 715–716.

Daar, A. S. (1992). Non-related Donors and Commercialism: A Historical Perspective. *Transplantation Proc.*, *24*, 2087–2090.

Darwin, C. (1872) The Expression of the Emotions in Man and Animals, as cited in Orlans, F. B., Beauchamp, T. L., Dresser, R., Morton, D. B., & Gluck, J. P. (1998). *The Human Use of Animals*. Oxford University Press.

Davis, R. (15 Nov. 1999). The trick to fighting organ mismatch. U.S.A Today. www.usatoday.com/life/health/transplan/lhtra022.htm. 1–4.

Descartes, R. (1968). Translated by Sutcliffe, F. E. Discourse 5. *Discourse on Method and the Meditations*. Penguin Books.

Dickens, B. M. (1990). Human Rights and Commerce in Health Care. *Transplantation Proc.*, *22*, 904–905.

Fox, C. (1999). Heartless. *Life Magazine*, Nov, 124–138.

Franchetti, M. (28May2000). Interpol hunts human kidney trade queen. *The Sunday Times* (U.K.).

Franklin, B. (1936). *The Autobiography of Benjamin Franklin*. The Spencer Press.

Gorman, C. (9March1998). Body Parts for Sale. Time, *76*.

Gutkind, L. (1988). *Many Sleepless Nights*. W. W. Norton & Co.

Hamilton, D. (1994). Kidney Transplantion: A History. In: P. J. Morris, *Kidney Transplantation, Principles and Practice*, (4th ed.). W. B. Saunders Co.

Hariharan et al. (2000). Improved Graft Survival After Renal Transplantation in the United States, 1988 to 1996. *N Engl J Med., 342*, 605–612.

HHS Fact Sheet (2000). HHS Guidelines for Xenotransplantation Safety. www.hhs.gov/news/press/2000pres/2000526.html.

Hume, D. (1920). *A Treatise on Human Nature*. Oxford University Press.

Humes, H. D., Mackay, S. H., Funke, A. J., & Buffington, D. A. (1999). Tissue engineering of a bioartificial renal tubule assist device: *In vitro* transport and metabolic characteristics. *Kidney International, 55*, 2502–2415.

Institute of Medicine. (1996) *Xenotransplantation: Science, Ethics, and Public Policy*. National Academy Press.

Kant, I. (1952). Translated by Abbott, T. K. *Fundamental Principles of the Metaphysics of Morals. The Critique of Practical Reason and other Ethical Treatises*. Encyclopedia Britannica, Inc.

Kant, I., (1975) Lectures on Ethics, as cited in Singer, P. *Animal Liberation*, below.

Lacoste et al. (2000). KHSV-like herpesviruses in chimps and gorillas. *Nature, 407*, 151–152.

Levinsky, N. G. (2000). Organ Donation by Unrelated Donors. *N Engl J Med., 343*, 430–432.

Lock, M. (1995). Contesting the Natural in Japan: Moral Dilemmas and Technologies of Dying. *Culture, Medicine, and Psychiatry, 19*, 1–38.

Michler, R. E. (1996). Xenotransplantation: Risks, Clinical Potential and Future Prospects. EID. wwwcdc.gov/ncidod/EID/vol2no1/michler.htm. 1–9.

Newman, A. (1988). *The Illustrated Treasury of Medical Curiosa*. McGraw Hill Book Company.

PHS Guideline on Infectious Disease Issues in Xenotransplantation (2000). www.fda.gov/cber/gdlns/xeno0500.txt

Rogers, L. (26 Mar. 2000). Organs go begging through NHS cuts. *The Sunday Times*: News (U.K.).

Rogers, L. (27 Aug 2000). British man is first to get electric heart. *The Sunday Times*: News (U.K.).

Rollin, B. E. (1992). *Animal Rights & Human Morality*. Revised Edition. Prometheus Books.

Singer, P. (1975). *Animal Liberation*. Avon Books.

Stolberg, S. G. (3 Oct. 1999). Could This Pig Save Your Life? *New York Times*.

Thomas, L. (1974). The Technology of Medicine. *The Lives of a Cell*. 35–42. Bantam Books, Inc.

United Network for Organ Sharing. www.unos.org.

USRDS. United States Renal Data Service.

Vanderpool, H. Y. (1999). Commentary: A Critique of Clark's Frightening Xenotransplantation Scenario. *Journal Law, Medicine, and Ethics, 27*, 153–157.

Weiss, R. A. (1998). Transgenic pigs and virus adaption. *Nature, 391*, 327–328.

9. PUBLIC POLICY MAKING IN ORGAN TRANSPLANTATION

Martin A. Strosberg and Ronald W. Gimbel

INTRODUCTION

Rationing is a controversial and confusing concept. Nevertheless, for almost 15 years, the federal government has successfully, and up until recently with relatively little public controversy, rationed organs for transplant. The National Organ Transplant Act of 1984 and subsequent acts and regulations established a centrally guided, explicit rationing policy for organ transplants. As one of the few examples of explicit government rationing of life-saving health services, it is worthy of study in its own right. Some have suggested that our national organ transplant policy serves as a model for national health care reform (Benjamin et al., 1994).

Rettig (1989), who has chronicled the evolution of the federal end-stage renal disease (ESRD) program, divides transplantation policy into three different areas:

(1) Status (whether the procedure is experimental or non-experimental), insurance coverage, and reimbursement;
(2) Organ acquisition and distribution;
(3) Facility certification (based on procedure volume and qualifications of providers).

In this chapter we will concentrate on the distribution of organs, although obviously related to the other aspects. The report of the federal Task Force On Organ Transplantation (1986), whose recommendations directly influenced the implementation of transplantation policy, declared organs to be a "scarce public

The Ethics of Organ Transplantation, Volume 7, pages 231–254.

ISBN: 0-7623-0764-1

resource" whose distribution should be governed "by criteria based on need, effectiveness, and fairness that are publicly stated and publicly defended (p. 86)".

The major focus of this study is to describe how organ transplantation policy is formulated and implemented. In spite of the centrality of objective (i.e. medical) criteria in allocating organs based on effectiveness, students of the public policy making process will recognize the actors and forces familiar to the American political arena: interest groups, politicians, bureaucracy, and ideology. Rationing, in spite of ethical imperatives, cannot be separated from Harold Laswell's definition of politics, "Who gets what, when, and how". The current national controversy over what to do about geographical inequities in access to organs (i.e. the debate over the so-called "Final Rule for Organ Allocation" promulgated by the United States Department of Health and Human Services) will be our lens for examining the public policymaking process.

Rationing and Public Policy in Context

A public policy is what government says and does about matters it wishes to influence. There are many ways of classifying public policies. Beyond categorization by substantive area, (e.g. foreign policy, economic policy, health policy/organ transplantation policy), one common way of classifying policy is on the basis of how they are designed to correct market deficiencies (Longest, 1998). When private markets do not function well, allocative policies provide benefits to distinct groups, often at the expense of others, in the interests of achieving certain public objectives. Regulatory policies are designed to influence actions and behaviors of others through interventions (e.g. market-entry restrictions, price controls, quality controls) also to achieve certain public objectives.

Transplant policy guiding organ distribution has both allocative and regulatory aspects, but it is generally referred to by the federal Department of Health and Human Services and other organizations as "organ allocation policy". Whereas allocative policy and regulatory policy are well understood and accepted analytical categories, "rationing" and "rationing policy" suffer from definitional imprecision. For clarification, Ubel and Goold (1998) have constructed a typology of definitions. Included in this typology is "explicit rationing of absolutely scarce resources of which the allocation of scarce organs is an example. Mechanic (1997) defines explicit rationing as "decisions made by an administrative authority as to the amounts and types of resources to be made available, eligible populations, and specific rules for allocation (p. 83)".

America's primary experience with explicit rationing occurred during World War II when certain scarce commodities were rationed (e.g. gasoline, and rubber tires). Citizens received a book of ration coupons which entitled them to a certain "ration", i.e. fair share. These commodities were not market goods; ability to pay was not a factor in allocation (although occasionally they could be illegally purchased on the "black market").

The National Organ Transplant Act of 1984 banned the purchase or sale of organs for transplant reflecting the prevailing national ethic that organs should not be considered a market good. As Blumstein (1989) pointed out, this ban, which represents one of the first times that the federal government undertook a regulatory measure unrelated to its role as payer, restricted consideration of market incentives even if they might increase the supply of organs. Organs are to be allocated on the basis of non-market criteria such as urgency of need and probability of success which allow for rank-ordering prioritization using a computerized point system. According to the Task Force (1986), "If two or more patients are equally good candidates for a particular organ according to the medical criteria of need and the probability of success, the principle of justice suggests that length of time on the waiting list is the fairest way to make the final selection (p. 89)".

The overall principle of rank-ordering access to organ transplantation based on medical-need criteria is generally well-accepted by the medical profession and the public at large. Contrast the organ rationing program with an early attempt in Seattle, painfully unsuccessful, to explicitly ration scarce life-sustaining kidney dialysis on the basis of "social worth criteria" (Fox et al., 1978). It soon became apparent that this was socially and politically unacceptable. In time, universal financing under Medicare (Social Security Amendments of 1972), unique to End-Stage-Renal Disease, alleviated the shortage of dialysis stations. Amendments to the act also helped to cover the financing of kidney transplants. However, the shortage of organs has not been alleviated.

In terms of the political feasibility of instituting an explicit rationing policy, one obvious lesson of the success of the system of organ allocation compared to the failure of the early Seattle experiment to ration kidney dialysis is that criteria must be perceived by the public to be fair, defensible, and legitimate. According to Benjamin et al. (1994), organ allocation embodies these characteristics:

> The participants – physicians, patients, and the public – know that an organ is denied to a potential recipient only for reasons of fairness and efficiency, not because of indifference

> or prejudice. Saying no to a particular patient is hard, but it means we can say yes to another. And the onus of making the painful judgment rarely falls on a single physician. The criteria for allocation, in which considerations of justice and efficiency are combined, have been developed and ratified by public bodies (p. 859).

Of course the social acceptance and political feasibility of explicit rationing is enhanced if the rationed resource is absolutely scarce (i.e. commodity scarcity). Like certain WW II commodities, organs are in scarce supply and are allocated in a zero-sum, closed system. They must be rationed, not because they are too costly, but because they are scarce. Nevertheless, managed care organizations and other third party payers including governments do make decisions on whether to provide insurance coverage for transplants. Without assured payment, most transplant centers will refuse to operate, even if organs are not in short supply and the patient ranks high on the priority list. Insurance coverage, reimbursement, and the determination of experimental and non-experimental status are important parts of overall public policy for organ transplantation but beyond the scope of this work.

The Current Controversy: The "Final Rule"

On April 2, 1998, Donna Shalala, Secretary of the Department of Health and Human Services (DHHS), issued a "Final Rule" – designed, according to a departmental press release, to improve fairness and effectiveness in allocating organs for transplantation. An administrative rule is a regulation that for all practical purposes has the force of law. As will be explained, "rulemaking" is an important phase in public policymaking. The issuance of a Final Rule is the culmination of the rule-making process, governed by the U.S. Administrative Procedures Act. In a nutshell, the Final Rule would require the Organ Procurement and Transplantation Network, the private sector system created by the National Organ Transplant Act of 1984, to develop revised organ allocation policies that will reduce the current geographic disparities in the amount of time patients wait for an organ. The OPTN Board of Directors would have considerable discretion in making allocation policies, subject to three broad "performance goals" spelled out by the Final Rule. These performance goals are:

- standardized listing criteria for placing patients on waiting lists, using objective and measurable medical criteria;
- standardized criteria for determining medical status, also based on objective and measurable medical criteria, sufficient to differentiate patients from least to most medically urgent; and

- organ allocation policies that give priority to those whose needs are most urgent, with the result that differences in waiting times for patients of like medical status will be reduced (U.S. DHHS, 1998, p. 3).

The Final Rule, which provides a framework for allowing DHHS to monitor and review OPTN actions, has generated a storm of controversy that has spilled over into national and state political arenas and has attracted national media attention. The debate over the promulgation of the Final Rule is now a high-profile conflict with political, economic, and ethical, ramifications. The vehemence of the controversy, as reflected in the following headlines, cannot help but threaten public confidence in the nation's explicit rationing system. The *New York Times* (1999), in an editorial entitled "Misguided Chauvinism on Organs" highlighted the inherent injustice of an allocation system where the "median wait for patients with blood type O for a liver transplant in New York City is 511 days while the wait a few miles away in New Jersey is 56 days. The *AMA News* (1999) in "Transplant Turf" has described the controversy as "turf wars between large and small transplant facilities fighting over prestige and profits". The *Wall Street Journal* (1998), in "With Livingston Adding Power as House Speaker, Fight Gets Tougher for Organ-Allocation Reform", described the fate of the Final Rule in terms of the waxing and waning of the power of various Congressional leaders, in this case former Louisiana Congressman Robert Livingston, whose state contained eight profitable transplant centers.

These headlines underscore the political forces involved in organ allocation and certainly challenge assumptions of rationality in our explicit rationing system. Nevertheless, seen in wider context, the ongoing debate over the Final Rule, although dramatic, is part of a public policymaking process that should not be considered unusual or even irrational. This process will be described in detail, but we will start at the beginning.

AGENDA-SETTING AND POLICY FORMULATION: NATIONAL ORGAN TRANSPLANTATION ACT OF 1984 AND THE TASK FORCE ON ORGAN TRANSPLANTATION

Policy analysts frequently describe the public policy-making process as a sequential pattern of activity made up of stages or phases. This process is depicted in the model by Longest (1998), Public Policymaking Process (Fig. 1). This model with the various policy phases will serve as a template for this study and its section headings.

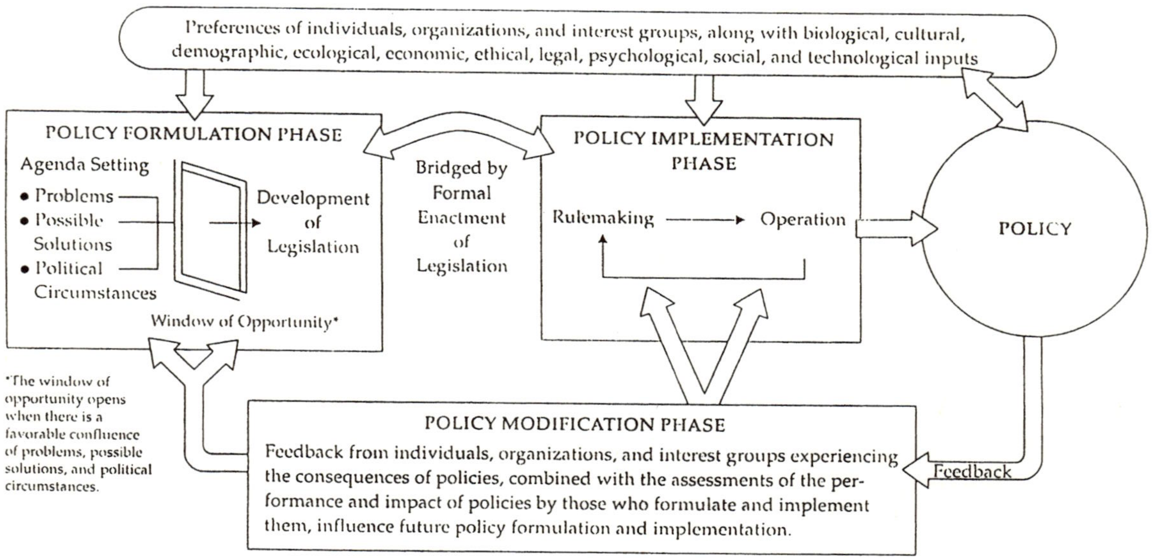

Fig. 1. Model of the Public Policymaking Process in the United States.
Source: B. B. Longest, *Health Policymaking in the United States*, Chicago, Health Administration Press, 1998.

The Agenda Setting Process

The concept of the public policy agenda and the agenda setting process has been introduced by John Kingdon (1995) in *Agendas, Alternatives, and Public Policies.* A government agenda is the list of subjects or problems to which government officials are paying some serious attention.

According to Kingdon, certain conditions must be present for an issue to receive spot on the policy agenda. In a nutshell, three processes – problem recognition, policy proposal generation, and the unfolding of political events – must converge at the right time and place in order for an issue to receive a spot on the agenda and then move forward to legislative action. At certain times, there are opportunities or "policy windows" when these three processes, which often operate independently from one another, meet. At this time, a policy proposal is chosen and action is taken in the form of legislation.

Problem Recognition. Up until a few decades ago, end stage liver and heart disease, were not a "recognizable problem" on the governmental agenda. They became a problem, in search of a solution, with the advent of life-saving organ transplantation. Without transplantation, patients died. Preventable death is indeed a very salient political fact. As with ESRD and kidney dialysis, advances in clinical capabilities created pressure on policymakers to take action, even if only symbolic.

What galvanized public concern and the attention of politicians most were the cases of individual children in need of transplants, often associated with public fund raising appeals and national media spotlight. In the early 1980s, President Reagan championed the cause of specific children through public appeals for liver donation. The personalization of the problem, magnified by media attention, focused public scrutiny not only on the lack of organs and the lack of financing, but on the chaotic and inequitable organ procurement and allocation system (Igelhart, 1984). The politicians responded. Rettig (1989) credits the publicity over children for triggering the Congressional hearings in 1983 chaired by Albert Gore of the Oversight Subcommittee on the House Science and Technology Committee, that led eventually to the enactment of the 1984 National Organ Transplant Act.

Possible Solutions: Political Actors and Policy Alternatives. The ESRD program and the institutional infrastructure of kidney transplantation provided ample precedent for dealing with many of the problems associated with organ procurement and allocation (Rettig, 1989). The various areas of federal organ transplantation policy mentioned at the beginning of the chapter (financing and reimbursement status, organ procurement and allocation, and facility certification) were to some extent constructed from the programmatic elements of the ESRD program.

The reason for the close tracking of the development of organ transplantation policy with the ESRD program experience is that most of the policy alternatives that were considered were generated by the same "policy subsystem". A policy subsystem is a small group of political actors, both governmental and non-governmental, that focus on a particular policy area and dominate policy formulation, implementation, and modification. Policy subsystems, ubiquitous on the federal governmental landscape, provide leadership and cohesion in the face of governmental fragmentation and the lack of strong, well-disciplined political parties. Sometimes referred to as a "triad" or an "iron triangle," they are typically composed of House and Senate Congressional committees and subcommittees that have jurisdiction over a particular policy area, governmental officials that manage programs carrying out policies, and non-governmental organizations and interest groups interested in a particular policy. The organ transplantation policy subsystem is composed of members from: various Congressional Committees and their staffs including the Senate Labor and Human Resources Committee, the House Energy and Commerce Committee and its Subcommittee on Health, the House Ways and Means Subcommittee on Health, and the Senate Finance Committee and its Subcommittee on Health; various bureaucratic sub-units of the Health Care Financing Administration and the Public Health Service, the two main components of the Department of Health and Human Services; interest groups and their lobbyists including transplant surgeons and other health professional groups, medical centers and transplant facilities, single disease associations such as the National Kidney Foundation, and the United Network for Organ Sharing (UNOS). UNOS is the private sector contractor that operates the Organ Procurement and Transplantation Network (OPTN), and whose members include many of the components of the health care delivery system as it relates to transplantation (see Fig. 2).

Interest groups and their representatives in the policy subsystem of course have vested interests in the types of solutions considered and chosen. They are prime beneficiaries of the allocative and regulatory policies produced by the system. One of the salient characteristics of policy subsystems is the extraordinary influence exercised by the non-governmental members. Ripley and Franklin (1991) note:

> American politics minimizes the distinction between governmental and non-governmental institutions and actors. The line between the two realms is easily crossed, a phenomenon widely approved of by those both inside and outside the government. A corollary is the

general belief that individuals most affected by governmental actions should have virtually continual access to governmental officials during the policy-making process (p. 8).

Kingdon (1995) points to the pivotal role of the "policy entrepreneur" in creating and taking advantage of opportunities to promote change by hooking "solutions to problems, proposals to political momentum, and political events

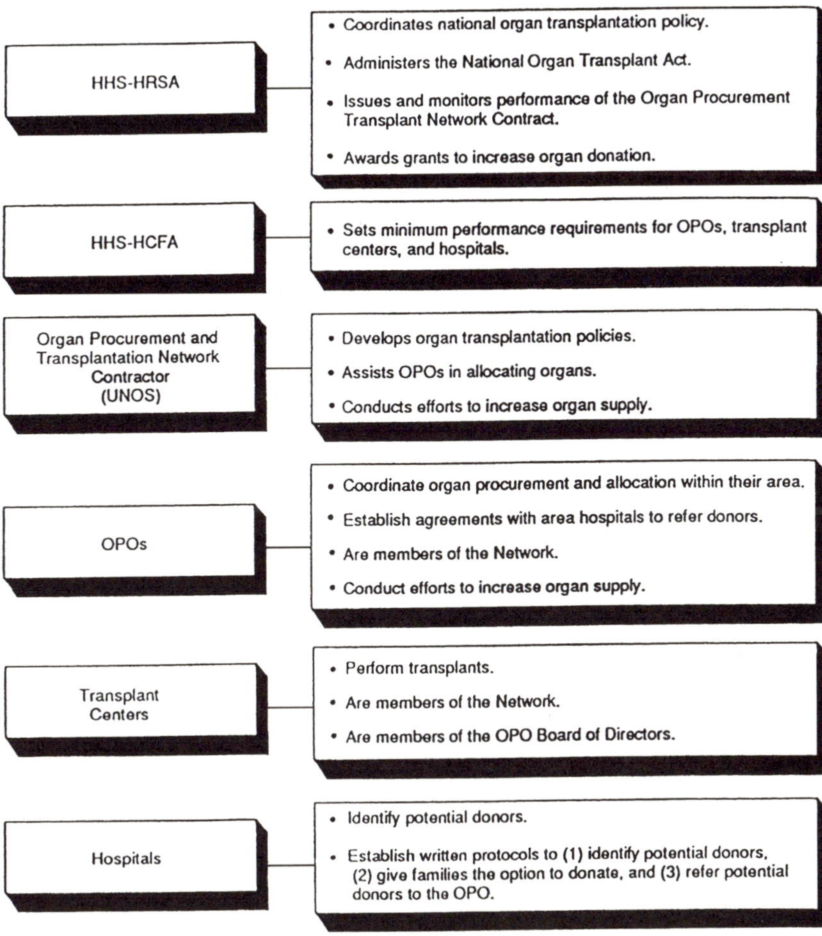

Fig. 2. Organ Transplantation Program.
Source: U.S. Government Accounting Office (1993). *Organ Transplants*. GAO/HRO-93-56. Washington.

to policy problems (p. 182)." Policy entrepreneurs originate in interest groups, research organizations and think tanks, and government itself. A typical operating mode of policy entrepreneurs is to advocate solutions and look for current problems to which to attach their pet solutions. In the case of interest groups, the solutions advocated usually advance the well-being of that group. On a personal basis, regardless of their origin, the policy entrepreneurs show:

> . . . a willingness to invest their resources – time, energy, reputation, and sometimes money – in hope of future return. That return might come to them in the form of policies of which they approve, satisfaction from participation, or even personal aggrandizement in the form of job security or career promotion (pp. 122–123).

Major policy change, however, is not the norm. Critics of public policymaking note that the coziness and insularity of the subsystem diminishes the ability of outsiders to influence policy. Ripley and Franklin (1991) describe three ways in which the normally low-profile operations of the policy subsystem can be opened up to outsiders:

(1) Disagreement arises among the normally friendly members of the subsystem that becomes publicized and stimulates attention and intrusion from non-members.
(2 The President or high administration official takes a particular interest into the functioning of the policy subsystem and brings the overwhelming resources of the Executive Office of the President to bear on the issue.
(3 A new issue that attracts attention from outsiders is introduced into the subsystems jurisdiction thus widening the set of interest groups (p. 8).

As we shall see, at least the first two of these methods are directly relevant to the controversy over the Final Rule for Organ Allocation.

Political circumstances. The debate in Congress over the National Organ Transplant Act of 1984 was over the level of government intervention, with the Republican Administration taking a minimalist approach and the Democratic House led by Representative Gore taking a more comprehensive approach. In the end, the compromise bill of the Republican Senate was the one that became the National Organ Transplant Act of 1984 (PL. 98-507) which amended the Public Health Service Act. Most significantly, the law prohibited the buying or selling of organs and established criminal penalties for violations. Support for this landmark regulatory policy came from both sides of the political aisle.

The law directed the Secretary of Health and Human Services to establish the national Organ Procurement and Transplantation Network to provide for the equitable and efficient allocation of organs, to establish a scientific registry of transplant recipients, and to report annually on the status of the organ transplantation program. The law also authorized grants to organ procurement organizations (OPOs).

Finally, the law established the Task Force on Organ Transplantation, a 25 member blue-ribbon commission composed of many persons closely associated with the policy subsystem as well as representatives from the health care industry in general. In charging the Task Force, Congress recognized that the National Organ Transplantation Act left many contentious policy and operational issues unresolved and there would be need for another round of legislation. The Task Force was designed to develop politically feasible solutions. However, most of the policy recommendations of the Task Force, regulatory in nature, were not to be legislated into law by Congress but "promulgated" into policies equivalent to regulation by UNOS, the private contractor responsible for operating the OPTN. The mechanism that would empower UNOS policymaking was provided by the 1986 Omnibus Budget Reconciliation Act which, among other things, added Section 1138 of the Social Security Act. The Act stipulated that all hospitals performing transplants, in order to be eligible to participate in the Medicare and Medicaid programs, had to abide by all the rules and requirements (i.e. policies) of the OPTN which would have effectively given them the force of regulation. In 1989, as will be explained below, compliance with OPTN rules and requirements became voluntary rather than compulsory.

In terms of our analytical framework, the development of the National Organ Transplant Act of 1984 sits squarely in the policy formulation phase of the Longest model. The statute-mandated Task Force Report is not only a key factor in policy formulation but also in policy implementation, the next phase in public policymaking (Of course the development of legislation, the product of policy formulation, is never completed; policymaking is an iterative process as shown in Fig. 1). In short, the Task Force Report is important for understanding the nexus between Congressional intent and operationalized policy, integral to the Final Rule controversy.

The Task Force Report (Organ Transplantation: Issues and Recommendations)

The Task Force issued a series of recommendations corresponding to the three major areas of transplantation policy delineated by Rettig and mentioned at the beginning of this chapter. Many of the recommendations were ultimately adopted by UNOS including a recommendation on facility certification, one of the most controversial issues in the 1983 Congressional debate (Iglehart, 1984, p. 868). During the hearings on Representative Gore's bill, which would grant the Secretary of DHSS authority under Medicare to limit the number of transplant centers and the types of procedures performed, representatives of the American Society of Transplant Surgeons (Drs. Norman Shumway of Stanford University and Thomas Starzl of the University of Pittsburgh) testified in favor of giving the Secretary decision making discretion. On the other hand, a representative of the AMA argued against federal intervention which he felt would constitute "improper intrusion into medical science and medical practice (p. 868)". The Task Force (1986), concerned with the over-expansion of transplant centers, recommended that federal and private sector reimbursement for transplant procedures "only be made to designated transplant centers that meet explicit criteria of experience, logistic medical support, volume, and graft and patient survival (p. xxi)". The tension over the level of federal intervention has never been fully resolved and would surface numerous times in the coming debate over the Final Rule.

Some Task Force recommendations did not become public policy, in particular the elimination of financial barriers (i.e. lack of insurance coverage) to equitable access to liver and heart transplants. This recommendation has unfortunately joined the ever-broadening stream of possible solutions that await the opening of another policy window for national health care reform, following the failure of President Clinton's managed competition plan.

The Task Force Report (1986) dealt extensively with the OPTN, the vehicle for carrying out its recommendations concerning the equitable allocation of donated organs among transplant centers and among patients medically qualified for an organ transplant. The OPTN and the OPOs can be considered elements of the national organ allocation "program", a set of activities, routines, and resources designed to accomplish the intended objective of a policy.

THE NEXUS BETWEEN POLICY FORMULATION AND IMPLEMENTATION

Rettig (1980), an expert on the implementation of the ESRD Medicare program, defines policy formulation and implementation:

> Policy formulation is the collective determination of a public policy and includes identifying, debating, and choosing among major policy alternatives. It may express or imply how the chosen policy is to be implemented. Implementation is the purposeful, organized activity undertaken to transform a policy into a program and the latter into program outputs corresponding to intended objectives (p. 11).

All too frequently in American public policymaking, the objectives of a law passed by Congress are imprecise; so too the route of implementation. Some of this imprecision is purposeful. It suppresses conflict and encourages consensus-building required for passing legislation. Some of it is due to the fact that Congress, because of lack of technical expertise, is incapable of detailing in legislation complex solutions to complex problems. It is up to the bureaucrats of the administrative agencies, the experts, to fill in the gaps. In doing so, public policy is made during the process of implementation. That non-elected bureaucrats are making public policy having the force of law is often disturbing to those who value a strict dichotomy between politics and administration where politicians, responsive to the voters, make policy and administrators faithfully execute that policy. The fact of the matter is that Congress, struggling with complex problems of a pluralist society, must give up some of its policymaking responsibility to the administrative agencies. However, policy-making by non-elected bureaucrats, who simultaneously exercise legislative, executive, and judicial powers, challenges American constitutional theory that goes to great lengths to separate these powers.

Rulemaking

One answer to this dilemma is supplied by the federal Administrative Procedures Act of 1946. In recognizing bureaucratic policymaking as a quasi-legislative function, the Act stipulates the formal procedures for making "rules". Rules, sometimes called regulations, are public policies just as surely as laws. The process of administrative "rule-making" generally requires publication of a draft of the proposed rule in the *Federal Register* as a "Notice of Proposed Rulemaking (NPR)". In publishing the draft rule, which may be used to guide the implementation of the law until the "Final Rule" is developed, administrators invite public comment from parties interested in the law's implementation. Public reaction may lead to changes in the Final Rule. Along the way, the administrative agencies may hold hearings and, of course, Congress may choose to intervene at any point. Needless to say, the rule-making process is subject to many of the same political forces that influence lawmaking.

The National Organ Transplant Act of 1984 required DHHS to contract with a private non-profit entity to establish and operate the OPTN. The challenge for DHHS, the administrative agency implementing the law, was to design an appropriate structure for the OPTN to carry out the law's objective.

The blueprint for the OPTN, which DHHS adopted, came directly from the Task Force Report. At the request of the DHHS and its Office of Organ Transplantation, the Task Force included in its report a section entitled "Model Organ Procurement and Transplantation Network" which detailed goals, composition of the board of directors with slots allocated to various constituencies and geographical regions, board responsibilities, organizational components, and membership requirements. The Task Force also intended the OPTN to play a regulatory role in carrying out its responsibilities. This role was not to be played on the stage of DHHS headquarters in Washington but at UNOS headquarters in Richmond, Virginia. UNOS, which began life as the Southeast Organ Procurement Foundation, was awarded the contract to administer the OPTN in 1986, and subsequently, guided by the Task Force model, assumed the right to become the chief policymaking body for organ procurement and allocation.

In making the case for the OPTN policymaking role, the Task Force (1986) "recognized the complex conflict between need for an organ (medical urgency) and the probability of success of the transplant, and did not presume to make recommendations in this sphere . . .". Instead, the Task Force recommended a "thoughtful process of development of policies for organ allocation, which takes into account both medical utility and good stewardship . . .". The OPTN, a "broadly representative body" would be the vehicle for the thoughtful process (pp. 8–9). Blumstein (1989), a critic of the implementation process, argued that Congress envisioned a coordinating and assisting role for OPTN, not "a top-down, command-and-control regulatory" role (p. 23). However the "top-down, command and control authority" of the OPTN over OPOs and transplant facilities was considerably blunted by actions taken by DHHS in 1989 which attenuated the linkage between eligibility to participate in Medicare and compliance with OPTN policies. The net effect of DHHS actions was to make OPTN policies voluntary (advisory) rather than compulsory. The Government Accounting Office (GAO) in its Report to Congressional Committees (1993), speculates on the motivation behind DHHS action. In an intriguing footnote, the GAO stated that officials from the DHHS Office of the Assistant Secretary for Planning and Evaluation indicated that, "DHHS was compelled to take this action because many of the policies adopted by UNOS were in conflict with other HHS requirements, otherwise misguided, or beyond the scope of the National Organ Transplant Act (p. 30)".

Ideally, according to the sequence of the Longest model, where rulemaking proceeds operation, DHHS should have promulgated the rules that guide the policymaking activities of UNOS and articulated the nature of the relationship between UNOS and DHHS. Unfortunately, technical complexity and political concerns often delay the promulgation of Final Rules, exactly the case with the OPTN. Meanwhile, as the clock ticks, the policy, with or without Final Rules, becomes an operational program producing outputs hopefully corresponding to intended objectives. If the administrative agency finds that the outputs do not correspond to intended objectives, it can revisit rulemaking in the policy modification phase. (Congress too can modify the policy by amending the law during reauthorization.) The Department of Health and Human Services, without ever having promulgated the Final Rule on organ allocation, found itself in such a situation.

Operations: The Program

At the federal level, the "home" of the transplantation program is in the DHHS Health Resources and Services Administration (HSRA), and the Health Care Financing Administration (HCFA). Federal program managers oversee the OPTN and the OPOs. However, not unlike many federal health care programs, implementation of federal policy takes place primarily "in the field", in the private sector health care delivery system. Needless to say, program managers, as contract administrators, facing a complex and decentralized program structure with few "command and control" tools at their disposal face formidable challenges in implementation. Furthermore they lack performance information on key programmatic activities. Figure 2 presents the various entities active in the national transplantation program.

The Institute of Medicine (1999), in its recent publication, *Organ Procurement and Transplantation: Assessing Current Policies and the Potential Impact of the DHHS Final Rule*, describes the policies guiding OPTN operations on liver transplants as they relate to DHSS's concerns over fairness and effectiveness:

> The process of organ procurement and transplantation begins when a patient in need of an organ transplant is referred to one (or more) of the 272 organ transplant programs (125 of which perform liver transplants) currently in operation in the United States. If accepted for transplantation by the transplant program, the patient is placed on the program's waiting list until a donated organ that is determined to be medically appropriate is available. Patients in need of a liver transplant are assigned to one of several classifications – status 1, status 2A, status 2B, or status 3 – depending on the nature and severity of the patient's illness. The retrieval and preservation of donated organs, and their transportation (if necessary) from the site of donation to the site of transplantation, is the responsibility of organ procurement organizations (OPOs). There are 62 OPOs currently in operation in the United States. Each is responsible for the retrieval and allocation of organs within a defined geographical area, and in accordance with organ allocation policies. These geographical service areas vary greatly in their size and population, as well as in the number of organs retrieved and the number of patients transplanted by the transplant centers in their service areas. The process of identifying which patient on a waiting list should receive an available organ is facilitated by the OPTN which . . . maintains a computerized listing of all patients, and certain vital data on such patients, on waiting lists for organ transplantation. When an OPO determines that an organ is available for transplant, it contacts the OPTN or more specifically the United Network for Organ Sharing (UNOS), which . . . then uses a complex, computerized

> algorithm to determine which patient is the most appropriate recipient of the available organ. There is general agreement that status 1 liver patients should be given first priority for an available organ and, if no suitable status 1 liver patient is identified, the organ should be offered sequentially to status 2A, status 2B, and status 3 patients. At the present time, this set of priorities is exercised first (with some exceptions) within the geographical area served by the OPO that retrieved the organ. The organ is offered to a patient outside the OPO's service area (using a similar set of priorities) only if no suitable transplant recipient is identified within the service area. Thus, despite the general consensus that status 1 patients should be given priority over other patients, the current allocation policies and practices may result in a status 2B or status 3 patients receiving an available organ because she or he is within the service areas of the OPO that retrieved the organ, while a suitable status 1 patient in a different OPO service area continues to wait for an organ. This is the basis for much of the debate about the fairness and effectiveness of the current system and one of the major concerns that the DHHS Final Rule was designed to address (p. 5).

At issue is the role of geography in organ allocation. In specific, which "community" has first claim on organs, a scarce national resource? The transplant facility? The local OPO service area where the organ was harvested? The region (the U.S. is divided up into eleven regions)? The state? The nation? Unfortunately, the Task Force Report provided no definitive guidance on this question. Childress (1989), Task Force vice-chair, acknowledged that the lack of clarity in the Report "affects many UNOS debates about procedural and substantive policies, insofar as they concern the relations among local, regional, and national communities (p. 103). In 1999, members of the organ transplantation policy subsystem are still searching for clarity. However the debate extends far beyond the subsystem.

POLICY MODIFICATION

According to Longest (1998), "policy modification results when the consequences of existing policies feed back into the agenda-setting and legislation-development stages of the formulation phase and into rulemaking and operational stages of the implementation phase and stimulate changes in legislation, rules, or operations (p. 208)." To a large extent, scientific progress drives a great deal of policy modification. Improvement in transplant success rates expands the number of potential candidates who could benefit and changes prioritization criteria. The increase in the time that an organ can be preserved also has obvious implications for the distance that it can be safely transported across state, and regional boundaries.

Policy modification is often associated with legislative and departmental oversight of the transplantation program in the form of reauthorization, oversight, and budgetary hearings, mandated GAO reports to Congress, reports from DHHS Office of the Inspector General, and reports prepared by private contractors performing evaluations. In addition UNOS prepares a variety of annual reports.

Through frequent amendments, Congress has changed the original National Organ Transplantation Act. Also, in part from pressure from DHHS, UNOS has made changes in many of its operational policies. The one area where DHHS has failed to bring closure has been in rulemaking. Since 1989, when DHHS announced that no OPTN policies could become legally binding, unless or until formally approved by the Secretary, the Department has been attempting through rulemaking to develop a framework for OPTN organ allocation.

The Consequences of Existing Organ Allocation Policies

Milford (1998) notes that, thanks to the establishment of various scientific registries under the National Organ Transplant Act, "solid organ transplantation is the only discipline in medicine in which complete demographic, risk, and outcome data are available on virtually all individuals with a specific medical condition. The availability of this information brings sharply into focus the ethical dilemmas involved in organ allocation, as well as donor and recipient selection (p. 1184)". Nevertheless, federal program managers have not always had access to the data that would demonstrate whether organs were being allocated equitably. A 1993 GAO Report found that a lack of measurement and monitoring systems impeded assessment of OPO allocation policies.

Even without the availability of sophisticated measurement systems, some very salient facts have been injected into the political arena with the help of the media. In 1998, some 5000 people – 14 people every day – die in the U.S. while waiting for a donated kidney, liver, heart, lung or other organ. Controlling for severity, waiting times for organs vary considerably across the nation. *The New York Times* (1999) and innumerable other publications have reported on the often-cited difference in waiting time for liver transplant between patients in New York City and those across the river in New Jersey. There are many other examples of differentials including longer waiting times for African-Americans. This type of news, especially when juxtaposed against the original aim of National Organ Transplant Act to produce a system that would allocate organs in a fair and equitable manner, mobilizes constituencies and energizes politicians. The very public consequences of organ allocation policy, as Rettig (1989) points out, cannot help but be felt in the political arena (p. 191).

Making the "Final Rule": The Chronology and the Controversy

As noted earlier, policy subsystems tend to operate in ways that are mutually reinforcing to its members. With interests converging, there is usually little conflict or media attention. However, the effort to develop the Final Rule ignited a storm of controversy within the organ transplantation policy subsystem that also involved President Clinton, Secretary Shalala, Congressional leaders, the courts, and even governors attempting to prevent organs from leaving the state. Listed in Fig. 3 is a chronology of some of the key dates in the history of the OPTN Final Rule.

The Department of Health and Human Services formulated the Final Rule to allow the OPTN considerable discretion in making allocation policies as long as they met the three performance goals described earlier. Why the controversy and the delay? UNOS and many of its members and their supporters have felt that the performance regulations, no matter how broad the delegation of policymaking responsibility, will ultimately lead to a single national waiting list. They have feared that the outflow of organs to distant locations containing the sickest patients will reduce the local donation rate, increase cost, jeopardize the financial viability of the smaller transplant centers, and increase organ wastage when sick patients fail to realize the benefits of transplantation. The Institute of Medicine Report, *Organ Procurement and Transplantation*, commissioned by Congress and released in July, 1999, addressed many of these issues. Nevertheless these concerns still remain.

Not all members of UNOS have opposed the rule. Some of the larger transplant centers with longer waiting lists of patients who tend to be sicker, most notably the University of Pittsburgh, strongly support the final rule. Ubel and Caplan (1998) characterize the controversy over the rule as a struggle "between the have and have-nots" and a "battle for supremacy among transplantation centers". Both UNOS and its supporters and the University of Pittsburgh have been actively lobbying Congress to intervene in DHHS rulemaking.

The splintering of the transplantation policy subsystem into warring factions was accompanied by the active involvement of high-level officials of the Clinton Administration, in particular Secretary Shalala. Usually rulemaking involves only governmental officials from the bureau level, regular members of the policy subsystem. Rarely do high-level administration officials take an active interest. Press accounts attribute the President Clinton's intervention and hence Secretary Shalala's to the lobbying efforts of David Matter on behalf of the University of Pittsburgh. In 1996, Matter, a long-time college friend of Bill Clinton, a major campaign contributor, and the president of a real estate firm with major connections to the University of Pittsburgh Medical Center wrote to Mr. Clinton at the behest of the president of the medical center advocating change in liver allocation policy (*The Washington Post*, 1996; *Pittsburgh Post-Gazette*, 1996).

- Sept. 8, 1994- Notice of Proposed Rulemaking (NPRM) issued with 90-day comment period.
- December 7, 1994 – Comment period on NPRM closes. Department begins to consider options to construct the final rule.
- November 13, 1996 – DHHS reopens comment period to 1994 NPRM with Federal Register announcement regarding public hearings.
- Dec. 10–12, 1996 – Public hearings held at the Natcher Center (NIH), Bethesda, MD, which discussed issues raised in 1994 NPRM as well as donation issues and organ allocation polices in general, and liver allocation policies in particular and comments considered in final rule development.
- April 2, 1998 – DHHS issues final rule on the OPTN with a 60 day public comment period. Rule is scheduled to become effective July 1, 1998,
- May 1, 1998 – President Clinton signs Public Law 105–174, which extends the comment period of the final rule to August 31, 1998, and delays the effective date to October 1, 1998.
- June 18, 1998 – Joint Congressional hearing (Senate Labor and Human Resources and House Commerce Subcommittee on Health and the Environment), entitled "Putting Patients First: Resolving Allocation of Transplant Organs", met in Washington, DC. Secretary Shalala, UNOS officials, invited members of the transplantation policy subsystem and vested external actors testify as to their perspective on the OPTN final rule.
- June 19, 1998 – Sen. Robert Toricelli (NJ) introduces rider to the fiscal year 1999 DHHS Appropriations Bill placing a one year moratorium on the effective date of the OPTN final rule.
- August 31, 1998 –Comment period ends for OPTN final rule.
- Sept. 17, 1998 – State of Louisiana, Louisiana Organ Procurement Organization, and transplant programs in Louisiana file complaint in the U.S. District Court for the Middle District of Louisiana challenging several provisions of the OPTN regulation and that state residents would be harmed by the new rule.
- Sept. 30, 1998 – U.S. District Court judge issues stay of the effective date of the regulation.
- October 21, 1998 – Consolidated Omnibus and Emergency Supplemental Appropriations Act, 1999 becomes law; places one year moratorium on effective date of the OPTN regulation (now 10/21/99); and requires a study of current allocation policies and new rules by the Institute of Medicine, National Academy of Sciences. The law also mandates that the IOM study issues such as access, impact on OPO performance and cost of transplantation services.
- November 3, 1998 – Louisiana law suit administratively closed without prejudice, allowing either party to re-open the issue in the future.
- February 24, 1999 – DHHS issues Sources Sought Announcement in the Commerce Business Daily seeking potential new sources for the OPTN and SRTR contracts.
- July 20, 1999 – Institute of Medicine releases its report entitled Organ Procurement and Transplantation: Assessing Current Policies and the Potential Impact of the DHHS Final Rule.
- July 20, 1999 – DHHS Secretary Shalala issues a statement in support of the recent IOM report and vows to move "vigorously" to implement the final rule with recommended improvements.
- October 20, 1999 – DHHS publishes amended Final Rule for the OPTN in the *Federal Register* scheduled to become effective November 19, 1999.
- December 17, 1999 – President Clinton signs the Ticket to Work and Work Incentives Improvement Act of 1999. Section 413 of the Act provides for a 90-day stay of the Final Rule for the OPTN which includes a 60-day public comment period, as announced in the *Federal Register* on December 21, 1999. The Department will consider public comments for 30 days prior to the effective date of the rule – March 16, 2000.
- March 22, 2000 – DHHS publishes Federal Register Notice response to the comment period for the Organ Procurement and Transplantation Network (OPTN) Final Rule. After considering the comments submitted, the Department has determined that no further amendments to the Final Rule are warranted at this time. The Final Rule published on April 2, 1998 and amended October 20, 1999, became effective March 16, 2000.

Fig. 3. Abbreviated Chronology of Key Events Related to OPTN Final Rule[1]

[1] *Source:* U.S. Department of Health and Human Services, Health Resources and Services Administration, Office of Special Programs. Chronology of Significant Events Relating to the OPTN Regulation Since 1996. http://www.hrsa.gov/osp/dot/chron.html, On-line December 28, 1999.

Consumer groups have also been vocal in the debate over organ allocation. There are dozens of such groups taking interest in virtually every aspect of organ procurement and allocation. Several consumer groups, such as the National Transplant Action Committee (NTAC), Transplant Recipients International Organization (TRIO), and National Minority Organ and Tissue Transplant Education Program (MOTTEP) have captured significant media attention and directly involved in the political arena. In general, groups affiliated with smaller transplant centers have reservations about the Final Rule, while those affiliated with large transplant centers tend to favor its implementation.

Political activity in opposition or in support of a rule is certainly not unusual. What is unusual is the vehemence of the antagonism between the supporters and opponents of the rule. In testimony before the Joint Congressional Hearing, "Putting Patients First: Resolving Allocation of Transplant Organs", Secretary Shalala made this extraordinary statement:

> Unfortunately, to this point, UNOS has failed to seize the opportunity by the rule to develop consensus about policy improvements. In fact, UNOS has gone to great lengths to preserve the current unfair system. It has launched a cynical political lobbying campaign against the April 2 rule. This campaign has been characterized by misinformation and outright falsehoods. The essence of the UNOS campaign has been to create phantom policies and use scare tactics that have hospital administrators and patients around the country up in arms. UNOS has sent form letters, part of a self-described "legislative action kit", to surgeons and patients across the country. UNOS has been loud and vociferous in its lobbying and is working with some of the highest priced public relations and lobbying firms in town. As a result of their slick lobbying campaign, you are hearing protests about the April 2 rule (p. 77).

CONCLUSION: PUTTING PATIENTS FIRST

Over thirty-five years ago, Don K. Price (1965) distinguished four broad functions in government and public affairs – the scientific, the professional, the administrative, and the political – each with its institutionalized estates. Each estate has its own internal logic and motivations. The four estates can be arranged along a continuum with truth and knowledge at one end, and power and action at the other. The scientific estate, driven by its pursuit of truth and the advancement of scientific theory, appropriately ignores all other purpose as irrelevant; the professional estate puts this scientific knowledge to social purposes in the service of clients; the administrative estate, not based on a special body of knowledge, attempts to advance the general purposes of its political superiors, governmental or corporate; the political estate makes decisions based on value judgments, compromise and power interests.

In the context of public policy making process, the issuance of the DHHS Final Rule for Organ Allocation can be understood as an exercise in policy modification, a discrete phase in a sequence of phases. However, the controversy generated by the rulemaking can be understood as a conflict between the second and third estates with DHHS and UNOS as the main antagonists. While the rhetoric of "putting patients first" constituted the leitmotif of The Joint Congressional Hearing on the Department of Health and Human Services Final Rule for Organ Allocation (1998), the real question being addressed was where on the truth to power continuum should policymaking responsibility lie for "putting patients first?" The rule attempted to shift the locus of policy making from the professional estate, its historic home, to the administrative estate. The tension between the two positions is illustrated by the testimony of the two antagonists. Secretary Shalala:

> As I have said, the National Organ Transplant Act gives the Department authority to oversee the network. The primary reason the Act was passed in the first place was because the unregulated network was rife with abuses . . . To say we have no basis to issue regulations when our authority is clear is a disservice to Congress, which created the network, and to the patients, whose transplant bills are paid by the taxpayers (p. 78)

Dr. Larry Hunsicker, outgoing UNOS President:

> It is our (UNOS) understanding of the Act (NOTA) that Congress specifically designed the system (OPTN) to be organized and run privately, shielding the government from direct involvement in the sensitive medical and ethical decisions associated with setting organ distribution policy. We must object to any implication that policy will be directed by the government rather than developed through consensus by physicians, patients, donor families and the many other important voices in the transplant community (Joint Congressional Committee, 1998, p. 136).

With regard to Dr. Hunsicker's last point, it is instructive to note that the Final Rule would change the makeup of the OPTN Board of Directors and the procedures for making policies. The net effect of the change would be to lessen the influence of the transplant surgeons.

Despite the current controversy between DHHS and UNOS, the initial decision by Congress and DHHS in the mid-1980s to locate organ allocation policymaking responsibility in the professional estate should not have been surprising to students of health care policy. If it were not located there, it would depart from a long-established pattern in health politics of ceding public policymaking authority to private sector professional associations, what Lowi (1969) calls interest group liberalism. The dominance of physicians over medical policymaking and subsequent administrative arrangements is based on the widely-shared belief that medical professionals are in fact the scientifically trained experts in the service of their patients who are removed from the power, politics, and action of the political and administrative estates. The Hippocratic tradition of patient advocacy places the professionals squarely on the truth side of the continuum. The further toward the truth side of the continuum an estate is, the more it can be trusted, the less the need for oversight. On the other hand, as Marone (1993) points out, the dominance of physicians over health policymaking and their autonomous position are also explained by the fact that physicians, through their professional associations, are active and effective in political arenas. He characterizes their activity as "exaggerated case of interest group liberalism – government authority wielded by an industry, generally for the benefit of its members (p. 726)".

Marone also argues that the United States, as compared to other Western industrialized democracies, lacks a stable and long-standing relationship between the administrative and professional estates where a unified physician leadership carries on high-level negotiation with high-ranking civil servants over the broad contours and budget of the national health system. Nor do we possess a respected and competent civil service capable of maintaining policy continuity while acting as a countervailing force to professional power. In our fragmented governmental system, Congress, as we have seen, is particularly responsive to the pleadings of special interests and is more than willing to thwart the initiatives of administrative agencies. For example, Representative Michael Bilirakis, chair of the House Commerce Subcommittee on Health introduced a reauthorization bill (HR 2418) in July, 1999 which would strengthen OPTN's policymaking autonomy. The bill, the Organ Procurement and Transplant Network Amendment of 1999, that passed the House on April 4, 2000, would neutralize many of the provisions of the Final Rule which went into effect on March 16, 2000. President Clinton has threatened to veto such a bill.

Ordinarily, Representative Bilirakis and like-minded colleagues should prevail in the political arena. But the debate about the Final Rule is not taking place under ordinary conditions. As we have seen, intense Presidential interest and concomitant Secretarial involvement, major dissension by an important player in the transplant community (University of Pittsburgh Medical Center) with good political connections, and an evolving and strengthening consumer group movement not necessarily allied with the professional estate make this an extraordinary episode in public policymaking.

Under these conditions, DHHS is making a credible claim that it is in the best position to "put patients first," and carry out the intent of NOTA. This is not to deny an important policy making role for UNOS and other professional and patient groups active in governing a decentralized organ procurement and transplantation network. But DHHS and its supporters claim that the responsibility for elicit rationing of a public good should rest with an accountable public body. Whether this claim will translate into the final say on organ transplantation remains to be seen.

REFERENCES

AMA News (1999). *Transplant Turf.* D. L. Shelton, April 1.

Benjamin et al. (1994). What Transplantation can Teach Us About Health Care Reform. *New England Journal of Medicine*, *330*(12), 858–860.

Blumstein, J. (1989). Government's Role in Organ Transplantation Policy. *Journal of Health Politics, Policy and Law*, *14*(1).

Childress, J. F. (1989). Ethical Criteria for Procuring and Distributing Organs for Transplantation. *Journal of Health Politics, Policy and Law*, *14*(1), 87–114.

Fox, R., & Swazey, J. P. (1978). *The Courage to Fail* (2nd ed.). Chicago: University of Chicago Press.

Iglehart, J. (1984). Health Policy Report: The Politics of Transplantation. *The New England Journal of Medicine*. *310*(13), 865–866.

Institute of Medicine (1999). *Organ Procurement and Transplantation: Assessing Current Policies and the Potential Impact of the DHHS Final Rule*. Washington, D.C.: National Academy Press,

Joint Hearing Before the Subcommittee on Health and Environment of the Committee on Commerce, House of Representatives, and the Committee on Labor and Human Resources (1999). *Putting Patients First: Resolving Allocation of Transplant Organs*, U.S. Senate. 105th Congress, Second Session. Government Printing Office. June 18, 1999.

Kingdon, J. (1995). *Agendas, Alternatives, and Public Policies, 2nd. Edition*. New York: HarperCollins College Publishers.

Longest, B. B. (1998). *Health Policymaking in the United States* (2nd ed.). Chicago: Health Association Press.

Lowi, T. J. (1969). The End of Liberalism: The Indictment. Reprinted from *The End of Liberalism, Ideology, Policy, and the Crisis of Public Authority*. W. W. Norton and Company.

Marone, J. (1993). The Health Care Bureaucracy: Small Changes, Big Consequences. *Journal of Health Politics, Policy and Law*. *18*(3), 723–739.

Mechanic, D. (1997). Muddling Through Elegantly: Finding the Proper Balance in Rationing. *Health Affairs*, *16*(5), 83–92.

Milford, E. L. (1998). Organ Transplantation – Barriers, Outcomes, and Evolving Policies. *Journal of the American Medical Association*, *280*(13), 1184–1185.

New York Times (1999). Fight Over Organs Shifts to States from Washington. By S. G. Stolberg, S. G. March 11.

New York Times (1999). Misguided Chauvinism on Organs. March 12.

Pittsburgh Post-Gazette (1996). Friend Faxes Clinton on Organ Dispute. S. Twedt. November 14.

Price, D. K. (1965). *The Scientific Estate*. Cambridge: Belknap Press.

Rettig, R. (1989). The Politics of Organ Transplantation: A Parable of Our Time. *Journal of Health Politics, Policy and Law*, *14*(1).

Rettig, R., & Marks, E. (1980). *Implementing the End-Stage Renal Disease Program of Medicare*. RAND: Santa Monica.

Ripley, R. B., & Franklin, G. A. (1991). *Congress, the Bureaucracy, and Public Policy*. Brooks/Cole Publishing: Pacific Grove.

The Washington Post. (1996). Who Should Get Liver Transplants?: As Demand Far Outpaces Donors, Federal Officials May Revamp the Rules. December 9.

Ubel, P. A. & Caplan, A. L. (1999). Geographical Favoritism in Liver Transplantation- Unfortunate or Unfair? *New England Journal of Medicine, 339*(18), 1322–1325.

Ubel, P. A., & Goold, S. D. (1998). Rationing Health Care: Not All Definitions are Created Equal. *Archives of Internal Medicine, 158*, 209–214.

U.S. Department of Health and Human Services, Health Resources and Services Administration, Office of Special Programs, Division of Transplantation (1998). *1998 Annual Report of the U.S. Scientific Registry for Transplantation Recipients and the Organ Procurement and Transplantation Network: Transplant Data: 1988–1997*. Rockville.

U.S. Department of Health and Human Services, Health Resources and Services Administration, Office of Special Programs. Chronology of Significant Events Relating to the OPTN Regulation Since 1996. *http://www.hrsa.gov/osp/dot/chron.html*, On-line December 28, 1999.

U.S. Department of Health and Human Services, Health Resources and Services Administration, Office of Organ Transplantation (1986). *Organ Transplantation Issues and Recommendations: Report of the Task Force on Organ Transplantation*. Washington.

United States Government Accounting Office (1993). *Organ Transplants: Increased Effort Needed to Boost Supply and Ensure Equitable Distribution of Organs*. GAO/HRD-93-56. Washington.

Wall Street Journal (1998). With Livingston Adding Power as House Speaker, Fight Gets Tougher for Organ-Allocation Reform. By L. McGinley, November 25.

10. AN INTERNATIONAL PERSPECTIVE TOWARD HUMAN ORGAN DONATION AND TRANSPLANTATION

Mario C. Deng and Hans H. Scheld

I. INTRODUCTION

I.1 Epidemiology of Heart Failure

Among the roughly 50 million annual human deaths worldwide, 15 million are due to cardiovascular diseases and a growing proportion of them is due to heart failure. The incidence and prevalence of heart failure is rising. This is largely a consequence of an increase of coronary artery disease during the second half of the 20th century in the industrialized countries and implementation of successful techniques aiming at restoring adequate myocardial blood flow. The latter development has been associated with a higher proportion of patients who survive acute coronary syndromes such as unstable angina and acute myocardial infarction albeit at the expense of irreversibly damaged areas of myocardium which undergo chronic remodeling with the clinical sequelae of chronic heart failure. Although the incidence and prevalence of coronary artery disease decreases owing to successful modification of risk factors associated with sedentary lifestyle, heart failure is the only cardiovascular disease entity rising in age adjusted mortality and morbidity rates. This holds true not only for the industrialized countries but also countries with economies in transition and in non-industrialized, so-called developing, countries. Heart failure is expected

The Ethics of Organ Transplantation, Volume 7, pages 255–276.

ISBN: 0-7623-0764-1

to be among the leading causes of death by the year 2020 (IHF White Book, 1999).

I.2 Development of Cardiac Transplantation

In parallel to this epidemiological development, research in the second half of the 20th century has generated a multitude of medically and surgically based heart failure treatment options including the concept of cardiac replacement by cardiac transplantation. Historically, following the first successful kidney transplant in 1954 (Peter Bent Brigham Hospital, Boston), successful pancreas transplant in 1966 (University of Minnesota, Minneapolis), successful liver transplantation (University of Colorado Health Sciences Center, Denver) and heart transplantation in 1967 (Groote-Schuur-Hospital, Kapstadt, South Africa), the first successful U.S. heart transplant was performed in 1968 (Stanford University, Stanford) (Table 1). In the meantime, more than 50.000 cardiac transplants have been performed worldwide in more than 300 hospitals (www.ishlt.org). The combination of reasonable surgical success rates and the presence of a growing number of well equipped cardiac transplant programs has created an enormous flux of heart failure patients towards these centers. The growing demand and the stagnant number of donor organs have inevitably led to the current waiting list problem.

Looking at the history of cardiac transplantation, we can somewhat arbitrarily distinguish four periods (Table 2): First, there was the long period in which mankind dreamt of replacing a terminally failing heart by a healthy one including the experimental period in the animal laboratory. This was followed by the second period of first clinical experience with mixed outcome results and a broad public debate over the ethical issues associated with brain death and outcome. With the introduction of cyclosporine and improvement of clinical results we can identify the beginning of the third period of establishment of heart transplantation as the perceived gold standard of advanced heart failure treatment. It coincides with the development of consensus guidelines and outcome databases. The fourth period is characterized by the redefinition of the role of cardiac transplantation from being the isolated gold standard to being an integrated part of advanced heart failure care. This coincided with reopening of the discussion on ethics of brain death, ethics of futile care at the end of life, and the cost-effectiveness of this mode of therapy. Although each of these four periods follow one another in a logical order as one step is born from the labor of the previous one, we currently witness an international scenario in which all periods of cardiac transplantation are simultaneously represented in different parts of the world.

Table 1. History of Organ Transplantation.

Year	Event
1954	First successful kidney transplant (Peter Bent Brigham Hospital, Boston, Massachusetts)
1966	First successful pancreas transplant (University of Minnesota, Minneapolis, Minnesota)
1967	First successful liver transplant (University of Colorado Health Sciences Center, Denver, Colorado)
1967	First successful heart transplant (Groote Schuur Hospital, Kapstadt, South Africa)
1968	Foundation of Eurotransplant International Foundation (Leiden, The Netherlands)
1978	First Medicare reimbursement of a kidney transplant
1981	First successful heart-lung transplant (Stanford University, Stanford, California)
1983	Use of cyclosporine approved by Food and Drug Administration
1983	First successful lung transplant (Toronto General Hospital, Toronto, Canada)
1984	First electrically driven implantable Novacor LVAD (Stanford University, Stanford, California)
1984	National Organ Transplant Act passed to establish a systematic national organ allocation system and a scientific registry of information on transplant recipients
1984	Establishment of the Division of Organ Transplantation in the Health Resources and Services Administration
1985	Report of the Department of Health and Human Services Task Force on Organ Transplantation with recommendations on national policy regarding donation and procurement, organ sharing, patient access, organ transplant technology and future research
1986	Establishment of the Organ Procurement and Transplantation Network
1987	Establishment of the Scientific Registry of Transplant Recipients
1990	Transplant Amendments requiring public release of transplant center-specific survival data
1991	First Medicare reimbursement of a liver transplant
1992	Release of first center-specific graft and patient survival rate report
1997	German Transplant Law requiring definition of necessity, urgency, and likelihood of success of organ transplantation in state-of-the-art guidelines

Table 2. Periods of Cardiac Transplantation.

Period	Characteristics
Before 1967	Cardiac transplantation as a vision and experiment
Before 1980	First clinical cardiac transplantation results & mixed public acceptance
Before 1990	Cardiac transplantation as an isolated gold standard
After 1990	Cardiac transplantation as integrated part of advanced heart failure therapy

Viewed against the background of the rapidly increasing numbers of heart failure patients, cardiac transplantation is serving only a very limited fraction of this patient cohort. It is playing a paradigmatically important rather than a quantitatively important role in the management of advanced heart failure. This role varies among societies. Practice of cardiac transplantation has developed heterogeneously in industrialized societies, societies with economies in transition and non-industrialized societies (Esmore, 1992; Tong, 1992; Hunt, 1993; Miller, 1995; Deng, 1997). But even among industrialized societies, there are appreciable differences in the public attitude and medical practice of heart transplantation. An analysis of this variation requires a sequential focus on different constitutive components of the cardiac transplantation process including:

(1) heart replacement paradigm
(2) brain death concept and donor recruitment
(3) recipient selection
(4) allocation criteria
(5) organizational structures
(6) quality control mechanisms
(7) alternative treatment research
(8) teaching and education
(9) societal policy making.

The comparison between countries requires detailed knowledge of the above processes within the respective societies. For this reason, the comparison will mainly focus on Germany and the United States of America which are best known to both authors (Table 3). An overview of different national policies and practices will be presented first.

I.3 Overview of Different National Policies and Practices

The role of heart transplantation in different countries can be assessed by surveys to national cardiology and cardiac surgery societies, by subanalyses of the International Society for Heart and Lung Transplantation (ISHLT), the Eurotransplant International Foundation (ET) and the United Network for Organ Sharing (UNOS) Registries, by literature searches on the topic in the relevant literature services, and by informal interviews with experts in the respective countries. After consulting all the above mentioned sources, the following results emerge: The heart replacement paradigm and the brain death

Table 3. Comparison of cardiac transplantation infrastructure between Germany and the United States of America.

Component	USA	Germany
Heart replacement paradigm	Introduced in 1968	introduced in 1981
Brain death concept	context of intensive care	context of transplantation
Recipient selection	consensus processes since 1980's: trend towards restriction to sickest	consensus processes since 1990's: trend towards restriction to sickest
Allocation criteria	regional waiting list combining urgency, waiting time, and distance, multiple listing allowed, regional audit	national waiting list combining urgency, waiting time, and distance, no multiple listing, national audit
Organizational structures	1 center per 2–3 million, variable center size	1 center per 2–3 million, variable center size, national audit
Quality control mechanisms	UNOS database, Regional audit	Eurotransplant and national database, national audit
Alternative therapy	active research	active research
Teaching and education	Certification available	no certification available
Societal policy making	federal rule enacted	federal rule enacted

concept seems to be the result of a Western approach of medicine (including North and South America, Western Europe, Australia) which is not universally accepted in African, Asian, Eastern European and Latin American countries. Reservations in these regions seem to be based on restricted health care related economic resources, religious backgrounds as well as philosophical attitudes which criticize transplant medicine as following a reductionist approach by neglecting the holistic aspect of the individual patient, his psychosocial environment, and the patient-physician encounter (Rowinski, 1996; Effa, 1998; Kimura, 1998). Opponents to organ transplantation in Japan, for example, criticize the brain-death concept as invalid, and demand a continued societal debate before transplantation medicine is started in Japan (Watanabe, 1994). Any solution of ethical controversies in the field of organ transplantation in these countries must consider the complex and significant impact of cultural and psychological factors on organ replacement therapies (Marshall, 1998). On the other hand, these countries seem to strive for acquisition of this new Western medical technology and to incorporate this approach into routine care as exemplified by the experience in Taiwan (Lee, 1996), Indonesia (Puruhito, 1998) and Japan (Tagaki, 1996). Donor recruitment policies vary greatly even within countries embracing organ transplantation, with Spain being the undisputed international leader based on a transparent policy and professional network with a cadaveric organ donation rate of close to 30 per million population (Miranda, 1998; Almenar Bonet, 1999) while in other European countries donation rates are falling (Pavie, 1996, www.eurotransplant.nl). In regions of public scepticism towards organ transplantation such as southern Italy a sophisticated program involving a large group of physicians and nurses directly involved in the care of endstage organ failure patients as well as a strategy of diffusing the "culture" of organ donation among the regional public media and lay people has been reported to successfully raise the donation rates (Roncone, 1996). Issues of recipient selection, allocation criteria, transplant center organizational structures, quality control mechanisms, and alternative advanced heart failure therapy are developed to differing degrees in countries actively pursuing cardiac transplantation as detailed in Chapter 2. For example, the practice of patient selection is highly different when comparing the United Kingdom and the United States. In one study, U.K. data were taken from an ongoing multi-center prospective study, the U.K. Cardiothoracic Transplant Audit. The U.K. population comprised 620 listings and 463 transplants. U.S. data were obtained from UNOS and comprised 3946 listings and 4704 transplants. There was a mean of 14 transplants per center per year in the U.S. compared with 34 in the U.K. Notable differences in practice included rarity of listing in the U.K. of patients >65 years (0.2% vs. 4.1% in U.S.) and patients with previous transplants (U.K. 0.9%, U.S. 3.2%). Patients listed in the U.S. were more likely to be on ventricular assist devices (odds ratio 8.0, 95% CI 3.0–21.7) or inotropes (odds ratio 4.9, 95% CI 3.7–6.4). Living donor (domino) transplants, although comprising 7% of transplants in the U.K., were virtually non-existent in the U.S. (1 domino in 4704 transplants). Heterotopic transplants were more common in the U.K. (4.4% vs. 0.5%). Indications for transplant were similar (except retransplantation). The donor age was >35 years in 43% of U.K. donors vs. 33% of U.S. donors. This study revealed substantial practice differences between the U.K. and U.S. The authors concluded that further studies were required to examine the reasons for these practice differences, the influence on transplant outcome, and their ethical and economic implications (Anyanwu, 1999). In addition to practice patterns, the degree of public debates and teaching, societal resource allocation, and policy making vary with the degree of consent with organ transplantation paradigms in the respective societies.

II. COMPARISON BETWEEN GERMANY AND THE UNITED STATES

II.1 Heart replacement paradigm

Although the revolutionary new paradigm was created on December 03, 1967 when Christiaan Barnard performed the first human heart transplantation in Kapstadt, South Africa, the United States can be regarded as the nation in which the concept of cardiac transplantation has been developed. This is due to the intensive research work mainly by the group around Norman Shumway at Stanford University in California after 1950. The societal struggles which cardiac transplantation encountered in the decade following its successful initiation at Stanford in 1968 has shaped its current important role in the U.S. medical system more than in any other country (Thompson, 1971). In 1998, according to the UNOS website there have been 2,345 heart transplants performed in the United States (www.unos.org).

More than decade after the initiation of cardiac transplantation in the U.S.A., in Germany the first cardiac replacement procedure was performed in 1981 although the concept was supported in Germany as early as 1969 by physicians active in the field (Messmer, 1969). During the last two decades, Germany has assumed an active role in cardiac transplantation. This is examplified by the annual data of the International Society for Heart and Lung Transplantation (www.ishlt.org). According to this registry, more than 10% of the >50,000 procedures performed so far have been performed in Germany (Hosenpud, 2000).

II.2 Brain Death Concept and Donor Recruitment

Cardiac transplantation requires societal consensus about the brain death concept since this is the prerequisite for the explantation of a functional heart from a dead organism. This concept has initiated societal debate in the border zone between medicine, ethics, and law (Price, 1997).

In the United States, the brain death concept has been originally developed more than 30 years ago. Its rationale originated from advances in intensive care medicine which rendered patient care undetermined with regard to ethical categories in borderline critical care situations and required a new operational definition of death in order to propagate a humane high tech medicine. To which extent the Harvard Ad Hoc Committee definition in 1968 has been influenced by the advent and prospect of transplant medicine has been reviewed recently (Giacomini, 1997). This historical development has at times been neglected in the context of the German public debate on brain death and transplantation.

While cardiac transplantation seemed to have been implemented into routine practice of advanced heart failure management in Germany, there have been considerable debates during the last decade with regard to the validity of the brain death concept. This is reflected in the debates preceeding the passing of the German transplant law in 1997. Relevant societal forces have questioned the brain death concept and consequently, organ transplantation (Deutscher Bundestag, 1996). Specifically, it has been called into question that the timepoint of brain death marks the timepoint of death of a person. Rather, it has been suggested by some that the process of dying extends beyond the timepoint of brain death, and, thus, explantation of organs for transplantation, would be ethically unacceptable because it would imply killing a dying person. At the same time, proponents of this view made the suggestion that if the dying person in question had consented prior to dying to the explantation of his/her organs and, thus, accepted the brain death criteria for him/herself, organ explantation should be ethically acceptable.

II.3 Recipient Selection

Recipient selection is crucial for achieving good posttransplant survival and quality of life outcomes for the individual recipient. First and foremost, the evaluation of the potential transplant candidate must establish an advanced heart failure condition with a high likelihood of death within the next one year period and the absence of comorbidities that would negatively impact on posttransplant outcomes. If a survival benefit and quality of life benefit are likely, the patient is presented with the recommendation of cardiac transplantation. One of the essential prerequisites for any iatrogenic intervention, and, thus, recipient selection, is the consent of the patient after being informed. Very few reports exist on cases in which cardiac transplantation has been performed in an emergency situation without informed consent of the patient (Grande, 1998). These situations understandably provoke intense public debates as recently witnessed in the U.K. While there has been international consensus that evaluation for transplantation must be done in a specialized heart failure/transplant center (Miller, 1998; Deng, 1999), no consensus exists whether cardiac transplantation should be preferably performed on stable or critically ill patients.

In the U.S., consensus processes have been initiated to establish guidelines on recipient selection and transplant management (O'Connell, 1992; Hunt, 1993; Miller, 1995, 1998). Recently, an initiative to accept older cardiac transplant recipients has been started at the University of California at Los Angeles using a so-called alternative waiting list and donor hearts which would have been considered unacceptable for transplantation, e.g. because of advanced age (Laks, 1997). In Germany, the consensus process on recipient selection has been started in the 1990s. The Working Group on Thoracic Organ Transplantation of the German Cardiac Society conducted surveys on current pretransplant and posttransplant practice patterns in Germany (Deng, 1997). In addition, to comply with the requirement of the new German transplant law which was enacted in 1997 to define necessity, urgency, and likelihood of success of cardiac transplantation, the Heart Committee of the German Transplantation Society – in close collaboration with the Eurotransplant International Foundation – conducted a study on comparative outcomes and clinical profiles in transplantation. In this study which is described in Section II.6, main results included a temporary benefit from transplantation in those patients who had a predicted high risk of dying on the waiting list for transplantation (Deng, 2000).

II.4 Allocation Criteria

Cardiac organ allocation can be organized locally, nationally, or internationally within a framework of an equitable rule. This rule should incorporate five factors relating to medical need including the likelihood of benefit to the patient, the impact of treatment on improving the quality of the patient's life, the duration of benefit, the urgency of the patient's condition, and the amount of resources required to achieve these goals. In contrast, the following non-medical patient-related criteria are believed to be unacceptable in the allocation process: ability to pay, contribution of the patient to society, perceived obstacles to treatment, contribution of the patient to his/her own medical condition, and past use of resources (Council AMA, 1995). In this regard, societal debate in the industrialized countries continues on issues such as allocation of cardiac transplants to criminals (Schneiderman, 1996). As to the medical criteria, patient related criteria such as medical urgency or waiting time may be used for prioritization. Alternatively, center-specific rotational allocation may be successfully used as demonstrated by the cardiac allograft allocation system in the U.K. (Haverich, 1997; Anyanwu, 1999).

The rules put forward by the U.S. Department of Health and Human Services (Federal Register 1998, April 2nd 1998; Ubel, 1998; Gibbons, 2000) reflect the attempt to reserve cardiac transplantation for the sickest patients but this point of view has been challenged. A similar conflictional scenario with regard to allocation rules prevails at this time in Germany (Deng, 1999).

The German transplant law requires all centers to utilize a uniform national waiting list in order to guarantee equitable organ allocation (Dt Aerzteblatt, 2000). As opposed to the U.S., multiple listing is not allowed in Germany because it is believed to contradict the principle of equitable access. To put this legal requirement into practice, all German heart transplant centers went through a period of intense debate. This debate was the consequence of a trend that had taken place in German cardiac transplant medicine in the years prior to the advent of the transplant law. During these years, a trend towards regional organization of donor recruitment, allocation, and transplantation has evolved in Germany (Schmid, 1999). This development seemed to be advantageous to most German transplant centers because of: (1) the expected improved outcome related to shorter ischemic times, (2) improved cooperation between regional centers sharing expertise and assist devices, (3) reduced transportation costs, (4) improved transparence of transplantation medicine in regions with more equitable access of patients to heart failure/transplantation medicine, and (5) enhanced acceptance of this medicine by the public in the region including the willingness to donate organs. Specifically, allocation was performed as a staged procedure within the Eurotransplant Organization, starting with high urgency requests on the ET level, then matching on the local, regional, and finally ET level. This allocation algorithm seemed to incorporate all benefits of a large distribution network for medical urgency cases as well as regional allocation whenever possible with the advantage of reducing ischemia time and costs and enhancing regional cooperation between centers. To balance the requirements of a national German waiting list with these historical accomplishments, the heart committee of the German Transplantation Society reached a consensus in May 1998 that a uniform German waiting list had to be created. Starting in the year 2000, for high priority transplantation of special urgency patients an estimated one third of cardiac transplants will be performed independent of previously accrued waiting time and regional distribution. Monitoring of adherence to predefined medical special urgency criteria will be accomplished by an expert audit group composed of experts with equitable regional distribution. This audit group reports to the heart committee by written records. Roughly two thirds of organs will be allocated according to waiting time and distance factor (Fig. 1). These two factors will be weighed equally. The allocation mode is to be reevaluated and further developed on the basis of the results of the clinical profile data base and other pertinent research updates. The proposed allocation rule will apply to lung and heart-lung transplantation as well. Within Eurotransplant, there will be a rule to account for national imbalances caused by net export of organs from one country associated with Eurotransplant (Germany, Belgium, Netherlands, Luxembourg, Austria) into

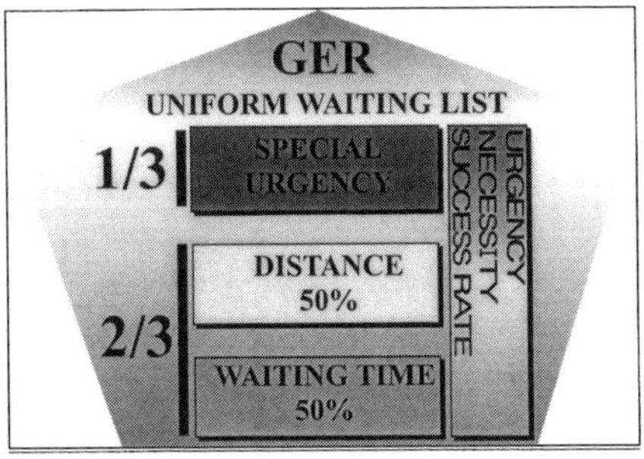

Fig. 1. Consensus allocation algorithm in the German transplant law.

another country. Issues to be resolved internationally include the quesions whether hearts should be allocated on a regional or a national basis and whether the sickest or to the more stable patients on the waiting list should have highest priority.

II.5 Organizational structures

Neither in the United States nor in Germany a federal oversight regulates the number of cardiac transplant centers. As a consequence, in the U.S. there are >160 transplant centers (300 million inhabitants) while in Germany there are >30 cardiac transplant centers (80 million inhabitants). This translates into roughly 1 transplant center per 2–3 million people inhabitants. As opposed to both of these countries, for example in the United Kingdom there are 8 cardiac transplant centers (56 million inhabitants) and in Italy there are 11 cardiac transplant centers (60 million inhabitants) regulated by federal oversight (Ministry of Health) (1 transplant center per 6–10 million people inhabitants).

With reference to data on the relation between center size and outcome (Hosenpud, 1994), a debate was initiated in Germany whether or not the number of >20 centers per 500 cardiac transplantations per year and 80 million inhabitants was too large to allow for a reasonable transplant volume and experience. This reasoning was in line with international guidelines (O'Connell, 1992). As of January 01, 1997, there were 31 cardiac transplant centers in Germany. Since it was felt that there should be some regulatory activity by the transplant centers themselves, two solutions were discussed, (i) a mere limitation of center numbers and (ii) the elaboration of criteria to which all centers should adhere if they wished to maintain a cardiac transplantation program. Arguments in favor of the former solution would have been that this might be the only way to effectively restrict center numbers; arguments in favor of the latter would include that a democratic consensus would facilitate a cooperative development in Germany. To facilitate the debate and consensus process, a questionnaire was distributed to all centers in 1996 on which the distribution of services was assessed. Consensus was reached on the following grounds in December 1996: In Germany, a cardiac transplant center structure is to be developed in which all aspects of care for advanced heart failure patients are incorporated. These include a sophisticated and specialized advanced heart failure management and organ preserving conventional cardiac surgery program (revascularization, mitral valve repair, aneurysmectomy, tachycardia operation, multisite pacing), a mechanical and antiarrhythmic bridging program, an active donor recruitment program, an elaborated post transplant care program according to international recommendations (Laffel, 1992), a teaching and education program in all aspects of care of advanced heart failure patients, the availability of basic research facilities commensurate with international points of view (Shumway, 1993; Oppell, 1994), active clinical research programs and quality control policies (Table 4).

II.6 Quality control mechanisms

In the U.S., the most consistent systematic, and detailed post transplant data bases have been established in an attempt to create an evidence-basis for rational decision making. Some of these data bases have become international registries (e.g. International Society for Heart and Lung Transplantation) while others have been maintained as a voluntary multicenter database (e.g. Cardiac Transplant Research Database at the University of Alabama in Birmingham).

After being awarded the contract by the federal government, the United Network for Organ Sharing (UNOS) established a registry in 1989 (UNOS,

Table 4. Transplant center infrastructure requirements in Germany.

heart failure management
high risk cardiac surgery
bridging devices
donor recruitment
post transplant care
basic/clinical research
teaching/education
quality control

1989). Although in the U.S. the United Network for Organ Sharing (in conjunction with the International Society for Heart and Lung Transplantation Registry) collects data on cardiac transplantation outcomes there is no analysis allowing assessment of outcomes based on specific clinical profiles at the time of placement on the waiting list. UNOS places region specific, state specific, and center specific outcomes on their internet web page (www.unos.org). An audit process within the UNOS regions has been initiated since 1991 in the U.S.

The German data base is maintained as part of the Eurotransplant data base (www.eurotransplant.nl). In Germany a clinical research project has been initiated by the Heart Committee of the German Transplant Society in 1997. It was named "Comparative Outcomes & Clinical Profiles In Transplantation (COCPIT)" study. This registry allows to estimate the transplant effect on outcomes in patient cohorts with comparable clinical profiles at the time of listing for cardiac transplantation, i.e. patients stratified for their heart failure severity and the associated risk of dying from heart failure. Specifically, all German transplant centers agreed to provide a set of prognostic data for the events "death before transplantation", "transplantation", and "death after transplantation" at the time of initial listing starting January 1, 1997. Prognostic information was generated by utilizing a multiparametric heart failure survival score which had been constructed at the University of Pennsylvania between 1986 and 1991 and had been validated in a second cohort at Columbia University in New York between 1993 and 1995 (Aaronson, 1997). It could be demonstrated that this previously validated score could be used in a cohort of 889 adult patients (all German patients listed for transplantation in 1997). In this observational cohort study, within 1 year after listing, patients with a predicted high risk had the highest global death rate (51%, 32%, 29% for high, medium and low risk patients; $p < 0.0001$), experienced the highest risk of dying on the waiting list (32%, 20%, 20% for high, medium, and low risk patients; $p = 0.0003$), and were more likely to undergo transplantation (48%, 45%, 41% for high, medium, and low risk patients; $p = 0.01$). Posttransplantation outcome differences between the risk groups did not reach significance ($p = 0.2$). While a mortality risk reduction by transplantation could not be demonstrated for the total cohort, a survival benefit was present for the high risk group. We concluded from this study that cardiac transplantation in Germany currently is associated with a survival benefit only in patients with a predicted high risk of dying on the waiting list and that patients with a predicted low and medium risk have no mortality risk reduction from transplantation and should therefore be managed with organ saving treatment approaches rather than with transplantation (Deng, 2000). The finding in the

German COCPIT study that heart transplantation is worthwhile only for a selected high risk group of patients suggests that heart transplantation listing should be limited to the sickest patients. In addition, these findings may have implications for heart allocation rules: Priority should be given to high risk patients. This rule which has been suggested by the German Transplantation Society (Deng, 1999) and the U.S. Department of Health (Federal Register, April 2, 1998), has been reinforced by the Institute of Medicine in July 1999 (Gibbons, 2000). In expanding the German COCPIT study, a six-month reevaluation procedure based on the initial data form with the exception of left heart catheterization derived parameters (e.g. pulmonary capillary wedge pressure) has been incorporated since 1998. Furthermore, a post transplantation follow-up form has been introduced. This form has been harmonized with Eurotransplant and the International Society for Heart and Lung Transplantation. These data will allow us to assess risk adjusted survival benefit of cardiac transplantation and regional differences in the management of patients with comparable clinical characteristics of advanced heart failure and allow us to draw conclusions with regard to center structure and organization.

A major advance in the cardiac transplant quality control mechanism in Germany is the introduction of an audit process. Monitoring of adherence to predefined medical special urgency criteria will be accomplished by an expert audit group composed of experts with equitable regional distribution. This audit group reports to the heart committee of the German Transplantation Society.

II.7 Alternative treatment research

The large discrepancy between the very small number of donor organs and potential transplant recipients has prompted intensive research into alternative therapies.

The U.S. is a country where the search for alternative heart replacement techniques namely mechanical circulatory support systems and xenotransplantation options are pursued most actively (Goldstein, 1998; Hunt, 1998). Other options such as high risk conventional surgery, ventricular volume reduction surgery, and multisite pacing are being evaluated. The National Heart, Lung, and Blood Institute (NHLBI) created a special emphasis panel in 1997 on research priorities in heart failure (Cohn, 1997).

Nevertheless, this research is increasingly being conducted in German university settings as well. Patients with ischemic cardiomyopathy, viable myocardium, and graftable vessels can be revascularized with acceptable risk. Since for these patients a standby of mechanical circulatory support must be anticipated perioperatively, this infrastructure should be established within the center. All other potential options including mitral valve repair, ventricular volume reduction, multisite pacing, and chronic ventricular assist device support are subject to intense clinical research.

II.8 Teaching and education

The qualification to manage patients with advanced heart failure, specifically after cardiac transplantation, requires specialization. While in the U.S., a specific process of certification has been initiated, this has not been recognized as a specific task in Germany.

The development of a continuing public dialogue has been recognized as a preeminent task and has to a large extent been supported and organized by lay organizations such as the American Heart Association (AHA) in the U.S. and the Deutsche Herzstiftung (DHS) in Germany.

II.9 Societal Policy Making

The successful establishment of cardiac transplantation as definitive treatment of endstage heart failure worldwide has led to an increase in awareness of physicians about this treatment option, in patients listed for transplantation, in centers performing this procedure but not in donor organs available. This has led to an increase in average waiting times, increased demand for bridging devices on the waiting list and a liberalization of donor criteria. Furthermore, this has triggered a public debate on equitable organ allocation according to medical urgency criteria.

In the U.S. in 1984, Congress passed the National Organ Transplant Act which created the Organ Procurement and Transplantation Network (UNOS). In 1986, UNOS was awarded a federal contract to administer the network as a private nonprofit corporation. UNOS was charged with developing, implementing, and monitoring national policies for transplantation. Its official mission statement is "to advance organ availability and transplantation by uniting and supporting its communities for the benefit of patients through education, technology and policy development" (www.unos.org). The 1984 act, along with the Omnibus Reconciliation Act of 1986, and the Transplant Amendment Act of 1990, is the legislative backbone of the U.S. national allocation system. As part of this legislation, the Health Care Financing Administration (HCFA) was given the authority to certify and recertify organ-procurement organizations. The U.S. is divided into service areas, each covered by a HCFA-designed non-profit procurement organization (the German equivalent being the

Deutsche Stiftung Organtransplantation DSO) which is responsible for acquiring and allocating solid organs as an intermediary among donor hospitals, histocompatibility laboratories, and transplantation centers. Over the past decade the activities of organ-procurement organizations have increased in scope and complexity and now include professional education, hospital development, and donor awareness campaigns (Hauptman, 1997). While an increasing percentage of the health care budget is spent on endstage patients in the U.S. and Germany, strategies for regulating expenditure have been different in both countries. In the U.S., health care providers have exerted a strong influence on the system of heart transplantation. The accreditation and reimbursement of transplant centers was based on the development of satisfactory performance. While in the U.S. there has been substantial support for a regionalization of cardiac transplant services during the last decade (Renlund, 1987), recent federal rules mandate a uniform national approach to the organization of cardiac transplantation (Federal Register, 1998).

In Germany, this debate has received renewed attention following enactment of the new transplant law in December 1997. Apart from establishing the criteria of brain death, this law which had long been anticipated required the transplant community to materialize the following requirements within a two year period:

> The organs subject to allocation are to be allocated for appropriate patients by the allocation agency in keeping with rules which correspond to state-of-the-art medical standards especially as regards the chances of success and the medical urgency of the procedure. In the process, the waiting lists of the transplantation centres are to be treated as a uniform waiting list. The decision regarding allocation is to be documented for each organ along with the grounds for the decision and shall be communicated to the transplantation centre and coordinating agency using the identification number.

To cope with these tasks, the German Transplantation Society asked its organ committees to provide consensus definitions with regard to the above issues. The process of reaching consensus within the heart transplant community has been cumbersome yet productive (Deng, 1999, 2000; Dt Aerzteblatt, 2000) and may serve as a model for international regulatory activities.

III PERSPECTIVES

III.1 Need for evidence based global approach

Based on the COCPIT study of the German Transplant Society, it is proprosed to initiate and maintain a global advanced heart failure registry (Deng, 1999). The three main purposes of such a registry are: (1) prognostication, (2) outcome analysis, and (3) assessment of differences in management which seem to vary substantially across and between nations. Not only can we learn from one another with regard to the impact of management protocols on outcome, but in addition, the most effective way of treatment may be assessed. One of the prerequisites to participate in this kind of registry is a consensus of all heart failure/transplant centers and their professional societies to contribute data. Another prerequisite is the establishment of a central data acquisition and analysis unit with decentralized expert units in each country. This registry must be maintained by all professional societies involved in advanced heart failure care and must obey the rules of transparent data acquisition and equitable access to data according to predefined consensus rules of all participating centers.

III.2 Internationally coordinated research

Besides established clinical options such as mechanical circulatory support, high risk conventional surgery, high risk valve repair and antitachycardia operation, other options such as ventricular volume reduction, multisite pacing as well as those at the stage of being implemented such as cell transplantation and xenotransplantation should be investigated internationally on a competitive yet coordinated basis. Since the resources required for intense research in this field are vast, it is suggested that an increased international cooperation not only in multicenter clinical trials but also in basic research areas is achieved. This has been already attempted. e.g. in the field of xenotransplantation (Cambridge University, Munich University).

III.3 Limits of high tech medicine & patient-physician encounter

High technology medicine approaches constitute a challenge for defining new boundaries. They demonstrate that even with replacement of the heart, although the cardiovascular function is restabilized, the recipient may not be able to bear the consequences of the intervention as well as the immunosuppressive therapy following this intervention. Thus, it is vital to understand our interventions in the context of the biology of the recipient. The differential therapeutic options that can be offered to a patient with advanced heart failure require continuing education and counseling to insure an educated decision-making process on the side of the patient. This requires a contemporary role of the physicain within an adequate framework of the patient-physician encounter (Uexküll, 1997; Koop, 1999; Weatherall, 1999).

III.4 Resource allocation

Cardiac transplantation is part of the high technology medicine approach that has been generated by scientific advances during the last century. Although the goal of cardiac transplantation is the restitution of full health and functionality, the procedure can, even if every recipient would return to work and participate in the tax paying process not be offered at neutral costs. Rather, it has been estimated that cardiac transplantation costs society roughly 25,000–30,000 U.S.$ per year of quality-adjusted life gained by the procedure (Scheld, 1994). In addition, it will be vital in the U.S. as well as Germany and all other countries utilizing cardiac replacement to initiate a broad and continued societal discussion (Council on Ethical and Judicial Affairs AMA, 1995) as to whether or not to allocate resources mainly to end stage heart failure care or to incorporate a major primary and secondary preventative approach into chronic heart failure management. This is even more important in light of the notion that while population growth has been enabled through increasing survivorship in infancy, improved sanitation, immunization programs, increasing economic productivity and trade as well as increasing food production and distribution, individual curative health care directed at a specific illness in the individual has played only a very small role in this trend (Daulaire, 1999). For this reason, most western countries are turning towards community health and disease prevention, with a special focus on noncommunicable diseases such as coronary artery disease. According to the "White Book" of the World Heart Federation on the "Impending Global Pandemic of Cardiovascular Diseases" published in 1999, this trend reflects the relative failure of high technology medicine to adequately address the needs of the population even in developed countries (White Book, 1999).

ACKNOWLEDGMENTS

We appreciate the comments on this manuscript by Jacqueline Smits MD, Eurotransplant Foundation, Leiden, Netherlands, Sharon A. Hunt MD, Director of Cardiac Transplantation, Professor of Medicine, Stanford University, California, and Sir Magdi Yacoub, Professor of Surgery, Chairman, Department of Cardiothoracic Surgery, Harefield Hospital, National Heart and Lung Institute, London, U.K.

ABBREVIATIONS

Abbreviation	Full name
AHA	American Heart Association
COCPIT	Comparative Outcomes & Clinical Profiles in Transplantation Study
CTRD	Cardiac Transplant Research Database
DHS	Deutsche Herzstiftung
DSO	Deutsche Stiftung Organtransplantation
ET	Eurotransplant International Foundation
HCFA	Health Care Financing Administration
ISHLT	International Society for Heart and Lung Transplantation
NHLBI	National Heart, Blood, and Lung Institute
UNOS	United Network for Organ Sharing

REFERENCES

Aaronson et al. (1997). Development and prospective validation of a clinical index to predict survival in ambulatory patients referred for cardiac transplant evaluation. *Circulation*, *95*, 2660–2667.

Almenar Bonet, L. (1999). The 9th official report of the Spanish National Heart Transplant Registry (1984–1997). *Rev Esp Cardiol.*, *52*, 153–158.

Anyanwu et al. (1999). Variations in cardiac transplantation: comparisons between the United Kingdom and the United States. *J Heart Lung Transplant.*, *18*, 297–303.

Council on Ethical and Judicial Affairs of the American Medical Association Report. Ethical considerations in the allocation of organs and other scarce medical resources (1995). *Arch Int Med.*, *155*, 29–40.

Daulaire, N. P. M. (1999). Global health, population growth, and United States policy. In: D. C. Grossman & H. Valtin (Eds), Great issues for medicine in the twenty-first century: ethical and social issues arising out of advances in the biomedical sciences. *Ann N Y Acad Sci.*, *882*, 192–199.

Deng et al. (1999). Development of cardiac transplant policy in Germany (editorial part 1). *Thorac Cardiovasc Surgeon*, *47*, 1–4.

Deng et al. (2000). Development of cardiac transplant policy in Germany (editorial part 2). *Thorac Cardiovasc Surgeon*, *48*, 183–185.

Deng et al. (1997). Management before and after heart transplantation in Germany: Results of two national surveys. *Tx Med*, *9*, 188–191.

Deng et al. (1999). Towards an evidence based perspective in advanced heart failure care (editorial). *Z Kardiol.*, *88* (Suppl III):III/1-III/3.

Deng et al. (2000) on behalf of COCPIT Study Group. The effect of receiving a heart transplant: analysis of a national cohort entered on to a waiting list, stratified by heart failure severity. *Br Med J., 321*, 540–545.

Department of Health and Human Services (April 2, 1998). Organ Procurement and Transplantation Network; Final Rule. *Federal Register.*

Deutscher Bundestag (German Parliament) (1996). Stenographic report of the 99th plenary session on April 19. *Bundesanzeiger.* 8817–8853.

Effa, P. (1998). Transplantation and xenotransplantation: legal perspectives for third world countries. In: J. Fishman, D. Sachs & R. Shaikh (Eds), Xenotransplantation: scientific frontiers and public policy. *Ann N Y Acad Sci, 862*, 236–236.

Esmore et al. (1992). Cardiopulmonary transplantation services established in the 1990s: Australia: a developing country? *Transplant Proc., 24*, 2007–2008.

Giacomini M. (1997). A change of heart and a change of mind? Technology and the redefinition of death in 1968. *Soc Sci Med, 44*, 1465–1482.

Gibbons et al. (2000). and other members of the Institute of Medicine Committee on Organ Procurement and Transplantation. Waiting for Organ Transplantation. *Science, 287*, 237–238.

Goldstein et al. (1998). Implantable left ventricular assist devices (review). *N Engl J Med., 339*, 1522–1533.

Grande et al. (1998). Heart transplantation without informed consent: discussion of a case. *Intensive Care Med., 24*, 251–254.

Hauptman et al. (1997). Procurement and allocation of solid organs for transplantation. *N Engl J Med., 336*, 422–431.

Haverich, A. (1997). Principles of heart allocation. In: G. M. Collins, J. M. Dubernard, W. Land & G. G. Persijn (Eds), *Procurement, Preservation and Allocation of Vascularized Organs* (pp. 209–216). Kluwer Academic Publishers.

Hosenpud et al. (1994). The effect of transplant center volume on cardiac transplant outcome. A report of the United Network for Organ Sharing Scientific Registry. *JAMA, 271*, 1844–1849.

Hosenpud et al. (2000). The Registry of the International Society for Heart and Lung Transplantation: Seventeenth Official Report 2000. *J Heart Lung Transplant, 19*, 909–931.

Hunt, S. A. (1993). 24th Bethesda Conference: Cardiac Transplantation. *J Am Coll Cardiol., 22*(1), 1–64.

Hunt et al. (1998). Frazier OH. Mechanical circulatory support and cardiac transplantation. *Circulation, 97*, 2079–2090.

Kimura, R. (1998). Organ transplantation and brain death in Japan. Cultural, legal, and bioethical background. *Ann Transplant, 3*, 55–58.

Koop, C. E. (1999). The top ten issues in health care today. In: D. C. Grossman & H. Valtin (Eds), Great issues for medicine in the twenty-first century: ethical and social issues arising out of advances in the biomedical sciences. *Ann N Y Acad Sci., 882*, 137–141.

Laks, H. (1997). The alternative recipient list for heart transplantation: does it work? *J Heart Lung Transplant., 16*, 735–742.

Laffel et al. The Relationship between Experience and Outcome in Heart Transplantation. *N. Engl J Med., 327*, 1220–1225.

Lee, C. J. (1996). Organ transplantation in Taiwan. *Artif Organs, 20*, 1270–1273.

Marshall et al. (1998). Cultural and psychological dimensions of human organ transplantation. *Ann Transplant., 3*, 7–11.

Messmer et al. (1969). Survival-times after cardiac allografts. *Lancet*, 954–956.

Miranda, B. (1998). International issues in transplantation: setting the scene and flagging the most urgent and controversial issues. In: J. Fishman, D. Sachs & R. Shaikh (Eds), Xenotransplantation: scientific frontiers and public policy. *Ann N Y Acad Sci., 862*, 129–143.

Miller et al. (1995). Medical management of heart and lung failure and candidate selection: Report of the consensus conference on candidate selection for heart transplantation – 1993. *J Heart Lung Transplant., 14*, 562–571.

Miller, L. W. (1998). Listing criteria for cardiac transplantation: results of an American Society of Transplant Physicians-National Institutes of Health conference. *Transplantation, 66*, 947–951.

OĆonnell et al. (1992). Cardiac Transplantation: Recipient Selection, Donor Procurement, and Medical Followup. *Circulation, 86*, 1061–1079.

Oppell et al. (1994). Heart transplantation – historical perspective and the need for a national policy. *S Afr Med J., 84*, 594–596.

Pavie et al. (1996). Cardiac transplantation: lack of donor organs. current status. *Arch Mal Coeur Vaiss, 89*, 43–46.

Price, D. P. (1997). Organ transplant initiatives: the twilight zone. *J Med Ethics, 23*, 170–175.

Puruhito, A. (1998). Availability and limits of intermediate cardiovascular technology. *Artif Organs, 22*, 237–242.

Renlund et al. (1987). Medicare-designated centres for cardiac transplantation. *N Engl J Med., 316*, 873–876.

Richtlinien zur Organtransplantation gemaess Paragraph 16 Transplantationsgesetz. Dt Aerztebl (2000). 97:B–352-B–367.

Roncone et al. (1996). Organ procurement: experience from a southern Italian region. *Transplant Proc., 28*, 239–241.

Rowinski et al. (1996). Factors limiting renal transplantation programs in Poland. *Ann Transplant., 1*, 18–22.

Scheld et al. (1994). Cost-effectiveness relationship in cardiac transplantation. *Z Kardiol., 83* (Suppl 6), 139–149.

Schmid et al. (1999). Impact of "local donor" and "regionalization" on a German transplantation center. *Transplant Int., 12*, 141–144.

Schneiderman, L. J., & Jecker, N. S. (1996). Should a criminal receive a heart transplant? Medical justice vs. social justice. *Theor Med., 17*, 33–44.

Shumway, N. E. (1993). Cardiac transplantation. *J Am Coll Cardiol., 22*, 6–7.

Tagaki, H. (1997). Organ transplants still too few in Japan and Asian countries. *Transplant Proc., 29*, 1580–1583.

Thompson, T. (1971). The tragic record of heart transplants: the year they changed hearts. *Life Magazine*, Sept 17, 56–70.

Tong, M. C. (1992). The establishment of a heart transplant program in Singapore. Presentation at the 1st International Congress on Transplantation in Developing Countries. Singapore.

Ubel, P. A., & Caplan, A. L. (1998). Geographic favoritism in liver transplantation – unfortunate or unfair (Sounding Board)? *N Engl J Med., 339*, 1322–1325.

Uexküll, T. V. (1994). Psychosomatic medicine (1st English edition). Urban & Schwarzenberg, Baltimore, 1997.

Watanabe, Y. Why do I stand against the movement for cardiac transplantation in Japan? *Jpn Heart J., 35*, 701–714.

Weatherall, D. (1999). The conflict between the science and the art of clinical practice in the next millenium. In: D. C. Grossman & H. Valtin (Eds), Great issues for medicine in the twenty-first century: ethical and social issues arising out of advances in the biomedical sciences. *Ann N Y Acad Sci., 882*, 240–246.

World Heart Federation (WHF) White Book (Editors Chockalingam A, and Balaguer-Vintro I) (1999). Impending global pandemic of cardiovascular diseases. *Prous Science*, Geneva, Switzerland.

11. THE RELIGIOUS AND SPIRITUAL PERSPECTIVE TOWARD HUMAN ORGAN DONATION AND TRANSPLANTATION

Laurence J. O'Connell

I. INTRODUCTION

Organ donation and transplantation continue to attract significant attention, especially in the fields of bioethics, medicine, law, and the humanities. Policy debates swirl around this highly charged area, commanding extensive media coverage and exciting wide-ranging public discussion (Milford, 1998). There are no simple answers. Embracing so many deeply personal, socially complex, and culturally ambiguous aspects of our humanity, transplantation taps into our deepest aspirations, while also playing into some of our most primal anxieties. It takes hold of us and inevitably draws us into the deepest recesses of our humanity, giving rise to very fundamental questions. What does it mean to repair and rebuild people through organ replacement? How do such practices resonate with our moral intuitions and commonly accepted standards of human decency and decorum.

Such basic questions inevitably intersect with the realm of religious speculation and spiritual sensibilities. Religious and spiritual traditions, after all, "strive to give symbolic access and concrete visibility to the deepest levels of human existence, especially at critical turning points like terminal illness and death, when the search for meaning becomes intense" (O'Connell, 1995).

The Ethics of Organ Transplantation, Volume 7, pages 277–292.

ISBN: 0-7623-0764-1

When persons confront the removal and re-implantation of human organs, either their own or someone else's, religiously motivated questions often move to the foreground as compelling and powerfully present considerations. How is such a procedure consistent with the Divine Plan? Is it legitimate stewardship or an affront to divine intentions? How does it square with the religious convictions of those who deny that life ends with physical death? Is the noble purpose of helping to save someone else's life possibly a defilement of one's own body? These and many other questions arise when religious individuals and communities confront the possibility of organ donation and transplantation (see Dorff, 1996 (2)). And, as specifically religious and spiritual perspectives on donation and transplantation are generated, they are directly or indirectly fed back into the broader cultural and socio-economic context. Their impact on public policy, then, should be neither underestimated nor ignored.

So an accounting of religious and spiritual perspectives constitutes an essential part of any comprehensive treatment of ethical issues in organ donation and transplantation. Obviously, religious and spiritual perspectives will influence moral attitudes towards transplantation. And these attitudes will in turn inform individual and communal judgments about what is ethically right or wrong, good or bad. It is important, then, to understand the character and dynamics of religious and spiritual conviction within the context of transplantation.

II. THE WORKINGS OF RELIGIOUS AND SPIRITUAL TRADITIONS

Religious and spiritual traditions play an important role in shaping the self-understanding of individuals and communities by creating frameworks for describing and interpreting human life and destiny. As mediators of self-understanding, religious and spiritual perspectives create markers of individual and communal identity. The meaning of health and healing, for instance, emerges from fundamental beliefs about human life and its relationship to whatever one considers divine. As Martin E. Marty has pointed out, "while each health-seeking individual is likely to improvise in order to meet current needs, he or she will tend to draw on a repertory of options made available in a spiritual heritage" (Marty, 1986). Approaches to organ donation and transplantation are then often quite naturally shaped by religious and spiritual perspectives. Japan provides a good example of how these religious and spiritual perspectives play and spill over into the thinking of the general public.

In Japan, the approach to organ donation and transplantation clearly resonates with traditional religious and spiritual beliefs. The lines connecting contemporary resistance to organ transplantation in Japan and traditional religious beliefs can hardly be denied (Lock, 1996). Three religious traditions still influence Japanese life and beliefs, i.e. Confucianism, Shintoism, and Buddhism. Each in its own way contributes to Japanese reluctance to embrace the technologically aided extension of human life. Confucianism, the ethical tradition on which Japanese social life was grounded for many centuries, prohibits all tampering with dead bodies. Organ procurement and transplantation are thus ruled out as a matter of principle. And adherents of Shinto, the indigenous religion of Japan, regard all contact with death as polluting; so again organ procurement would be religiously objectionable and something to be avoided. Finally, the Buddhist tradition, which is quite prominent in Japan, holds that dying is not complete until post mortem services are held on the seventh and forty-ninth days. This practice offers philosophical resistance to the speedy removal of organs. Further complicating the prospect of taking organs is the Buddhist practice of engaging in a years-long process of converting dead relatives into ancestors. In a culture where actual death is not over and done with in a clinical split second, organ donation and transplantation can be an unsettling prospect.

Specific religious values and more general cultural values take shape within traditions. The word tradition is rooted in the Latin word, "tradere," i.e. to hand over. Traditions are all about handing over the lived experience of individuals and communities, handing over from one generation to another a basic view of the world and how one engages it. Tradition is the reservoir of customs, norms, and values that integrate individuals into families, communities, professions, religious congregations, and indeed nations. In each succeeding generation a tradition remains the same, yet different. In other words, a tradition grows and develops; it builds upon the living past in light of current circumstances. Contemporary cultural influences – advances in medical technology, for instance – find their way into religious circles and open them to new ways of understanding. In light of contemporary circumstances, practices, which have been forbidden in the past, may gradually become acceptable. Consequently, most of the world's major religious traditions have found ways and means of accommodating organ donation and transplantation. Few religious traditions prohibit transplantation outright, yet several are marked by lingering hesitancy. In general, though, there seems to be more and more receptivity to the practice. The varying sensitivities of religious traditions about organ procurement and transplantation are best illustrated by reviewing a range of current opinions. In these examples, generalities about religious and spiritual influences become concrete and clearly identifiable.

III. RELIGIOUS PERSPECTIVES ON ORGAN DONATION AND TRANSPLANTATION

African American Churches

The African Methodist Episcopal and African Methodist Episcopal Zion churches view organ and tissue donation as an act of neighborly love and charity. They encourage all members to support donation as a way of helping others (see www.transweb.org).

Anabaptist

Mennonites do not have a formal position on organ donation, but they are not opposed to it. They tend to leave decisions about organ donation up to the individual and/or his or her family, but they are concerned about larger social justice issues. Theological principles that guide their consideration of organ donation include those of stewardship and mutual aid. The *Mennonite Mutual Aid Organ Transplant Task Force* has issued a statement raising social justice concerns about the expensive and resource-intensive nature of the procedures. They also expressed concerns about the efficacy of these procedures, given the critical nature of the underlying condition and the associated risks and side effects of the surgery itself. For these reasons, the task force recommended that transplants not be considered a health care priority. The Amish approve of organ transplantation, but raise questions about the effectiveness of the procedures. They are inclined to approve the procedure in cases where the recipient would clearly benefit, but they are reluctant where the outcome is questionable. The Church of the Brethren has issued resolutions supporting and encouraging organ donation in order to help others out of love for Christ (DuBose, 1996 (1)).

Baptist

The Baptist churches do not have official statements on organ donation, but they support organ donation as an act of charity. They actively encourage their members to become organ donors, but the decision to donate is ultimately left up to the individual. The more conservative Southern Baptist Conference has, through its *Southern Baptist Ethics and Religious Liberty Commission*, opposed the use of fetal tissue for transplantation. It has also called for a permanent, worldwide ban on the cloning of entire human beings, but it does support the production of tissue and organs for transplantation. It has also criticized policies that would deny organ transplants to some people based on an assessment of inadequate, post-operative quality of life due to lifestyle, disability, and other conditions (see www.transweb.org; Strode, 1999).

Buddhism

While Buddhism emphasizes compassion and the elimination of suffering, Buddhism is not particularly concerned with the body, which it views as transitory in nature. No part of the body, living or dead is considered intrinsically sacrosanct or holy and there are no prescribed rituals for the disposition of the dead body. Official Buddhist response to the issue has been negligible in most cases. Varying Buddhist analyses of brain death, which must be established prior to harvesting organs, demonstrate tensions within the tradition itself. Some Buddhist arguments, for example, emphasize the body's development from an original mass, such that no particular organ like the brain should take priority in determining death. Given this lack of hierarchy, some would argue that the dissipation of heat after the last breath favors criteria based upon the cessation of cardio-pulmonary activity rather than brain death criteria. Other Buddhists begin with the concept of the human being as a storehouse of consciousness, arguing that consciousness is the only reality and that its loss, along with the accompanying loss of integrated functioning and social relationships, is equivalent to death. They are thus quite comfortable with the brain death criteria. It should be noted that there is no official consensus among Buddhist communities as to the determination of death or the permissibility of organ donation and transplantation. Overall, there is little in the Buddhist tradition specifically to affirm organ transplantation, but most Buddhist communities permit organ donation as a matter of individual conscience and consider it an act of compassion and generosity that can serve as a condition for realizing nirvana (Sagunasisri, 1990; Hardacre, 1994).

Christian Church (Disciples of Christ)

The church does not prohibit organ and tissue donation, but considers it a personal decision to be made in conjunction with family and medical personnel (see www.transweb.org).

Christian Science

Christian Scientists reject organ transplantation for the same reasons that they reject other forms of medical treatment. These reasons are premised in a theology that views the material world as a construct of the human mind, and that sin, sickness, and disharmony can be overcome through a deeper understanding of divine truth (Harris-Abbott, 1996 (1)).

Episcopal Church

The Episcopal Church has passed several resolutions recognizing the life-giving benefits of organ, blood, and tissue donation. It encourages its members to become organ, blood, and tissue donors as part of ministry to others in the name of Christ. The church emphasizes that the decision to donate should be made well ahead of time to ensure prompt donation. Its *Standing Commission on Human Affairs and Health* has raised questions about the moral permissibility of attempts to avoid death and the risk to living donors. Accordingly, it has recommended careful reflection about the issue (DuBose, 1996 (2)).

Evangelical Christian

The Assembly of God church has no official policy on organ and tissue donation, but is strongly supportive of organ donation. The decision to donate is left largely up to the individual. Pentecostal churches also support organ donation as an individual choice (see www.transweb.org).

Hinduism

In practice, Hindus are said to permit organ donation and transplantation as a matter of individual choice. The issue does, however, seem to be somewhat problematic within the tradition. Some Hindus argue that having a part of one's body remain alive forestalls the achievement of spiritual liberation, or nirvana. This concern is said to underlie the Hindu requirement of cremation and to prohibit cloning. The same concern about karmic entanglement in the attainment of nirvana is said to apply in the cases of organ donation and even the donation of blood (Hinduism Today, 1997; Amritanandamayi, 1997; Subramuniyaswami, 1999).

Islam

Muslims generally approve of organ donation and transplantation out of a belief in the principle of saving human lives, but the issue is not unproblematic within the tradition. Concerns about organ donation and transplantation in Islam stem, first of all, from the tradition's emphasis on the integral relationship of body and soul and the doctrine of bodily resurrection on the Day of Judgment. According to the latter doctrine, God has the power to bring the dead back to life to account for their deeds. Some Muslims consider the concern about bodily integrity and the requirement that one be whole before God to be a constraint, if not an outright prohibition, on the donation of organs. These concerns are also reflected in the Islamic practice of burying a person as soon as possible after death and the prohibition against mutilating or cremating the dead body. While compassion for others and responsibility to family and community may serve as arguments for organ donation in Islam, some Islamic scholars raise concerns that the social indebtedness of a recipient to a living donor may be morally problematic. Despite these concerns, Islam approves of organ donation in most circumstances. Donation from a living donor is approved when the donor's consent is obtained in advance and in writing and the probability of saving the recipient's life is substantially greater than the risk to the donor's life or health. Where the donation is from a cadaver, Islamic law requires the will and testament of the decedent or the unequivocal permission of the family. Some Islamic jurists argue that, in the case of donation from a Muslim to a non-Muslim, there should be a condition providing that the organ will be separately buried if the recipient is cremated at the end of life. The tradition is clear that donors should not receive payment for their organs (Sachedina, 1988; Waugh, 1999).

Jehovah's Witnesses

Jehovah's Witnesses find no direct warrant for or against organ donation and transplantation in the Bible, so decisions about donation and transplantation are left to the individual. Because of their adherence to the biblical command to "abstain from blood" and their belief in the special ritual and symbolic meaning of blood in their relationship with God, Jehovah's Witnesses do require that transplanted organs be completely drained of blood so as not to result in a transfusion of the recipient. Organ transplants are thought to be different from blood transfusions, since they do not have the capacity to suppress the recipient's own immune system. Jehovah's Witnesses have also expressed concerns about the possibility of contracting HIV and other blood-borne diseases from donated organs. Otherwise, Jehovah's Witnesses do not make distinctions between living or cadaveric donors, nor do they appear to have taken any positions on the use or organs from anencephalic newborns or human fetuses (DuBose, 1995 (1)).

Judaism

The two principles that govern Jewish consideration of organ donation and transplantation are the principle of honoring the dead (kavod ha-met) and the principle of saving life (pikkuah nefesh). The Jewish prohibitions against desecration of the dead, deriving benefit from the dead, and delaying burial do not, as is sometimes thought, constitute a barrier to organ donation. There is some variation in treatment of this issue, with Orthodox raising more objections to organ donation than their Conservative, Reform, and Reconstructionist counterparts. In general, Judaism permits organ donation as an act of special kindness (hesed), and it may even consider donation a positive moral obligation (hovah) and an honor to the deceased person when transplantation would save a life. Indeed, absent an advance directive, the default assumption is that a person would have wanted to donate organs, so as to help another person live. The definition of "saving a life" is broad, and it includes the transplantation of corneas, since the restoration of the crucial sense of sight is considered life-saving in nature. In the case of living donors, the tradition requires that Jews preserve their own lives, thus they are encouraged to donate only where the procedure can be accomplished without major risk to their own life or health. Though the default assumption is that a cadaveric donor would have wanted his or her organs to be used to save another's life, some rabbis adhere to a restrictive requirement that there be a specific patient before them (lefaneinu) who would benefit and that the person's life or an entire physical faculty be at stake. Most rabbis, however, would expand both the eligibility of potential recipients and the causes for which an organ may be taken. All Jewish authorities insist that the family agree to the donation of their loved one's organs. Since the traditional determination of death through cessation of breathing and heartbeat, would rule out the harvesting of some organs, some Conservative rabbis have allowed, over the objection of some of their Orthodox counterparts, the cessation of spontaneous brain activity to be the determining factor. The use of animal organs is also permitted within Judaism, and they do not even have to come from a kosher animal, since saving a life takes precedence over dietary laws. The use of animal or artificial organ would also eliminate any problems with determining the time of death, and solve some of the significant social justice issues in organ donation by providing more and cheaper sources of organs (Dorff, 1996 (1); Kroot, www.transweb.org).

Latter Day Saints

The LDS tradition permits and supports organ donation and transplantation. Both the Church of Jesus Christ of Latter-Day Saints and the Reorganized Church of Jesus Christ of Latter Day Saints deem this to be an individual decision made in conjunction with family and medical personnel, and that it should be confirmed through prayer. The LDS tradition emphasizes the importance of the body for salvation, the body's status as an essential part of the soul, and that the experience of bodily life on earth for salvation and eternal life with Jesus Christ – all of which might suggest that the tradition would have reservations about organ donation and transplantation. However, the LDS faith is also premised on a belief that earthly bodies perish and believers will be given new, spiritual bodies at the resurrection, which would relativize the importance of the earthly body after death. While procurement of tissue and organs from living fetuses would be considered an unacceptable interference with their eternal progression toward the embodiment that is necessary for salvation, organs may be taken from severely deformed and/or anencephalic children, provided that the action does not hasten death. In such cases, the fact that the child has attained embodiment, however short the duration, is considered sufficient for salvation (Harris-Abbott, 1995).

Lutheran

Both the Evangelical Lutheran Church in America (ELCA) and the Lutheran Church-Missouri Synod (LCMS) affirm organ donation as a contribution to the well-being of humanity and as an expression of sacrificial love for a neighbor in need stewardship of life's resources. The ELCA calls on its pastors to include as part of its healing and stewardship education ministries active discussion and education on organ donations, within the context of respect for the sanctity of life. Lutheran congregations encourage their members to consider donation and to make necessary family, legal, and medical arrangements to permit donation in case of death, particularly through signing Universal Donor Cards. The LCMS would, however, object to the procurement of organs from anencephalic newborns or human fetuses, if death were the result (Evangelical Lutheran Church of America, 1989; Harris-Abbott, 1996 (2)).

Orthodox Christian

The Orthodox Christian believes in the wholeness of human beings, respect for the human body, and the need to preserve the integrity of a person's bodily life. The tradition does not oppose organ donation and transplantation, provided that the procedures are intended to contribute to the restoration of health, are motivated by philanthropy and concern for the welfare of both recipient and donor, are the result of genuine and uncoerced decision on the part of the donor, and are done in such a way that the body remains intact for Orthodox burial rites. Donation of the entire body to science for experimentation and research is not permitted within the tradition (Harakas, 1999).

Presbyterian

The Presbyterian Church (USA) supports and encourages organ donation to save life, improve health, and improve quality of life. It is also thought to be a positive outcome of a seemingly senseless death and source of comfort to family members of the deceased. The church does not accept the abortion of fetuses solely to obtain parts for transplantation (Harris-Abbott, 1996 (3)).

Roman Catholic

The Roman Catholic tradition encourages organ donation as a noble and meritorious act of charity and human solidarity, particularly when motivated by the compassionate principle of neighbor love. Pope John Paul II has been particularly supportive of organ donation, which he frames theologically in the concept of gift. Donation is a very personal decision made by the donor with free and informed consent; however, it should not deprive the donor of life or the integrity of an organ system. Under the moral theological principle of proportionality, there should be an acceptable proportion between the good of the recipient and the harm of the donor. Church teaching on organ transplantation and respect for the dignity of the human person would prohibit the removal of organs from living, anencephalic children and human fetuses, especially where removal would cause the child's death. Though the church would not permit the use of anencephalic children merely as a source of organs, it would allow the use of organs from anencephalic newborns that have died. The church also condemns the use of fetal tissue in scientific experimentation and the sale of organs as a reductive, materialist, and instrumental use of the person (Hamel, 1996; Teo, 1992).

Seventh Day Adventist

The Seventh Day Adventist tradition strongly encourages organ donation out of a belief in the centrality to their faith of helping and serving others. The Adventist-owned Loma Linda University in California, in fact, has been a pioneer in organ transplantation surgeries, including infant heart transplant surgery, using the hearts of anencephalic infants in some cases. The university has a Transplantation Institute, which continues to do cutting edge research in this area. Adventist philanthropic organizations and congregations have also been instrumental in raising funds to bring needy people around the world to North America for organ transplants (DuBose, 1996 (3)).

Shinto

The Shinto tradition, native to Japan, is premised on the idea of the dualism of body and soul. The Shinto tradition considers the dead body to be impure, dangerous, and very powerful. Folk customs prohibits the injuring of a dead body. There is also particular concern within the tradition about injuring relations between the dead person and his or her grieving relatives. Death rituals include customs that attempt to call the soul back to the body and allow for a waiting period in order to determine that the soul will not return to the body. While death is considered to be the point at which the soul leaves the body, death rituals recognize the continuing attachment of the deceased's relatives to his or her body and their need for these funereal rituals aimed at launching the soul on a new journey. Shinto followers deem the injury to the body in organ donation procedures to be a violation of filial piety and their duty to treat the bodies of the deceased with stewardship and care. The Shinto tradition, while not forbidding organ donation in any formal or official way, is very solicitous of the concerns of the survivors and is usually viewed as clearly opposed or extremely cautious about organ donation. These religious and cultural factors have made it difficult to obtain consent from bereaved families for organ donation or dissection for medical or scientific research in Japan (Hardacre, 1994).

Society of Friends

The Society of Friends does not have an official statement on organ donation, but Friends generally support organ and tissue donation as an individual decision (see www.transweb.org).

Unitarian Universalist

The Unitarian Universalist denomination has no official statement on organ donation, but its members widely support organ and tissue donation as an act of love and selfless giving (see www.transweb.org).

United Church of Christ

The United Church of Christ has not made any official statements on organ donation and transplantation, but it supports and encourages organ donation as stewardship of the gift of life. It has expressed concern about social justice issues in organ donation and transplantation and about the relatively low rate or organ donation among people of color (Nehring, 1999).

United Methodist

The United Methodist Church officially encourages donation as a part of love and ministry to others in need and urges pastoral care persons to explore these options as a normal part of conversation with patients and families. Paragraph 66 of the 1996 edition of the Book of Discipline, the church's major statement of doctrine, recognizes the life-giving benefits of organ and tissue donation and encourages donation as an act of charity, agape love, and self-sacrifice for another, a source of comfort for survivors, and a positive outcome of what might otherwise seem to be a senseless death. Its only concerns are that the procedure does not hasten death, is carried out using reliable criteria for death, and that request of family members are made in an environment of respect for the deceased or living donor and for the benefit of the recipient and following protocols which will carefully prevent abuse to the donor and their family. The church participates in National Donor Sabbaths organized by the Department of Transplantation at Health and Human Services to dispel some of the myths about organ donation and religious perspectives on it (DuBose, 1995 (2); United Methodist Church, 1996).

IV. THE CENTRAL POSITION OF RELIGIOUS AND SPIRITUAL PERSPECTIVES

The foregoing review of twenty-three religious traditions underscores the variety and delicate shading of opinion with reference to the retrieval and transplantation of human organs. The generous spirit, yet haunting hesitancy of many religious traditions should come as no surprise. Religious traditions, as we pointed out, are the vessels of unfolding insight into the deepest recesses of human life and destiny. These traditions, while seeking to support good and decent behavior, also experience the weight of precedent and already-received wisdom. Put simply, they tend to move into the future with an eye to the past.

Although the insistence and reliance of religious individuals and groups on traditional moorings sometimes frustrate the more impetuous secular and scientific communities, they can and often do play a pivotal role in the reasoned advance of societies. And in any case, whether or not they are a welcome voice in scientific conversation and public discourse, they always seem to make their way to the forefront of debate. For example, as the field of genetics advances, especially in the area of cloning not only of animals but specific body parts, the voice of religious traditions will undoubtedly make themselves heard.

The particular relevance of religious and spiritual perspectives to the general debate about the moral propriety, practical advisability, and social impact of organ transplantation takes a very different turn when individuals and families personally confront the specter of inevitable death. Yet, despite – and perhaps because of – the existential dread associated with sober thoughts of mortality, the prospect of transplantation almost always excites religious sensibilities in a country like the United States where more than ninety percent of the population claims to be believers. The moral imagination and practical reach of the American people still slosh about in the religious breeding pool of the Republic's birth.

Anyone who has worked with those who have been forced to contemplate the possibility of donating the organs of loved ones has encountered the pervasive influence of religious and spiritual perspectives. Specifically religious or more general spiritual themes emerge quite naturally, often in secular dress but nonetheless religiously resonant. Stewardship, charity, and co-creative duty are the most commonly mentioned religious themes that help families overcome their reluctance and even revulsion at considering retrieval and donation. A quick review of the twenty-three religious traditions reviewed above will reveal the prominence of these three themes.

There is something very deep within the human spirit that recoils at the idea of taking organs (see Youngner et al., 1996). Religious and spiritual perspectives help people to contextualize and universalize what is experienced as a uniquely personal and deeply private event. Often, religious and spiritual perspectives move inconsolable and self-centered pain to a place where incipient grief can take hold and healing can begin, especially in cases where young children or adolescents die unexpectedly. Family members fall back upon their beliefs to find meaning and some consolation. In offering organs for donation, they feel that there is some higher good served by the unexplained and enigmatic death of a youngster, for example. Their religious beliefs or general spiritual inclinations provide a framework for understanding and action.

These beliefs also provide specific moral guidance or an ethical vision that many people find reassuring. The normative guidance afforded by religious doctrine or less prescriptive spiritual belief systems often provides support for the notion that one is doing the right thing. And it also helps assuage guilt that can often develop in the wake of a failed attempt or unanticipated outcomes of a successful transplantation. For everyone involved, life after transplantation is sometimes every bit as emotionally harrowing, physically stressful, and morally ambiguous as pre-implantation. Religious and spiritual resources are thus often in high demand and richly appreciated by many people.

V. CONCLUSION

Religious and spiritual perspectives can help in understanding and navigating the mental, moral, social, and medical eddies that swirl about the constellation of issues related to organ transplantation. There are no simple and unequivocal answers. Each person, each community, and indeed each nation will seek out culturally attuned and morally responsible responses to the fundamentally ambiguous practice of repairing and rebuilding people through organ replacement. Religious and spiritual points of view cannot make absolute claims on where the truth may or may not lie. History, however, has proven – despite some glaring evidence to the contrary – that religious and spiritual insight can disclose dimensions of our shared humanity that might otherwise go unnoticed or untapped. It is this positive role and inherent potential that should illumine the inescapable influence of religion and spirituality on the web of complicated issues that surround organ retrieval and transplantation.

REFERENCES

Amritanandamayi, M. (1997). Hindu Spiritual Leaders Respond to the Question of Whether the Cloning of Human Beings is Ethically Permissible According to Sanatana Dharma. *Hinduism Today.*

Dorff, E. (1996 (1)). *The Jewish Tradition: Religious Beliefs and Health Care Decisions*, 12–13.

Dorff, E. (1996 (2)). *In Organ Transplantation: Meanings and Realities*, 168–193.

DuBose, E. R. (1995 (1)). *The Jehovah's Witness Tradition: Religious Beliefs and Health Care*, 5.

DuBose, E. R. (1995 (2)). *The United Methodist Tradition: Religious Beliefs and Health Care*, 4.

DuBose, E. R. (1996 (1)). *The Anabaptist Tradition: Religious Beliefs and Health Care Decisions*, 4–5.

DuBose, E. R. (1996 (2)). *The Episcopal Tradition: Religious Beliefs and Health Care Decisions*, 7.

DuBose, E. R. (1996 (3)). *The Seventh-Day Adventist Tradition: Religious Beliefs and Health Care*, 5.

Evangelical Lutheran Church in America. Division for Church in Society. "Organ Donation." Assembly Action CA89.7.72 (1989).

Hamel, R. (1996). *The Roman Catholic Tradition: Religious Beliefs and Health Care Decisions*, 13–14.

Harakas, S. S. (1999). *The Orthodox Christian Tradition: Religious Beliefs and Health Care Decisions*, 7.

Hardacre, H. (1994). Response of Buddhism and Shinto to the Issue of Brain Death and Organ Transplant. *Cambridge Quarterly of Healthcare Ethics*, *3*(4), 585–601.

Harris-Abbott, D. (1995). *The Latter-Day Saints Tradition: Religious Beliefs and Health Care Decisions*, 11.

Harris-Abbott, D. (1996 (1)). *The Christian Science Tradition: Religious Beliefs and Health Care Decisions*, 6.

Harris-Abbott, D. (1996 (2)). *The Lutheran Tradition: Religious Beliefs and Health Care Decisions*, 9.

Harris-Abbott, D. (1996 (3)). *The Presbyterian Tradition: Religious Beliefs and Health Care Decisions Center*, 5–6.

Kroot, K. *A Jewish Perspective on Organ Transplantation*. At www.transweb.org/reference/articles/religion/shalomarticle.html

Lock, M. (1986). In: *Organ Transplantation: Meanings and Realities*, pp. 142–167.

Marty, M. E. In: R. L. Numbers & D. W. Amundsen (Eds), *Caring and Curing: Health and Medicine in the Western Religious Traditions* (p. viii). New York: Macmillan Publishing Company.

Milford, E. L. (1998). Organ Transplantation – Barriers, Outcomes, and Evolving Policies. *Journal of the American Medical Association*, *280*, 13, 1184–1185.

Nehring, A. K. (1999). *United Church of Christ: Religious Beliefs and Health Care Decisions*. Chicago: Park Ridge Center,.

O'Connell, L. J. (1995). Religious Dimensions of Dying and Death. *The Western Journal of Medicine*, *163*, 232.

Sachedina, A. A. (1988). Islamic Views on Organ Transplantation. *Transplantation Proceedings*, *20*(1), Suppl. 1 (February), 1084–1088.

Sagunasisri, S. H. J. (1990). The Buddhist View Concerning the Dead Body. *Transplantation Proceedings*, *22*, 3 (June) 947–949.

Satguru Sivaya Subramuniyaswami. How Do You Know? (February 18, 1999) (cybertalk on karmic entanglements of organ and blood donation from Kauai's Hindu Monastery, U.S.A) at http://www.gurudeva.dynip.com/~htoday/today/Archives/Past/1999/February/February181999/satguruspeaks.html

Strode, T. (1999). Reports of Trade in Fetal Body Parts Fuel Call for Congressional Hearings. *Baptist Press* (November 15).

Teo, B. (1992). Organ Donation and Transplantation: A Christian Viewpoint. *Transplantation Proceedings*, *24*(5) (October), 2114–15.

Transweb.org website at <http://www.transweb.org/qa/qa_txp/faq_religion.html>

A Hindu Perspective for the President, Mr. Bill Clinton: Hindu Spiritual Leaders Offer Their Faith's Unique Voice to the Ethical Debate on Human Cloning. *Hinduism Today* (April 7, 1997).

United Methodist Church. (1996). Organ Transplantation and Donation. In: *The Book of Discipline*. Nashville, TN: United Methodist Publishing House. Par. 66R.

Waugh, E. H. (1999). *The Islamic Tradition: Religious Beliefs and Health Care Decisions*. Chicago: Park Ridge Center. 12–13.

Youngner, S. J., Fox, R. C., & O'Connell, L. J. (1966). *Organ Transplantation: Meanings and Realities*. Madison: Wisc.: University of Wisconsin Press.

12. THE ROLE AND RESPONSIBILITY OF THE MEDIA IN RELATION TO ORGAN DONATION AND TRANSPLANTATION

Elisa J. Gordon

INTRODUCTION

In 1997, local and national news media alerted the public to The Cleveland Clinic's ethically questionable protocol to procure organs from non-heart-beating donors (NHBD) by "hastening death." The transplant community believed that the media's reports were sensationalized and that they chilled local willingness to donate. Consequently, the transplant community made efforts to ameliorate the resulting public distrust (Mazzolini, 1997).

This chapter explores how transplant professionals' fear of sensationalized news media coverage influences their decisions when they anticipate public controversy over unusual transplant situations. American cultural values, reinforced by news media, have provided the public with a negative opinion about controversial transplant issues. Maintaining a favorable public opinion about transplantation is important since it can influence organ donation practices (Slapak, 1997; Slapak et al., 1997). This chapter contends that transplant physicians' treatment decisions based on the fear of the media may pose a serious ethical problem in the form of rationing at the bedside. In the context of scarce organs for transplantation, physicians must decide to protect

The Ethics of Organ Transplantation, Volume 7, pages 293–315.

ISBN: 0-7623-0764-1

either the interests of their patients or the interests of their hospital and transplant community.

This ethical dilemma is explored through one case analysis which highlights how historical, political, cultural, and economic factors influenced one transplant team's decision making about placing a foreign national patient on the national transplant waiting list. To understand the impact of the news media on the transplant team's decisions, I review the ethical and legal status of foreign nationals seeking transplants, and of the media's coverage of transplant issues. The chapter then presents an ethical analysis of choices transplant professionals can make in the context of media attention. I argue that it is unethical for transplant physicians in the U.S. to turn away foreign nationals before reaching the legal limit on transplanting them.

THE UNITED NETWORK FOR ORGAN SHARING (UNOS) POLICY ON TRANSPLANTING FOREIGN NATIONALS

A growing international demand for transplantable organs has led to a worldwide exodus in search of available kidneys. In most countries, the demand for kidneys far outnumbers the supply because of various factors, including: (a) cultural or ethnic beliefs against donating organs, as among the Japanese and African Americans (Lock, 1996; Callendar et al., 1982), (b) a lack of well-organized infrastructures to procure organs (Land & Cohen, 1992), and (c) clinical practices that undermine presumed consent policies (Caplan, 1984). Many people with end-stage renal disease now seek kidneys outside of their own country (Ikels, 1997; Bandini et al., 1991). However, the local responses to foreigners in their quest for kidneys cannot always be characterized as welcome. Anecdotal evidence shows that foreign patients are sometimes turned away from transplant lists partly because of xenophobic policies and beliefs (Gordon, 1999).

The United States' policy on this issue, as stipulated by UNOS, allows transplant centers to transplant up to 5% of their yearly volume on foreign patients (both resident aliens and foreigners) (UNOS, 1997). While kidney recipients in the U.S. pay for the transplant surgery and hospital stay through Medicare, Medicaid, or private insurance, foreigners pay by cash up front. The financial incentive to transplant many foreign patients constitutes one reason why there is a 5% cap.

Despite the UNOS policy, bioethicists and transplant professionals continue to debate the pros and cons of allowing foreign nationals access to American transplant waiting lists. Proponents of transplanting foreign nationals contend that people are equally deserving of a chance to preserve their life through organ transplants (Davis, 1993). The central reason for limiting the number of foreign nationals who may receive organ transplants in the U.S. is that 'they' take a limited resource away from Americans (Office of Inspector General, 1986). An organ that goes to a foreigner is one less organ that goes to an American. Some scholars posit that Americans should get American kidneys first because they are members of a "giving community" that donates organs (Prottas, 1986; Jonasson, 1986). Scholars also justify an Americans first position because, as citizens and residents, Americans pay taxes which subsidize the costs of public education campaigns encouraging organ donation and of organ acquisition (Prottas, 1986; Jonasson, 1986).

Foreigners who seek transplants in the U.S. benefit or suffer from inequality in access to transplantation based on their financial means. The value of fairness that is woven in the UNOS allocation system (i.e. equal access to all regardless of financial capacity to pay) is undermined when foreigners seek kidney transplants in the U.S. If foreigners do not have enough resources, then they have no access to American organs.

Another key factor limiting transplants to foreign nationals is the assumption held by the transplant community that Americans will stop donating organs if they perceive the allocation system as unfair. Accordingly, a 1986 report, The Access of Foreign Nationals to U.S. Cadaver Organs, stated that:

> Organ donation in the U.S. rests on a fragile foundation. People donate organs with the assumption that the system for distributing them will be a fair one. When they learn that foreign nationals receive organs instead of U.S. residents and that they generally do so in a shorter period of time, they begin to question the fairness of that system and may very well become less inclined to donate. Indeed, in some communities where there has been much publicity about foreign nationals receiving transplanted kidneys, there has been a subsequent reduction in donation levels (Office of Inspector General, 1986).

UNOS and transplant professionals place considerable emphasis on ensuring the fairness of the allocation system since without organ donations, many people's lives would be lost. The transplant community – made up of health care and public relations professionals involved in donation and transplantation activities and (potential) organ recipients and donors – has consequently cultivated a defensive stance against misinformation about donation and transplantation. Misinformation can be perpetuated by the public through urban legends and myths, and by the mass media (Matesanz & Miranda, 1996). Negative news reports about brain death, organ trafficking, or fairness in access to transplantation can adversely affect public opinion about organ donation (Ohler, 1997; Brady, 1990). According to Linda Ohler, a transplant coordinator and editor of *The Journal of Transplant Coordination*, perceptions of transplantation as unethical and unfair that emerge in news reports persist among the public long after the details of a story are forgotten (Ohler, 1997). Although the news media can be useful in promoting organ donation,[1] it can also be harmful when it reports incorrect or imprecise information (Cuzin & Dubernard, 1995; Barnard, 1972). According to Arthur Caplan, "Nothing is more threatening to the integrity of the present system for obtaining organs and tissues than the perception that bias and inequity prevail within the allocation process" (Caplan, 1987: 18).

MEDIA COVERAGE OF TRANSPLANTATION

The news media have covered numerous stories of patients' triumphs with organ transplantation (e.g. Bray, 1997; Riley, 1997; Trent, 1984). But these are not the stories that trouble the transplant community. Rather, transplant professionals are cautious of media reports of controversial issues, e.g. foreign transplants and definitions of death, because they greatly affect public opinion of and trust in organ donation and transplantation. Transplant professionals are apprehensive that popular opinions are based on non-expert understanding of ethics, scientific facts, and legal policies, as presented within sensationalized news media reports. Transplant professionals engaged in public relations and education spend considerable energy clarifying the public's misinterpretation of inaccurate news media reports by community programs and paid advertising campaigns, among other activities. Transplant professionals rely on the public's delicate acceptance of their expertise and work in transplantation and in the organ allocation system in order to advance their humanitarian cause of increasing organ donation and transplantation. When members of the news media report inaccurate or sensationalized information about donation and transplantation, the transplant community has little control over the discourse on these ethical issues. Consequently, the transplant community must face the havoc of the resulting misguided public opinion, which, in effect, counters their ability to get work done (Kesten, 1998). The work of transplant professionals, especially those involved in public education, is therefore centered on controlling information to the public. Such apprehension, public education, and "damage control" are integral features of the culture of organ donation and transplantation.

Here I describe how the news media, specifically newspapers and a television news magazine, reported on two transplant-related stories. I will illustrate the popular opinions conveyed and perpetuated therein. Also, I will show how three separate news agency reports on those stories were sensationalized and perceived by the transplant community as threatening. Both stories had considerable impact on transplant professionals' decision making for the case of the foreign national patient discussed below.

On May 12, 1985, *The Pittsburgh Press* began a series of over thirty articles on kidney transplantation focusing on foreign patients and international organ trade. This series opened with articles demonstrating conclusively that Presbyterian-University Hospital in Pennsylvania had been denying kidneys to Americans and providing them to foreigners instead for financial gain (Schneider & Flaherty, 1985). Recurrent themes implicitly conveying the idea that transplanting foreign nationals was inherently unethical included, how American patients were bypassed by foreign patients who "jumped the line," how foreign patients receiving transplants were wealthy, and how such patients financially benefited transplant hospitals.

The Pittsburgh Press series framed the discussions about foreign patients receiving kidney transplants in the U.S. in terms of them receiving "American kidneys" for "non-medical reasons." The emphasis placed on the reasons transplant surgeons provided for transplanting foreign patients indicated that the reporters believed this practice to be unethical and therefore required explanation. For example, the journalists covering the story reported that: "Among the reasons surgeons gave for the special treatment was that the foreign patients were the children of doctors or members of the Saudi royal family" (Schneider & Flaherty, 1985). The repetitive use of the term "non-medical" also reflects the reporters' focus on the unfairness of this practice. Furthermore, by assigning social identity to kidneys according to the national identity of the donor reinforces the idea that organs should be the sole property of the nation from which they came.[2] The series also conveyed the notion that American donors trust the transplant system to allocate kidneys to American rather than to foreign patients. As the reporters perceptively wrote, "Worried about public opinion, most hospitals talk gingerly about transplanting scarce *American kidneys* into foreign patients" (Schneider & Flaherty, 1985: 26; emphasis added).

The articles' negative representation of foreigners 'jumping the line' strikes a nerve with the transplant community because it perpetuates the public's commonly misunderstood notion of the "waiting list." Whereas the public generally perceives the waiting list as a single, long list of patients waiting *in line* for a transplant, transplant professionals acknowledge that such a list is nonexistent. Rather, short, new lists of the best recipient matches are generated as each donor organ becomes available. Based on the present allocation system, foreign patients in the U.S. receive cadaver kidneys because they are the best match. Jumping the list is thus an inaccurate perception of how kidneys are allocated. However, the combination of the public's perception of the waiting list and the news media's presentation of foreign nationals as 'jumping the line' contribute to the public's misunderstanding and distrust of the transplant system and to physicians' apprehension of loss of control over ethics discourse.

The Pittsburgh Press series significantly influenced several agencies: Presbyterian-University Hospital revised its policy to exclude foreign patients, UNOS adopted its "Americans-First" policy, and the Office of Inspector General was prompted to conduct a study on the access of foreign nationals to U.S. cadaver organs (Office of Inspector General, 1986).

Just as the news media's reports on foreign nationals significantly influenced hospitals and policies, the news media also greatly concerned the transplant community with their heightened attention to the Cleveland Clinic's protocol. The transplant community perceived the newspaper and television coverage of this protocol as inaccurate and the debate it generated as overblown. Understanding why the transplant community perceived the news reports on the protocol as sensationalized is important since these perceptions directly influenced the case of the foreign national presented below.

In April 1997, a Cleveland State University bioethics professor, Mary Ellen Waithe, alerted the Cuyahoga County prosecutor's office that The Cleveland Clinic's test protocol for preparing severely brain-injured patients for organ donation amounted to "homicide." The protocol, which had not yet been implemented, would entail bringing these patients (who are often in a persistent vegetative state) into the operating room, withdrawing "life support," administering two drugs – Heparin and Regitine, and then waiting two minutes after the heart had stopped beating to remove organs. Heparin stops blood from clotting, and Regitine is a vasodilator that increases blood flow to the organs and consequently reduces blood pressure; both are used to keep organs healthy for organ transplantation. While the protocol would require physicians to test for death based on irreversible cessation of cardiac functioning by the absence of a carotid pulse, it was standard practice in the hospital to also use an electronic heart monitor (Funk & Mazzolini, 1997). The protocol was intended to be implemented only for those families with durable power of attorney over the patient who had specifically requested to donate their loved one's organs. Unlike cases of donation from people who are brain dead, transplant coordinators would not have approached families for donation unless families had initiated the request.

The news media covering this story included local and national newspapers, such as *The Plain Dealer* as well as a television broadcast of a segment on CBS's *60 Minutes* (Schneider & Flaherty, 1985; Wendling et al., 1997; Dempsey & Bray, 1997; *60 Minutes* April 13, 1997). The newspaper journalists were correct to point out that using non-heart-beating donors for organ donation raises important ethical issues (see Arnold & Youngner, 1993a, b). However, their reporting style led professionals within the transplant community to perceive the coverage of the protocol as slanted and inaccurate thereby contributing to public confusion (Debbie May-Johnson, Executive Director, Lifebanc, personal communication 5–3–00; Ohler, 1997).

First, both newspaper articles and CBS's broadcast on the protocol in the *60 Minutes* segment entitled, "Not Quite Dead," were selective in what they reported, highlighting the ethical and legal opposition to the protocol. For example, the journalists presented negative views of the protocol while lending credence to these through their association with authority figures, e.g. "what some *doctors* say is a *life-shortening drug*" and "a local *prosecutor* continues to regard it as *homicide"* (Wendling et al., 1997, emphasis added). The framework of featuring initially and primarily the opponents of the protocol conveyed an unbalanced idea that the protocol is unethical.

The news media reports of the protocol were sensationalized also through their lay use of language. For instance, the newspaper and televisions reports failed to use technically appropriate language, including, "family consent" (Ohler, 1997), and "double effect." The reports also commonly used the term "life support," rather than "ventilator," which conveyed the idea that its removal constitutes an active form of killing. The titles of the reports were also alarming, e.g. " 'Murder,' She Wrote of Clinic's Donor Plan . . ." (Wendling, 1997). Using such selective language contributes to transplant professionals' apprehension that the news media's reports would generate and reinforce the public's fears.

The provocative tone of these reports is best illustrated by Mike Wallace's opening line, "Are surgeons taking organs from patients who are not quite dead? And in some cases, giving them drugs that might hasten death?" While interviewing Mary Ellen Waithe, Mike Wallace led the audience to believe his overblown conclusion. He does so by responding to Waithe's comment "What are they trying to do, kill them?" with "That's the question that you – that has to occur to you if you read this [protocol]."

There were also several inaccuracies in the content of all the news reports on the protocol. The most striking example was that opponents consistently claimed that the drugs are *intended* to "hasten death" therefore using them constitutes "murder." Consequently, the news media reports played into public fears that doctors killed people to get their organs. These fears were reinforced by the failure to specify that the protocol would have been applied only when families requested to donate their loved one's organs. What also frustrated the transplant community was that the accusations were unwarranted and generated unnecessary public concern since the test protocol had not yet been put into practice (Debbie May-Johnson, Executive Director, Lifebanc, personal communication 5–3–00).

Another source of inaccuracy pertained to definitions of death. Although there are two legally acceptable definitions of death, Wallace was quick to discount the use of the heart definition. He stated that it is an "older, less precise method" and relied on the authority of one physician to back this up who then claimed that it is a "much more complex and difficult state to diagnose . . ." Yet, what Wallace failed to recognize is that even brain death is culturally shaped, subjective, and value-based in definition and diagnosis and was originally conceived to facilitate organ donation (Farrell & Levin, 1993). In addition, the drugs were perceived as the immediate cause of death rather than the removal of the ventilator from brain-injured patients. The closest a newspaper report came to clarifying the ethics of the protocol was a quote by bioethicist Tom Tomlinson: "There's (*sic*) all kinds of ways we're hastening the patient's death: Regitine, morphine, as well as taking the patient off the ventilator" (Funk & Mazzolini, 1997).

Mike Wallace concludes the television segment by ironically creating the fear of being a victim of the protocol through a rhetorical strategy of allaying the public's concerns as he states, "The chance of this happening to you or your family are minuscule. And now that this controversy is out in the open, the chances are nil." This rhetoric affirmed *60 Minutes's* role as the news team who stopped a harmful process by educating the public of its danger.

The transplant community in the U.S. expressed alarm at the news reports, but not because they believed The Cleveland Clinic's protocol constituted homicide. They feared that the heightened media attention and its inaccurate coverage of The Cleveland Clinic's protocol would adversely affect the public's willingness to donate cadaveric organs and would spur distrust in organ procurement. In actuality, transplant professionals' fears were partly realized. A local radio station reporting the story created an "air of crisis" and countless concerned listeners called The Cleveland Clinic and the local organ procurement organization (OPO), Lifebanc (Wendling et al., 1997). Organ donation rates plummeted in Lifebanc's catchment area of 65 hospitals: no referrals were made for six days following the *60 Minutes* television newscast (Debbie May-Johnson, Executive Director, Lifebanc, personal communication

5–3–00).[3] Hospitals served by Lifebanc feared that reporters from *60 Minutes* and newspapers would appear on their door-step. Public educators from Lifebanc still receive questions from the public about the protocol, indicating that public distrust of the procurement process, heightened by these news reports, continues today. Most OPOs in the U.S. experienced little if no impact from the *60 Minutes* report. Yet at least one OPO in the U.S. (in West Virginia) suspended for one year its non-heart-beating donor protocol out of fear of media-related "bad press" (Pam Silvestri, Association of Organ Procurement Organizations, personal communication 4–26–00). Despite this heightened public apprehension, organ donation rates did not decline in the following period nationally (Pam Silvestri, Association of Organ Procurement Organizations, personal communication, 4–24–00; UNOS, 2000).

Do the outcomes of this episode mean that transplant professionals' fears are fully warranted? Yes. Transplant professionals' apprehension with the media stems from their lack of control in providing the public with accurate and complete information sufficient for understanding the complexity of delicate ethical issues. The problem is that the news media, as shown above, may misinterpret, slant, and/or magnify views of those who are not expert in transplant ethics, thereby perpetuating misperceptions of organ procurement and allocation. Transplant professionals witnessed aw just how journalists used inexpert language and unrefined distinctions in their reports to advance their agenda of protecting the public against what news reporters believed to be a harmful policy. In response to media coverage of The Cleveland Clinic's protocol, Thomas Murray said that organ donation will be adversely affected because the non-heart-beating donor protocols don't pass the "next-door neighbor test." He explained the test: "You ought to be able to explain this to the person next door, and if you can't you've got a problem" (Davis, 1997).

How then, did transplant professionals decide whether to wait-list and transplant foreign nationals in this context of increased media attention to transplant-related issues? The following case analysis shows how one transplant team's decision making was responsive to these negatively-toned media reports of foreign nationals receiving U.S. kidneys and of organ procurement.

The data for the case study were collected through direct observation of fifteen monthly transplant selection meetings at one academic hospital, "American Hospital" (AH) in Ohio. During these meetings transplant professionals, including surgeons, nephrologists, nurses (transplant coordinators), and social workers, discussed and decided whether to place patients on the national transplant waiting list.[4] Informal interviews with the head transplant surgeon supplemented these observations. All names are pseudonyms. This study was approved by AH's institutional review board.

THE CASE

Vittorio Moreno is an Italian man who originally sought a kidney transplant in Italy and in other Western European countries, but was rejected because the waiting lists were extremely long. Although his family offered to donate to him, Vittorio declined their offers for unknown reasons. Subsequently, Vittorio learned from his nephrologist that a hospital in Ohio, AH, would be willing to evaluate him for a transplant. Vittorio traveled from Italy to the AH transplant center and was evaluated by the transplant team. Vittorio's case is discussed in the following interchange:

Surgeon:	This is the guy from Italy. His nephrologist is in Italy. Ken (The nephrologist) knows Dr. Lombardo (the Italian nephrologist). Sarah Burke (the hospital CEO) doesn't want to transplant any more foreigners. People [foreigners] already on the list we'll keep on [the list]. It's an ethical issue since we called him over – should we list him? In the U.S., most families try to get a living-donor and this guy doesn't want to take from his family even though his family is willing. Is it ethical to do it? [Otherwise, *The Plain Dealer* (the local newspaper) will find out].
Team:	[It's important to 'take care of one's own.' Americans will be upset to learn about transplanting a foreigner with American organs in times of scarcity.]
Nurse:	We're not obligated because he came here.
Surgeon:	We have to be careful because *The Plain Dealer* is looking for new stories. There is no problem with transplanting foreigners with live donors . . . In Italy nobody donates. European countries are clamping down on Italy because they don't donate. Other centers in Europe already turned him down. Sarah said we're not supposed to do it.
Nephrologist:	[I'm not in favor of doing foreigner transplants].
Surgeon:	[We transplanted an Italian patient 3–4 years ago who had AB blood. I felt 'comfortable to do it ethically' because there is no shortage of AB donors. I've done a half dozen foreign transplants.] But this guy is blood type O.
Team:	Oh![5]
Nurse:	My vote is no.
Surgeon:	I agree. I'm sorry he had to spend all that money coming here [even though AH is under the 5% foreign UNOS limit. I told the Italian patient that there has been a political change in the last three months] (regarding his talk with Sarah). I had told Sarah that doing a foreign transplant is not a Medical Director decision but a hospital decision so I told her to decide on the policy and she said 'no' against doing foreign transplants.

The transplant team's decision against wait-listing Vittorio was clearly influenced by sociocultural, political, and ethical considerations. The transplant team buttressed their decisions on the cultural value of helping Americans first in times of scarcity, or "taking care of one's own." This value took precedence because of the team's fear that Americans would be upset to learn about transplanting a foreigner with scarce "American organs."

Although AH was at that time well below the 5% legal cap on foreign transplants, the surgeon feared that the local news media, given recent events at The Cleveland Clinic, would 'expose' transplant practices that the public might dislike, thus generating further mistrust in the transplant establishment. The surgeon was leery of *The Plain Dealer's* sensationalized reporting of The Cleveland Clinic's protocol for preparing brain-injured donors. The surgeon stated that wait-listing Vittorio would constitute yet another opportunity for the news media to sensationalize a sensitive issue.

If the news media reported on foreign transplants occurring at AH, several problems could result. First, the public might perceive kidney transplants as unfairly distributed when foreigners: (a) receive American kidneys, and (b) pay cash for transplants. The public might misinterpret the direct payment of kidney transplants as a form of purchasing organs. While paying for services involved to secure an organ and perform a transplant is legal, purchasing organs per se violates the federal law established in 1984 by the National Organ Transplant Act. Second, distrust of the allocation system might lead to the decreased rate of organ donation. Lowered donation rates would result in fewer patients receiving kidneys and other organs.

In addition, local backlash by the public might mean that the transplant hospital loses patients to other transplant centers, which could have deleterious results. For example, such backlash may ultimately result in the disaccreditation of AH's transplant center by UNOS and subsequently, disruption in the continuity of care of transplant recipients. Thus, to prevent harm to the hospital from a potential exposé, the hospital CEO directed the surgeon to avoid placing foreign nationals on the waiting list in the future. At the expense of denying a single patient access to the waiting list, the team therefore decided in favor of protecting the public, the hospital, and the transplant community.

Despite the team's decision that day, the surgeon continued to debate the ethics of not wait-listing Vittorio. He was still concerned with having initially told Vittorio that the team would be willing to list him, and then reneging on the offer after Vittorio had expended considerable resources to travel to the U.S. for the evaluation. Because the surgeon had not resolved this ethical quandary, the case was discussed again at the next monthly meeting.

Surgeon: Vittorio Moreno. He's medically perfectly OK. I subsequently talked to Sarah, who instructed me not to transplant any foreign people. I brought it up with her because of more requests for foreign transplants. I told her I'm not going to [figure out the policy on it.]

Social Worker: The question is National policy.

Surgeon: We can do up to 5% of the list but there's no mandate to do foreign transplants.

Nurse: This guy wants a cadaver-donor kidney even though he has a living donor.

Surgeon: I felt this was a CEO position. Personally I don't feel comfortable. I can't justify doing them with 30,000 Americans on the list. I wouldn't know how to justify it to *The Plain Dealer.* Are we obliged to do a transplant for him because he spent all this money before we made a decision? (Rhetorically), Sarah, are you prepared for *The Plain Dealer's* next exposé on foreign transplants? That's the only downside, when Americans are dying on the list.

Nephrologist: My conscience tells me we should put him on.

Nurse: I have a problem because he has other family members willing to be evaluated. That bothers me.

Surgeon: I agree with [the Nephrologist]. I'd feel uncomfortable if we didn't list him after he made the trip and spent money. This is strongly debated at UNOS. America has always shown the rest of the world how to do medicine as a gesture of citizenship . . . I don't feel comfortable to not list him when we told him to come. I agree to put him on the list, but this is the last one.

This time, however, the surgeon decided to wait-list Vittorio by appealing to another cultural value to override his and the team's concerns with the media. The surgeon justified his position by recourse to the American value of humanitarianism and goodwill toward others (Davis, 1993). According to the surgeon, the U.S. holds a tradition of allowing people to come to the U.S. for the best health care. Additionally, the surgeon's moral conscience as well as that of the nephrologist led them to wait-list Vittorio because they had originally welcomed him.

DISCUSSION

This case raises several ethical problems for the practice of health care. Should transplant professionals make treatment decisions out of fear of the news media's responses? I argue that doing so can harm patients, and violate medical ethical principles and American cultural values. The transplant team had several choices. First, they could have refused to transplant all foreign nationals to avoid any popular perception of impropriety on the part of the hospital. Second, they could have selectively transplanted some foreign patients to intentionally perform less than 5%, their legal limit, as they initially did. Third, they could have accepted as many foreign patients as they could up to the legal cap to take full opportunity of helping people worldwide regardless of their nationality.

OPTION NO. 1: TRANSPLANT NO FOREIGN NATIONALS

The first option is the most ethically problematic since denying all foreigners access to kidney transplants violates the most and upholds the fewest medical and American cultural values. According to health care professionals' standards of conduct, such as the American Medical Association's Principles of Medical Ethics (1989) or the World Medical Association's Declaration of Geneva of 1948 (1989), the health of the patient is the primary consideration. However, by denying foreign patients access to transplantation, transplant professionals fail to respect the best interests of such patients. Thus transplant professionals' decisions in this scenario are based not on the health of the patient, but upon external factors, e.g. the news media. However, as with any system for allocating scarce resources, some patients will benefit while others do not. Accordingly, attending to the health of the immediate patient may be to the detriment of future patients. Learning that health providers may not respect patients' best interests may consequently undermine patients' trust in and relationship with healthcare professionals.

This option also violates an American cultural value of humanitarianism. Americans have a tradition of altruism (O'Connell, 1983). Screening the kinds of people Americans are willing to help threatens such core values. A similar value within biomedicine is that all people should receive health care regardless of identity. This value is expressed clearly in the Declaration of Geneva when it states, "I WILL NOT PERMIT considerations of religion, nationality, race, party politics or social standing to intervene between my duty and my patients" (World Medical Association, 1989). This value is even more compelling for treatment of end-stage renal disease because the current allocation system is continually being revised so as to ameliorate unfairness in access to transplantation by geography and race. Turning away patients from transplantation due to their nationality violates this principle and constitutes a form of discrimination.

Although denying transplants to foreign patients may be ethically problematic, the harsh reality is that this option constitutes fairness according to the current national standard. More conservatively, this choice may be fair considering that the U.S. routinely ships organs to other countries (Ota, 1997; UNOS, 1999; Schneider & Flaherty, 1985).[6] Shipping organs (usually marginal kidneys discarded in the U.S.) to foreign countries, but denying foreigners access to the U.S. waiting list, constitutes fairness in that it upholds the value of "Americans first" and a compromised form of humanitarianism (by donating the unused, marginal organs). The international exchange of organs decreases the pool of less usable organs available, while minimizing the number of people on the waiting list and thus competition for the best match.

With regard to international exchange, the transplant surgeon noted his willingness in the past to transplant Italian patients with uncommon blood types for which more organs were available, since doing so did not threaten the pool of scarce blood type O organs for other Americans to use. This thought process clearly reflects a priority accorded to Americans. But the concept of "Americans first" arguably undermines the core notion of fairness established by UNOS in its allocation system. Specifically, while the allocation system stresses the equal opportunity of all to gain access to organ transplants, the transplant team undermines this system by according foreign patients secondary consideration for treatment. Also, refusing to transplant foreigners who may be the most medically suitable for a transplant counters UNOS's effort to maximize *medical efficacy* in allocating kidneys. Consequently, transplants arranged by physician interference, rather than by the chance availability of organs according to blood type and best antigen matches of donor to recipient, results in foreign patients receiving biased care. This argument can be used to justify the elimination of the 5% cap. I argue instead, however, that even within the current allocation system, foreign nationals are not being treated fairly because hospitals, such as AH, intentionally limit transplanting kidneys in foreign nationals below the 5% cap out of fear of the news media.

OPTION NO. 2: TRANSPLANT FEW FOREIGN NATIONALS

The second option, which is what the transplant team actually chose to do, is ethically questionable since the transplant team avoided helping a person because of his nationality despite their legal capacity to do so. Like the first option, healthcare professional values are undermined, but to a lesser extent. In addition, this option risks some public distrust in the allocation system and consequently upsets some transplant community values. As a middle of the road course of action, the hospital's reputation is unlikely to be affected.

The team chose this option because of political and cultural factors. In the initial meeting about Vittorio, the surgeon was unwilling to counter the CEO's directive despite past experience in transplanting foreign nationals without public protest. In the wake of recent events, he preferred to protect the hospital from *The Plain Dealer's* bad press, as experienced by The Cleveland Clinic, rather than make decisions in favor of the patient. In addition, the surgeon was clearly influenced by cultural notions of fairness that involve allocating kidneys to American patients first.

Yet interestingly, the surgeon exhibited enough ambivalence about the prospect of transplanting foreign nationals to later accept the patient for wait-listing. In an interview with the surgeon after the case had been finalized, he said that as a transplant surgeon, he was generally in favor of doing foreign transplants. But as an American citizen, he felt that organs should go to Americans first. The surgeon's experience of two conflicting consciences with regard to transplanting foreign patients contributed to his ambivalence. His ambivalence may also stem from his already developed relationship with the patient: it is legally and ethically (and likely psychologically) easier to refuse care to patients whom one has not yet managed than to refuse care to those whom one has already begun to manage.

OPTION NO. 3: TRANSPLANT AS MANY FOREIGN NATIONALS AS LEGALLY POSSIBLE

Unlike the first two options, the third option upholds more and violates fewer values and principles. Transplanting foreign patients would be ethically beneficial because it respects the best interests of patients in their need for a transplant, it is humanitarian, and it enables access to health care regardless of identity.

The value that may be jeopardized is fairness in organ allocation. Fairness is questioned when people perceive the allocation of kidneys to foreigners as unjust because it increases the demand for scarce kidneys and thus the waiting time for Americans. Jeopardizing this value carries some risk to organ transplantation because negatively-toned media coverage can shape public opinion on organ donation (Slapak, 1997; Slapak et al., 1997; Brady, 1990; Ohler, 1997; Kesten, 1998). Public opinion has been shown to influence organ donation in both negative and positive ways (Slapak, 1997; Slapak et al., 1997). Since the news media (newspaper and television) represent the only source of information on transplantation for 72% of the U.S. population (Garcia et al., 1997), it is understandable that transplant professionals, like those at AH, are fearful of transplanting foreigners because of a potential media exposé and consequent decrease in organ donation. Although positive news media coverage increases organ donation rates, it does so for only a short period of time (Slapak, 1997; Slapak et al., 1997). Despite Linda Ohler's (1997) observation that negative news reports have a long-lasting effect on public perceptions of transplantation, no studies have empirically examined the duration of their negative perceptions.

News media exposure, therefore, does not necessarily result in negative public opinion. The news media are conduits for conveying ideas about fairness, and a mechanism that can shape these ideas. That is, the news media affect public opinion through selective reporting (Entwistle et al., 1996; DeVries, 1988). Case stories tend to grab the heart of individual readers. If the news media were to report on the case of Vittorio above, journalists could write the story in such a way that supports the hospital for transplanting them, as a humanitarian practice. This would probably generate public sympathy and support for transplanting foreign patients. Of course, journalists could just as easily disparage the hospital for helping foreigners as a breach of fairness in the allocation system.

The risks posed by this third option entail generating public distrust of transplant center practices and jeopardizing the transplant hospital's reputation. Such risks force us to question the ethics of transplanting foreign patients when doing so may turn public opinion against the hospital. However, fear of public reprisal is not a sufficient reason to discount this option. Making complex medical decisions based on a fear of public reprisal is irresponsible if the hospital can anticipate public outcry and has the mechanisms to educate the public.

Another perspective in support of transplanting foreign nationals pertains to public notions of fairness, particularly in light of the patient-physician relationship. Transplant professionals have a duty to transplant patients fairly. While the allocation process requires transplant physician discretion in selecting patients for the waiting list, it is unfair for them to use their discretion out of fear of public perception. The bases for doing so are grounded on tenuous assumptions. First, transplant physicians assume to know in advance public opinion on controversial transplant topics. Second, by making decisions that accede to public opinion, transplant physicians assume that they can avoid controversy. However, as Dr. Solinger, the chair of the transplant service at the University of Wisconsin and president of the American Society of Transplant Surgeons, clarified for Mike Wallace in *60 Minutes*, the entire transplant endeavor is laden with controversy. Thus, whichever decision transplant physicians make will likely upset some people. While transplant centers are not mandated to transplant foreign patients, there is no reason to allow biased values, reinforced through the media, to alter the allocation process. Ironically, should the public come to learn through the media that transplant professionals make medical decisions based on fear of public reprisal, they might come to see the allocation policies and system as untrustworthy. And we know what happens when the public distrusts the allocation system . . .

IMPROVING THE RELATIONSHIP BETWEEN THE TRANSPLANT COMMUNITY AND THE NEWS MEDIA

Hospitals and the transplant community can engage in a variety of measures to ensure that the news media have an accurate understanding of bioethical issues relating to organ transplantation. Hospitals should prepare well-articulated, targeted press releases through pamphlets, posters, editorials, articles, etc., to openly explain their position on transplanting foreign patients or other issues, and to guide popular perception of controversial decisions. Hospitals usually maintain public relations personnel who can shape public opinion about the treatment practices performed by the hospital. Educating the public has been shown to be a helpful way to resolve some ethical dilemmas (Callender et al., 1982).

Highly effective means of interacting with the news media are illustrated well in Spain's successful efforts to increase organ donation, which now has the highest rate in the world (Romay, 1996). Spain's National Transplant Organization established guidelines for the content of messages about transplantation to provide to the media (Matesanz, 1996). These include: (a) clear, concise, and well-argued messages, (b) consistency in manner of presentation of information, (c) always providing positive messages, (d) encouraging participation by the population in a common undertaking, e.g. donation, (e) specializing in the message of donation, (f) avoiding contradictory information, (g) avoiding conflicting topics such as doubt about brain death, (h) highlighting an unfractured organizational system, and (i) making clear distinctions between local situations and elsewhere (Matesanz, 1996). Matesanz specifically explains that "... tear jerking messages focusing specifically on the personal plight of someone chained to a machine or on the verge of dying if a suitable organ cannot be found, are not only of little use but are often counter-productive" (1996: 119). Should the media choose to report Vittorio's case in a melodramatic fashion, the positive message would be lost since, as Matesanz points out, it gives the population the feeling of anguish stemming from a desperate situation, impotence in being unable to solve the situation, and consequently rage against the transplant system. Transplant organizations and professionals can help improve the media's coverage of transplant issues by providing short, well-prepared messages that convey an energetic tone without doubt (Matesanz, 1996: 121). While Spain's high donation rate can be attributed to many factors, its highly-effective methods of public education have served them well, and the American transplant community can learn from their success.

Although in Vittorio's case we saw how health professionals perceived the news media as inclined to publish incorrect and sensationalized information to run a story, many other physicians are receptive of media exposure to increase the public's recognition of and confidence in their practices and institution (DeVries, 1988; Cohen & Morgan, 1988). But how do journalists feel about advancing this cause? Although journalists such as the scientific press and media communicators do not perceive themselves as "educators" or "advocates" but as "conveyors" of information to the public (Engel, 1990; Hollobon, 1990), information "can be educative, if it is accurate, balanced, and complete" (Hollobon, 1990). As one physician noted, "It is up to the scientist whose material is being reported to make sure that the reporters get a succinct press release or abstract delineating the results, their meaning, the overall purpose of the presentation and its relevance to everyday people (if any!)" (Engel, 1990).

OTHER ETHICAL ISSUES RAISED BY VITTORIO'S CASE

Vittorio's case raises other important ethical issues that must be addressed. My intention in this section is not to engage in extensive analysis of these issues, but rather to call our attention to them and suggest avenues for further research. One ethical dilemma that emerged, though the team did not explore it, was whether it is ethical for patients to receive cadaver donor kidneys when they already have living-donor kidneys offered to them. This dilemma can also be framed medically, as whether it is ethical for physicians to offer less effective treatment, e.g. cadaver donor kidneys, when a more effective treatment, e.g. living donor transplant, is available. Using kidneys from living donors would help decrease the high demand for cadaver donors. However, important sociocultural factors may impinge on attaining this ideal situation. Patient preferences, informed in part by sociocultural values and beliefs about gift-giving and interpersonal dynamics, may lead patients to decline offers of living-donor kidneys (Gordon, in press). Transplant professionals may find it helpful to explore patients' reasons for turning down living-donor kidney offers in order to clarify any misconceptions of the process.

Another ethical issue is that foreign nationals may experience difficulty or "triple jeopardy" in gaining access to transplantation in the U.S. First, they are accorded lowest priority by dint of the 5% cap in the U.S. Second, some transplant centers transplant into foreign patients organs that do not pass standards for American patients (Schneider & Flaherty, 1985). Third, organs exported to other countries also fail to pass standards for use in American patients, despite reports that the success rate of such organs approaches 80% (Schneider & Flaherty, 1985: 31). Scholars and policy makers should reevaluate their policies on foreign nationals to better address concerns about fairness. Proposals should strive to curb prevailing American public perception that only wealthy foreigners can receive kidneys. This perception is detrimental to notions of fairness in the allocation system because of its focus on wealth as a factor influencing the receipt of kidney transplants.

The idea of according organs social identity, particularly national identity, raises the broader question of ownership of organs. Are "American organs" the property of United States citizens? While the debate over ownership of organs focuses heavily on organ trade and commerce, scholars have paid virtually no attention to the role of national boundaries. How do proprietary conceptions of organs affect organ donation and transplantation? Does according organs national identity influence the public's disposition toward altruism and views about which strangers (Americans vs. non-Americans) should benefit from their donated 'gifts of life'? Just as increasing geographic ranges in the organ allocation system have generated considerable debate among the U.S. government and transplant professionals (Ubel, 1998; Milford, 1998), the idea of increasing the geographical ranges across national boundaries is likely to be controversial. Much remains to be explored on these issues.

Vittorio's case raises the general question of the news media's responsibilities in reporting issues in transplantation. Whether medical news reporters seek out medical news or physicians seek attention by the news media, as was the case in the Cleveland Clinic's protocol, both have the responsibility to ensure that the medical facts are accurate and not misleading. This is especially the case in media reports of transplantation, which can significantly affect organ donation rates. However, accurate reporting may be difficult to do since medical publishing and medical reporting maintain competing values (Johnson, 1998). While the former prioritizes collective and accurate data, the latter emphasizes individual anecdotes, and being the first to report the information, despite on-going developments in medicine. Physician and medical journalist, Timothy Johnson (1988) suggests that discrepant values can be minimized when medical-news reporters receive training or credentials in biostatistics and epidemiology to learn how to accurately analyze and represent medical news. It is unknown whether the reporters of the transplant stories described herein had such credentials, however, their reports would have likely benefited from them and minimized their sensationalized tone. In sum, the news media should make great efforts to foresee how their reports on transplantation can affect public perceptions of transplantation and donation.

CONCLUSION

Transplant professionals inescapably must make controversial decisions. As well, the knowledge they use to arrive at their decisions is specialized and not readily available to the public. We have seen in this chapter just how transplant professionals' fear of sensationalized news media coverage and anticipated public controversy influences their treatment decisions. However, if transplant professionals and hospitals concede the management of public discourse to news media, they will always be at the mercy of non-experts who easily generate public panic. Moreover, if transplant professionals and hospitals decide against treating patients because of anticipated controversy, they have neglected their ethical responsibility to care for patients in a fair manner. Because the supply of available organs relies to some degree on public opinion, transplant professionals and the hospitals they work for must learn to present controversial subjects in ways that inform the public so that controversy is managed through education.

NOTES

1. There was an international media blitz when bandits in Italy killed American boy Nicholas Green and his family donated his organs to Italians. The news of this event led to a major cultural change: the rate of organ donation in Italy increased by 400% in the days following Nicholas' death (People Magazine, 1994).

2. It is interesting that scholars and the media accord kidneys different social identities relative to the ethical debate. In regard to the issue of disparities among minorities in gaining access to transplantation, the discourse centers on matches between "black kidneys" or "white kidneys" and black or white recipients (Gordon, 1999).

3. Lifebanc received, on average, 384 calls per week in 1999. Seeing this rate is helpful in contextualizing the impact of the media on donation in 1997. Yet it is likely that this rate would be slightly different than the rate in 1997 because the Health Care Financing Administration's policy for hospitals to report each death was implemented in 1998 (Debbie May-Johnson, Executive Director, Lifebanc, personal communication 5–3–00).

4. A note about quoted statements: phrases within brackets indicate that the words may not be precisely those used by the respondent, although they are quite close in meaning. Such slight inaccuracies are the inevitable result of verbatim documentation of interviews and observations that were not audio tape recorded (Switzer et al., 1997).

5. The team responded this way because blood type O is most common thus there is greater demand for such organs.

6. Kidneys are discarded if there are problems relating to: the age of the donor, length of ischemic time, a positive crossmatch, causes of death of the donor, viral and

bacterial infection, problems with the recipient, and institutional difficulties associated with the availability of beds and/or doctors (Ota, 1997; UNOS, 1999).

ACKNOWLEDGMENTS

I thank the Health Care Financing Administration for financial support, No. 30-P-90882/5-01. I am grateful to the AH transplant team for allowing me to observe their decision-making process. I wish to thank Dr. C. K. Daugherty for helpful comments on an earlier draft. A poster version of this chapter was presented at the American Society for Bioethics and Humanities, October 1999.

REFERENCES

American Medical Association. (1989). Principles of medical ethics. In: R. Veatch (Ed.), *Cross Cultural Perspectives in Medical Ethics: Readings*. (pp. 39–40). Boston: Jones and Bartlett Publishers.

Arnold, R. M., & Youngner, S. J. (1993a). Back to the future: Obtaining organs from non-heart-beating cadavers. *Kennedy Institute of Ethics Journal*, *3*, 103–111.

Arnold, R. M., & Youngner, S. J. (1993b). The dead donor rule: Should we stretch it, bend it, or abandon it? *Kennedy Institute of Ethics Journal*, *3*, 263–278.

Bandini et al. (1991). Foreign versus one's own country waiting list in the case of organ shortage. In: W. Land & J. B. Dossetor (Eds), *Organ replacement therapy: Ethics, justice and commerce* (pp. 368–372). Berlin: Springer-Verlag.

Barnard, C. N. (1972). Medicine and the mass media. *American Journal of Cardiology*, *30*, 579–580.

Brady, W. J. (1990). The role of the media in organ donation. *Transplantation Proceedings*, *22*, 1047–1049.

Bray, D. (1997). The Gift. (Series reprint) *Dayton Daily News* (November 9–27) 1–24.

Callender et al. (1982). Attitudes among Blacks toward donating kidneys for transplantation: A pilot project. *Journal of the National Medical Association*, *74*, 807–809.

Caplan, A. (1984). Organ procurement: It's not in the cards. *Hastings Center Report*, *14*, 9–12.

Caplan, A. (1987). Equity in the selection of recipients for cardiac transplants. *Circulation*, *75*, 10–18.

Cohen, L., & Morgan, P. P. (1988). Medical dramas and the press: Who benefits from the coverage? *Canadian Medical Association Journal*, *139*, 657–661.

Cuzin, B., & Dubernard, J. M. (1995). The media and organ shortage. In: J. L. Touraine, J. Traeger, H. Betuel, J. M. Dubernard, J. P. Revillard & C. Dupuy (Eds), *Organ shortage: The solutions*. (pp. 287–293). Dordrecht, The Netherlands: Kluwer Academic Publisher.

Davis, D. S. (1993). Those who don't give. *The Mount Sinai Journal of Medicine*, *60*, 59–63.

Davis, D. (1997). Need for organs prompts new donation strategies. *The Plain Dealer* (April 5) 12A.

Dempsey, L., & Bray, D. (1997). The Gift. *Dayton Daily News* (November 9–27) 1–24.

DeVries, W. C. (1988). The physician, the media, and the 'spectacular' case. *Journal of the American Medical Association*, *259*, 886–890.

Engel, J. (1990). Improving media interaction with medical scientists. *Transplantation Proceedings*, *22*, 1052–1053.

Entwistle et al. (1996). Media coverage of the child B case. *British Medical Journal*, *312*, 1587–1591.

Farrell, M. M., & Levin, D. L. (1993). Brain death in the pediatric patient: Historical, sociological, medical, religious, cultural, legal, and ethical considerations. *Critical Care Medicine*, *21*, 1951–1965.

Funk, J., & Mazzonlini, J. (1997). Clinic puts controversial transplant plan on hold. *The Plain Dealer* (April 4) 1A.

Garcia et al. (1997). Mass media and organ donation. *Transplantation Proceedings*, *29*, 1618–1621.

Gordon, E. J. (1999). *If it's not broke, don't fix it: Patients' and clinicians' decision making for treatment of end-stage renal disease in the United States*. Unpublished dissertation in Anthropology. Case Western Reserve University, Cleveland, Ohio.

Gordon, E. J. (In press). They don't have to suffer for me: Why dialysis patients refuse living donor kidney offers. *Medical Anthropology Quarterly*, *15*.

Hollobon, J. (1990). The public, the media, and the professions: Perceptions of reality. *Transplantation Proceedings*, *22*, 1050–1051.

Ikels, C. (1997). Kidney failure and transplantation in China. *Social Science and Medicine*, *44*, 1271–1283.

Johnson, T. (1998). Shattuck lecture – medicine and the media. *Journal of the American Medical Association*, *339*, 87–92.

Jonasson, O. (1986). In organ transplants, Americans first? Commentary. *Hastings Center Report*, *16*, 23–25.

Kesten, S. (1998). Mass media and transplantation. *Journal of Heart & Lung Transplant*, *17*, 654–655.

Land, W., & Cohen, B. (1992). Postmortem and living organ donation in Europe: Transplant laws and activities. *Transplantation Proceedings*, *24*, 2165–2167.

Lock, M. (1996). Deadly disputes: Ideologies and brain death in Japan. In: S. Youngner, R. Fox & L. O'Connell (Eds), *Organ transplantation: Meanings and realities* (pp. 142–167). Madison, WI: University of Wisconsin Press.

Matesanz, R. (1996). Transplantation and the mass media. In: R. Matesanz & B. Miranda (Eds), *Organ Donation for Transplantation: The Spanish Model* (pp. 111–125). Madrid: Grupo Aula Medica, s.a.

Matesanz, R., & Miranda, B. (1996). Organ donation – the role of the media and of public opinion. *Nephrology, Dialysis, and Transplantation*, *11*, 2127–2128.

Mazzolini, J. (1997). Guidelines sought for taking organs from patients not declared brain-dead. *The Plain Dealer*. (December 20) 1.

Milford, E. L. (1998). Organ transplantation – barriers, outcomes, and evolving policies. *Journal of American Medical Association*, *280*, 1184–1185.

O'Connell, B. (1983). *America's Voluntary Spirit: A Book of Readings*. B. O'Connell (Ed.). New York: The Foundation Center.

Office of Inspector General (1986). The access of foreign nationals to U.S. cadaver organs, P-01-86-00074 (Washington, D.C.: Office of Analysis and Inspections, U.S. Department of Health and Human Services Publication).

Ohler, L. (1997). Organ transplantation and the media: The good, the bad, and the ugly. *Journal of Transplant Coordination*, *7*, 52–53.

Ota et al. (1997). Transplantation of kidneys donated from the U.S.A: Long-term results and viability testing using 31P-MRS. *Transplantation International*, *10*, 7–12.

People Magazine, (1994). The gifts of Nicholas: Italian bandits snuff out an American boy's life but not his legacy of hope. *People Magazine*, *42*, (24 October) 61–64.

Prottas, J. M. (1986). In organ transplants, Americans first? Commentary. *Hastings Center Report*, *16*, 23–25.

Riley, M. (1997) Marrow match gives girl hope to live as a 6-year old likes to. *St. Louis Post – Dispatch* (December 31) B3.

Romay, J. M. (1996). Prologue. In: R. Matesanz & B. Miranda (Eds), *Organ Donation for Transplantation: The Spanish Model* (pp. xi–xii). Madrid: Grupo Aula Medica, s.a.

Schneider, A., & Flaherty, M. P. (1985). The challenge of a miracle. *The Pittsburgh Press*.

Slapak, M. (1997). Organ donation: Transplant games, the 'island effect,' and other successful methods. *Transplantation Proceedings*, *29*, 3047–3049.

Slapak et al. (1997). Do the transplant games help organ donation? *Transplantation Proceedings*, *29*, 1479–1480.

Switzer et al. (1997). Donor ambivalence and postdonation outcomes: Implications for living donation. *Transplantation Proceedings*, *29*, 1476.

Trent, B. (1984). Is media hype necessary for organ transplants? *Canadian Medical Association Journal*, *130*, 774–780.

Ubel, P. (1998). Geographic favoritism in liver transplantation – unfortunate or unfair? *New England Journal of Medicine*, *339*, 1322–1325.

United Network for Organ Sharing. (1997). Transplantation of foreign nationals. UNOS policy 6.0.

United Network for Organ Sharing. (1999). UNOS OPTN Data as of 4/5/99.

United Network for Organ Sharing (2000). Number of U.S. organ donors by organ and donor type: 1988 to June 30, 1999 by year donor recovered. Critical Data: Donor statistics.

Wallace, M. (1997). Not Quite Dead. CBS *60 Minutes*, April 13.

Wendling, T. (1997). 'Murder,' She wrote of clinic's donor plan professor started state review of transplant policy. *The Plain Dealer* (April 13) 1A.

Wendling et al. (1997). Clinic will modify contested organ-procurement procedure. *The Plain Dealer* (5 April) 1A.

World Medical Association (1989). Declaration of Geneva. In: R. Veatch (Ed.), *Cross cultural perspectives in medical ethics: Readings* (p. 24). Boston: Jones and Bartlett Publishers.

13. WOMEN, MINORITIES AND ORGAN DONATION IN TRANSPLANTATION

Etienne Juarez Phipps and Gala True

INTRODUCTION

Women and members of minority groups have had a troubling and complex place in the history of American medicine. For the most part, neither has occupied a position of power or privilege in the medical establishment, either as patients or providers. Ethical concerns regarding fair treatment and respect for persons who are members of these populations extend to many aspects of organ transplantation: from identification of a patient as a transplant candidate to the use of living donors. In addition, because organ transplantation involves limited, scarce resources and heightened scrutiny over allocation decisions, it also provides a window into how societal values about individual and social worth are embodied in American medicine.

The experiences of powerlessness and, at times, outright abuse of women and minorities as patients and research subjects, set an uneasy stage for examining the organ transplantation enterprise. Negative health effects as a result of poverty, decreased access to health care and lack of familiarity with mainstream medicine, all have consequences – social and medical – for how organ transplantation is situated as a complex arm of organized medicine.

The consideration of beliefs and experiences of both patients and providers is essential to any discussion involving diverse populations and organ transplantation. For physicians, who in the case of organ transplantation are

The Ethics of Organ Transplantation, Volume 7, pages 317–337.

ISBN: 0-7623-0764-1

mostly white and male, subjective views about individual patients or ethnic groups figure strongly in opinions about who "deserves" an organ or who is likely to be an organ donor (either living or deceased). For potential organ donors and recipients, subjective views, from cultural and religious beliefs regarding removal of body parts to perceptions of the trustworthiness of providers in the health care system, can affect willingness to consider transplantation and many other issues involving individuals and families who become part of this process.

BACKGROUND

Issues in organ donation and transplantation for women and minorities are inextricably linked to health status, access to care, and individual and collective experiences within the history and organization of American biomedicine. Today, women constitute slightly more than half of the general U.S. population, while minorities constitute roughly 29% (1998 U.S. Census). Women and people of color are more likely to be living in poverty, with the relationship between lower socioeconomic status and poor health being well documented (Yergan et al., 1987; Blendon et al., 1989; Wenneker & Epstein, 1989; Schwartz et al., 1990; Burstin et al., 1992; Pappas et al., 1993, 1997; Whittle et al., 1993; Kahn et al., 1994; Carlisle et al., 1995; Lee et al., 1997; Andrulis, 1998).

Data from the Commonwealth Fund Survey of Minority Health Care show that minority adults are twice as likely as white adults to be uninsured. In addition, minority adults are more likely to experience difficulties obtaining appropriate and necessary medical care, have less choice in where they receive care and less access to regular sources of care, and report more negative experiences with the health care system (Commonwealth Fund, 1995).

Women, particularly members of minority communities, also have less access to quality health care. According to the 1998 Commonwealth Fund Survey of Women's Health, one in four women is uninsured during all or part of the year, with African American, Hispanic, and Asian American women being more likely to be uninsured than white women. Women without continuous insurance coverage are more likely to have problems with access to care, particularly quality care, and are less likely to visit a physician for preventive care (Collins et al., 1998). Lack of access to quality, continuous care for many women and minorities obviously increases the vulnerability of these groups to health problems, of which organ-related damage is but one.

Women and Minorities in Medicine

Women and members of minority communities have been and continue to be under-represented in key areas of medicine, from student and faculty representation in medical schools (Palepu et al., 1998; Cantor et al., 1998) to inclusion in clinical drug trials and the study and treatment of disease. Over time, the result of this exclusion is that more of what is known about specific diseases and effective treatments is based and focused on non-minority males.

Historically, both women and minorities have been excluded from many clinical trials because of researchers' desire to maintain the homogeneity of subjects and out of the belief that the effects of any drug in white males will be predictive of the effects in women and minorities (Angell, 1993; Bennett, 1993; Merkatz et al., 1993). The treatment and study of disease has also tended to favor men; for example, women have been notably absent from studies of cardiovascular disease, which affects both men and women equally (Wenger et al., 1993). Although women suffer more chronic conditions such as obesity, diabetes, respiratory ailments, and gastrointestinal problems, the vast majority of research has focused on male subjects (Rodin & Ickovics, 1990; AMA Council on Ethical and Judicial Affairs, 1991; Angell, 1993).

The past decade has seen increased efforts and commitment of federal funds and monies from private foundations to address the health status of women and members of minority communities and to ensure that women and minorities are appropriately represented in clinical research. Both the Federal Drug Administration and National Institutes of Health have revised their policies to require that researchers justify any exclusion of women or members of minority groups from research trials, stipulating that under most circumstances studies must actively recruit women and minorities as research participants (Baird, 1999). As a result of these efforts, more attention and funds are being directed toward the health and health care of women and minorities. Still, the inequities of the past continue to shape concerns about equality of inclusion of women and minorities in the processes and practices associated with organ transplantation.

Issues of Distrust

The experiences of members of minority communities in the United States – African-Americans, Asian-Americans, Hispanics, and American Indians, among others – with medicine are unique and cannot be stereotyped; however, there are similarities and common themes. Events, actions, and episodes in the history of American medicine and research, initiated by institutions and individuals alike, as well as the realities of social and economic discrimination, have played an important role in the relationship of minority communities with the health care system. Medicine's treatment of minority groups has often reflected the status and perceived value or disvalue of these communities in other areas of American life.

For minority communities in the U.S., distrust in the medical community is often rooted in experience and historical fact. In the case of African-Americans, slavery, segregation, and racism create a unique shared history and experience different from other American groups. Abuses in the historical and recent past, from the use of slaves as subjects in medical experiments to the Tuskegee Syphilis Trials, provide a disturbing context for African Americans as patients (see Thomas & Quinn, 1991; Jones, 1992, 1993; Corbie-Smith et al., 1999).

Women of color in particular have been the targets of unethical treatment by the medical professions. For a period in the early 1970s, over 100,000 low-income minority women annually were coerced into undergoing sterilization under a federally funded program (Apple, 1990; Gamble & Blustein, 1994). Another case in the 1970s, where a number of low-income, non-English speaking Hispanic women were sterilized after signing consent forms written in English, led to changes in federal guidelines for informed consent (Rosser, 1994). As recently as the mid-1980s, a study of the contraceptive Norplant was conducted with Mohawk and Navajo women without full disclosure of possible risks and contra-indications. Nor were procedures in place for taking the women off Norplant when the study was concluded. Diabetics in this study, who should have been excluded initially from the protocol because of anticipated complications from the use of Norplant with these patients, suffered additional health problems as a result of their participation. In addition, many of the women enrolled in the study still had Norplant implants five years after the study had been terminated (Rosser, 1994).

Distrust in medicine and the health care system has a number of consequences, not the least of which involves a preference *not* to participate in organized medicine, not to confide in providers, and to 'resist' the use of medications and treatments for fear of being experimented on. Research conducted by the authors has also identified skepticism concerning the motives of providers around end-of-life care among members of minority populations. Specifically, community members were concerned that providers might hasten the death of a minority patient in order to obtain organs for transplants, as well as remove body parts without family knowledge for use in organ transplants (Phipps & True, 1999).

In sum, many issues related to women and minorities in organ donation and transplantation arise in a context where the subjective figures strongly. Social and economic realities heighten the vulnerability of these populations to poor health – all of which yield significant medical, social and economic, as well as ethical challenges for the parties involved.

TRANSPLANTATION

Though sometimes controversial, organ transplantation is often the last hope for an individual with major organ damage. In order to become a "player" in this process, however, one must enter into the medical system and pass through a myriad of procedures and evaluations before becoming "listed" to receive an organ. Thus, barriers and facilitators to a patient's ability to access care represent the starting point for any informed discussion about gender and ethnic differences.

Access to the Health Care System

With organ transplantation and donation, access means that individuals must first enter into the system and then be able to stay in it and participate in the protocols and régimes. Access to medical care assumes that an individual has the economic, social, cultural, and linguistic resources and skills to enter into and successfully navigate the complex system of organ donation and transplantation. For some minority populations, staying engaged in such a process carries with it additional difficulties. For example, the ability to communicate with one's healthcare provider affects a patient's ability to understand health information and treatment options. When discussing organ donation and transplantation, already a complex topic for many patients and families, language differences and linguistic miscues can lead to greater apprehension for patients and families who are non-English speaking or who speak English as a Second Language.

Access issues also arise from the health care system, where providers make assessments and judgments every day about potential organ recipients; what kind of person is the patient, will they comply with treatment regimens; do they have a stable or protective home environment. There are many issues at each stage of the transplantation process, from identification of disease, evaluation and work-up, to listing, waiting, transplant, and post transplant régimes, where the interactions between health providers and patients are complicated by the values and beliefs all parties bring to the table.

Selection and Choice of Transplant as a Treatment Option

It is well documented that minorities and women are less likely to be the recipients of certain organs than are white males (Kjellstrand, 1988; Kasiske et al., 1991, 1998; Delano et al., 1997; Eckhoff et al., 1998; Klassen et al., 1998). However, it is difficult to know the reasons for these differences without additional data about incidence and prevalence rates of diseases for specific groups or a clear identification of the social, economic, and cultural dynamics that may contribute to the different recipient rates. For example, numerous studies have documented differences in referral rates of white and non-white (usually African American) candidates for transplantation, with white patients being referred more frequently than non-whites. It is safe to suggest that discriminatory practices play a role here. However, few studies have investigated aspects of the process such as: how many individuals might wish to become candidates for organ transplantation if presented with the option? How many patients have chosen not to undergo a transplant when provided appropriate information in language they can understand? How many have been discouraged from becoming a registrant on a waiting list, either subtly or explicitly? And how many have gone along with the process without adequate informed consent? In addition, there is an assumption in most studies investigating social or ethnic bias, that the option *in favor of* transplantation is the preferable choice for positive outcome. Whether or not transplantation listing should always be considered the desired outcome or an indicator of improved justice in healthcare is debatable. At best, studies that report data on socio-demographic differences of who gets transplants and who gets listed provide us with the barest of details about transplantation. Additional research is needed to obtain a fuller picture of what really goes on in the clinical setting between patients, families, and providers, and to look at the range of factors that affect patient decision making in favor or against transplantation.

Views on Organ Transplantation

Views about organ transplantation vary greatly among all sectors of the population. Many members of minority populations come from backgrounds – social, religious, and ethnic – in which health, illness, death and dying, and views about the meaning of the body and specific organs are intertwined with individual, family, and/or community religious, social and spiritual views. For many communities, beliefs about organ donation and transplantation are concerned with boundaries and crossing boundaries: the boundaries of life and death and the afterlife, of the physical body, of appropriate topics for discussion, and of what is acceptable or valued in a community.

Initiating a conversation about organ transplantation requires that people discuss the serious illness and/or death of themselves or their loved-ones in hypothetical terms. This can be seen as inappropriate, foreign, unacceptable, and even dangerous according to the beliefs and values of a number of religious and cultural communities. For some Asian cultures, conversations about death are to be avoided, and it would be particularly inappropriate for a child to discuss the death of a parent (Joun et al., 1997; Cheung et al., 1998). For members of other communities, including the Navajo, conversations about death are avoided because words are believed to have power and consequences, and talking about a person's death is seen as wishing for or hastening their death (McCabe, 1994; Carrese & Rhodes, 1995). In working with patients who hold these beliefs, this can present difficulties for providers who want to discuss organ transplant as an option but are cognizant of the conflicts open discussion can pose for patients and their families.

For some communities, the concept of prolonging life through organ transplantation is foreign and may be at odds with deeply held religious or cultural values. For many Christian and other religious communities, only God or another higher power can determine and control the time of death (Ferguson et al., 1998). For cultures in which predestination is a central concept, as in many Southeast Asian cultures, the length of a person's lifetime is predetermined and cannot be altered by humans (Chindarsi, 1976; Bliatout, 1982; Thao, 1986). For members of these communities, it may be difficult to reconcile religious and cultural beliefs with medical advances that prolong life, such as organ transplantation.

Beliefs about the Body

Beliefs about the sacredness of the body and a desire to keep the body intact, both throughout life and after death, are present in most religious and cultural communities. According to Judaic Law, the physical body is God's creation, and as such it should not be mutilated or desecrated (Dorff, 1996). For other religious communities, there is a strong proscription against touching a dead body, or cutting or altering a body for fear that spirits and ancestors will become angry and punish the living (Irish et al., 1993; Doniger, 1996). Of course, religious and cultural communities are heterogeneous, and individuals may vary in how closely they follow such proscriptions, especially in the context of a health crisis. Many religious and cultural communities adapt to developments and availability of new medical technologies such as organ transplantation by lifting proscriptions or making exceptions in cases where a patient would die without a transplant. Furthermore, systems of traditional beliefs and practices may co-exist with western allopathic and other medical systems, and individuals within communities may draw more on one system or another depending on the circumstances. In addition, though some members of a minority group may hold traditional beliefs about the body, others may be comfortable with the co-existence of traditional and mainstream biomedical views and approaches.

Beliefs about Organs

A number of cultural and religious communities have beliefs about specific organs – organs can be seen as containing the soul, the essence of a person, facets of an individual's personality, a person's memory and emotions. For example, many Hmong refugees from Southeast Asia believe that each person has a number of souls, some of which are located in specific organs (Bliatout, 1982; O'Connor, 1995).

For many people, specific organs themselves may have special meaning or symbolism, making it difficult to deal with the idea of losing one's own organ and replacing it with an organ from another. Witness, for example, the special meaning with which many of us imbue the heart. The same is true for other organs: for many Hmong, the liver is seen as the seat of essential elements of an individual's personality, and being a liver transplant recipient could result in changes to one's personality (O'Connor, 1995). Belief in karma, central to Hinduism and other religious belief systems, means that organ transplant recipients can "inherit" the good or bad karma of the donor (Doniger, 1996). This belief is found among organ recipients across cultural and religious communities; that organ recipients will lose some essential aspect of themselves, or take on aspects of the donor's personality or memories (Youngner, 1996).

From a broader socio-cultural perspective, societies where religious and cultural traditions might be opposed to donation and transplantation have been forced to deliberate about the removal of body parts from individuals, both dead and alive, and the morality and meanings attached to those actions. In general, the more technologically developed countries with established medical professions have come to view the practices and procedures associated with organ transplantation and donation more secularly, as offering benefit to an identifiable person. Religious opposition may still exist in these countries though it may not restrict the practice. In other nation states, opposition to organ transplantation and donation may be based on religious, spiritual, cultural, or economic factors. In developing nations, the cost alone of transplantation, e.g. the technology, medications, and expertise required, may be sufficient to preclude this treatment modality altogether.

DATA ON ORGAN TRANSPLANTATION

In 1997 there were just over twenty thousand organ transplants, including kidney, liver, pancreas, kidney-pancreas, heart, lung, and heart-lung transplants in the United States. Of these, approximately 35% were women and 31% were minority recipients. Of minority transplant recipients, 17% were African American, (unchanged from 1988), 9% Hispanic (up from 7% in 1988), and 5% Asian/Other (up from 4% in 1988) (Annual Report OPTN/SR AR, 1998).

For certain organs, whites accounted for a significantly higher percentage of recipients. For example, white patients received 91% of all pancreas transplants (down from 96% in 1988), 83% of all kidney-pancreas transplants (down from 95% in 1988), and 89% of all lung transplants (down from 97% in 1988) (Annual Report OPTN/SR AR 1998). With regard to the 2292 heart transplants conducted in 1997, 74.8% of recipients were male and 80.7% were white; white women, Hispanics, and Asians were under-represented as recipients relative to their numbers in the general population, though African Americans were not (Annual Report OPTN/SR AR, 1998).

Kidney and Liver Transplants

With kidney transplants, while African Americans comprised 35.5% of registrants on the waiting list, they accounted for 27.1% of those receiving cadaveric transplants and 13.9% of those receiving a transplant from a living donor. Women constituted 43.1% of those on the waiting list, and accounted for 39.1% of those receiving cadaveric transplants and 41.8% of those receiving "living" transplants. Males constituted 56.9% of registrants on the waiting list, and comprised 60.9% of recipients of cadaveric transplants and 58.2% of those receiving living transplants. In sum, the majority of recipients of kidney transplantation (7769 cadaveric and 3669 living donors) were white and male (57.3%, and 60.9% respectively for cadaveric and 71.2% and 58.2% respectively for living donors), even though minority populations constituted slightly more than half of the 38,270 registrants on the kidney waiting list (Annual Report OPTN/SR AR, 1998).

In the case of kidney transplantation with cadaveric donors, minority recipients historically have been at a disadvantage due to a federally mandated system that calls for a high degree of HLA matching between donor and recipient. Higher quality of HLA matching is thought to increase graft survival based on antigenic similarities between donor and recipient. White populations are more likely to have well defined HLA antigenic specificities, resulting in a higher likelihood that an organ will be matched with a white patient rather than with a patient of color (Gaston et al., 1993).

Liver transplant data show that there were 4168 transplants conducted in 1997 and 9647 individuals on the waiting list. More males than females received liver transplants (58.1% vs. 41.8% respectively) and whites constituted the predominant group receiving liver transplants (76.2%) compared with all minority recipients combined (Annual Report OPTN/SR AR, 1998). It is not clear from the data what factors might account for why white patients receive more liver transplants than do minority patients.

Many investigators have reported on the inequalities and inequities in the transplant process that relate to the care provided to minority populations. It is not our purpose to review them here, but rather to mention a few illustrative studies. It has been demonstrated that other areas of medicine suffer from bias and that members of minority communities and women are often underserved (Schulman et al., 1999). There is no reason to think the situation is any different in the area of organ transplantation.

While the data continue to demonstrate that transplant recipients include more white males than any other group, there are many factors that are not easily measured or concluded from the available reported data. For example, Alexander and Sehgal in a prospective cohort study of four stages of the transplantation process followed 7125 patients beginning long-term dialysis over a three-year period (Alexander & Sehgal, 1998). They reported that, after adjusting for age, sex, cause of renal failure, years receiving dialysis, and median income, black patients were less likely than were white patients to: (1) be definitely interested in transplantation (OR 0.68; 95% Confidence Interval [CI]. 0.61–0.76); (2) complete the pre-transplant work-up (OR 0.56; 95% CI, 0.48–0.65); and (3) move up the waiting list and receive a transplant (OR 0.50; 95% CI, 0.40–0.62). They also found that women were less likely than men to complete all four identified stages of the transplantation process: (a) medically suitable and possibly interested in transplantation (OR 0.90; 95% CI, 0.82–0.99); (b) definitely interested in transplantation (OR 0.89; 95% CI, 0.80–0.99; (c) complete work-up (OR 0.80; 95% CI, 0.70–0.92); and (4) move up waiting list and receive transplant (OR 0.82; 95% CI, 0.68–0.99). Lower socio-economic status patients were also less likely than higher SES patients to complete the stages of the process identified above, with ORs of 0.67 (95% CI, 0.59–0.76); 0.78 (95% CI, 0.68–89); 0.77 (95% CI, 0.64–0.92); and 0.83 (95% CI, 0.77–0.91), respectively.

Inequities in Organ Transplantation

Obviously the enrollment process is a critical step towards receiving a transplant. Many investigators have found white patients are more likely to be evaluated for transplants and placed on waiting lists than minority patients (Soucie et al., 1992; Eggers, 1995; Alexander & Seghal, 1998). Randall has also reported that African Americans wait almost twice as long as whites for a transplant (Randall, 1996). Kasiske and colleagues conducted a large ($n = 41{,}596$) study of patients registered for kidney and kidney-pancreas. Transplantation patient and center factors predicting dialysis status at time of registration were examined. The authors found patients from racial and ethnic minorities, less educated patients, and those with fewer financial resources were less likely than their counterparts to be listed for renal transplantation before dialysis. In other words, the less advantaged patients were identified and listed at a later point in time in the course of their disease when they were likely to be sicker than were the more advantaged patients (Kasiske et al., 1998).

Addressing the why of low enrollment is complicated. Increased concerns about bias against minority patients in transplantation have been raised in an important study by Ayanian and colleagues (1999). The investigators examined the association between race and patients' preferences regarding transplantation. In their interviews with 1392 patients (384 black women, 354 white women, 337 black men, 317 white men), with End Stage Renal Disease (ESRD), they found that black patients were less likely than white patients to want a transplant (76.3% of black women reported such a preference for transplantation vs. 79.3% of white women and 80.7% of black men vs. 85.5% of white men), and they were less likely to be very certain about this preference (58.3% vs. 65.3% and 64.1% vs. 75.7%, respectively, $p < 0.01$ for each comparison with both sexes combined). Thus, uncertainty about the transplantation – clearly an important factor in patient decisionmaking, was stronger in black patients than in whites.

In addition, Ayanian and colleagues found larger differences in the rates for referral for evaluation at a transplantation center (50.4% for black women vs. 70.5% for white women, and 53.9% for black men vs. 76.2% for white men; $p < 0.001$ for each comparison) and placement on a waiting list or transplantation within 18 months after the start of dialysis therapy (31.3% for black women vs. 56.5% for white women, and 35.3% for black men vs. 60.6% for white men; $p < 0.001$). The differences between blacks and whites remained significant after adjustment for patients' preferences and expectations about transplantation, sociodemographic characteristics, the type of dialysis facility, perceptions of care, health status, the cause of renal failure, and the presence or absence of coexisting illnesses. The authors concluded that the patients' preferences alone did not account for the differences between the populations studied and suggested that "physicians need to provide information and refer patients who desire transplant accordingly" (Ayanian et al., 1999). The implications of this study are that physicians' subjective views about patients who are black account for why these patients are rejected for a procedure that the physicians would otherwise offer to white patients with similar disease severity.

More evidence of ethnic bias of providers in the evaluation process, is given by Narva and colleagues (1996) who analyzed a large data set of kidney transplantation and ESRD in the Southwestern United States, comparing transplant rates for Native Americans and whites. Native Americans had a slightly earlier onset of ESRD than whites, and diabetes mellitus was the primary ESRD diagnosis for 63–73% of Native Americans and for 34–39% of whites. In reviewing the transplant rates for patients with the primary diagnoses of diabetes mellitus and glomerulonephritis, the two most common causes of ESRD, the investigators found a large difference between the Native American and white rates. They found that Native American women were transplanted at lower rates than men, and Native Americans experienced a greater delay from onset of treated ESRD to transplant than whites. As with the implications of Ayanian's study (1999), the authors concluded that the lower transplant rates in Native Americans versus whites could *not* be explained by age-specific or diagnosis specific factors (Narva et al., 1996).

While sometimes difficult to prove through quantitative data alone, there is mounting evidence that biases, whether they be gender or ethnically based, can influence use of diagnostic work-ups and referral patterns. Assumptions made about an individual's social worth, ability to comply with treatment regimens, willingness to consider transplantation as an option, etc., can contribute to the use of informal rationing in organ transplantation decisions, in spite of established procedures and guidelines. At the same time, patients' perceptions of providers as 'untrustworthy,' language and cultural differences, and negative experiences with the healthcare system, hinder cooperation and trust between providers and patients, with direct impact on a range of outcomes that are part of the organ transplant process.

ORGAN DONATION

Organ donation is a procedure where one person's organs are removed and transplanted into another. Images of donation as the ultimate "gift of life" are used by organ transplant programs to encourage individuals to complete donor cards and to foster a (more) positive image of the organ donation enterprise. Stories of strangers as living donors volunteering to give their organ either to an anonymous or identified patient, and families donating the organs of a child who has died unexpectedly support this image.

While "gift giving" is the positive view about donation; the truths and fictions regarding removal of organs, referred to clinically as 'harvesting,' also shape societal perceptions. Reports of the marketing of organs in other countries, urban legends claiming that medical personnel will keep people "on machines" in order to get their organs, and the auctioning of organs on the Internet, whether real or hoax, contribute to a disturbing picture of an underworld of organ donation and transplantation. Research conducted by the authors, along with that of others, has identified a concern on the part of minority families that agreeing to donate a loved one's organs will lead medical personnel to "let the patient die sooner," or as has been mentioned earlier, that any discussion about end of life support is a cover for providers wanting to procure organs from minority families (Phipps & True, 1999).

These beliefs and urban legends are so pervasive and powerful that UNOS has created a web site listing a number of urban legends about organ theft and debunking each one. The distrust that results from these stories and concerns about organ donation has been cited as a component of negative views toward donation and a possible reason for lower rates of completion of donor cards among minority populations (Siminoff, 1997).

Discussion of Organ Donation

Members of specific religious and cultural communities may be less likely or resistant to discussing organ donation for a number of reasons. A recent study of reasons for lower rates of organ donation among African-Americans as compared to whites found that African-Americans were more likely to donate a relative's organs if that relative expressly stated a desire to be an organ donor, but less likely than whites to discuss preferences about organ donation with their families (Creecy et al., 1992; Siminoff et al., 1995). Similar findings have been reported in Hispanic families; they are less likely than whites to discuss organ donation (Daniels et al., 1998).

Beliefs about Organ Donation

In the medical language of cadaveric organ donation, death is determined by brain death, the cessation of all brain activity. With the advent of non-heart beating donation, the picture becomes even more complicated, as it also becomes possible to control a severely damaged patient's time and manner of death in order to make him or her a suitable donor. However, this medical demarcation between life and death does not hold for many cultural and religious communities. In Judaism, for example, "death does not occur in one, definite, clearly recognizable moment; rather, it is a process that begins before a person's heart and lungs stop functioning and continues well after that time" (Dorff, 1996). For other religious and cultural communities, the concept of medically defined death and medically controlled time of death may be fundamentally opposed to deeply held beliefs.

Other beliefs about the body relevant to organ transplantation include religious and cultural communities where a viewing of the body is an essential element of a funeral, as in Catholicism and in Filipino culture. For members of these communities, there may be a concern that organ donation will result in a mutilated body and thus interfere with the viewing and mourning process (Cheung et al., 1998). For religious traditions where reincarnation and the afterlife are central, organ donation is seen as an unthinkable desecration of the body that will have serious consequences in the afterlife and future incarnations. For example, Japanese Buddhists, Indian Hindus, and Southeast Asian Hmong animists all believe that the state of the body in this life (and at death) mirrors the state of the body in the afterlife and future incarnations. For those who hold these beliefs, any cutting to the body or removal of organs could result in scars, illness, and missing organs in the next life (O'Connor, 1995; Doniger, 1996).

DATA ON CADAVERIC DONATION

Cadaveric donation takes place when a patient is declared brain dead or following the withdrawal of mechanical ventilation with those categorized as 'non-heart-beating' donors (Arnold & Youngner, 1993a, 1993b). In the ten-year period between 1988 and 1997, the majority of cadaveric donors were both white and male. The numbers have been changing during that period: in 1997 minorities accounted for 24.4% of cadaveric donors, up from 16.6% in 1988 (Annual Report OPTN/SR AR, 1998). African American and Hispanic donors had the largest increase from 1988 to 1997, and account for nearly all minority donors during that ten-year period. The data show that the majority of cadaveric donors are men: in 1988, 62.4% of cadaveric donors were male and only 37.6% female, and by 1997 the gap had closed to 59.3% male and 40.7% female (Annual Report OPTN/SR AR, 1998).

DATA ON LIVING DONATION

The number of living donations has been steadily increasing, doubling in the period from 1988 to 1997. In 1997, the majority of living donor organs were kidneys (72%), and in 85% of those cases the donor and recipient were related.

The picture for living donors is somewhat different than cadaveric donors when it comes to gender, with women constituting the majority of living donors. In 1988, women accounted for 54.7% of living donors and men for 45.3%. The gap has been increasing over a ten-year period, so that in 1997 57.1% of living donors were women and 42.9% were men (Annual Report OPTN/SR AR, 1998).

In terms of ethnicity and living donors, the data are much the same as that for cadaveric donors. Whites continued to constitute the majority of living donors for the ten-year period from 1988 to 1997. While there was an increase across all minority groups in living donation during that period, minorities continued to account for less than 25% of living donors in 1997 (Annual Report OPTN/SR AR, 1998).

Reasons for Differences

We can only speculate about the factors that may account for differences in donation figures, which may include, in the case of cadaveric donors: cause of death (e.g. more men die violent deaths than women – often the circumstances in which cadaveric organs are obtained); views about appropriate treatment of the female body (e.g. families may be more reluctant to give permission to 'cut' a female open to remove organs than to do so with a male); knowledge about patient wishes; provider relationship with family; provider views about appropriateness of patient as donor; and provider comfort with discussion of patient as a donor candidate. With both brain-dead and non-heart-beating cadaveric donors, consent to donate is almost always sought from the patient's family, even in circumstances where the patient had a signed donor card. Thus, differences in numbers of female versus male cadaveric donors may have more to do with societal forces and pressures rather than whether or not a patient is a viable candidate for donation.

Clinicians have reported a number of reasons for being biased toward potential donors who are white and male, and thus approaching the families of those potential donors more frequently, although little research has been done in this area. Some clinicians in the transplant field report a preference for male donors over female donors based on physical size – the larger organs of many adult males can be used for adult recipients of almost any physical size.

Off the record, providers and transplant coordinators have also reported biases towards white male donors over minority male donors due to the assumption that white males are less likely to have a past medical and social history complicated by drug and alcohol abuse and high-risk sexual practices. Some studies have demonstrated that physicians, the majority of whom were white, were more reluctant to approach families from ethnic minorities about donation than they were to approach white families (Hartwig et al., 1993; Guadagnoli et al., 1999). Whether this is because of sensitivity to ethnic or cultural differences or because of ethnic stereotyping has not been established. However, it is apparent that providers' perceptions and stereotypes about the health status of potential donors and about which families are most likely to donate strongly influences the frequency with which patients and families from minority communities are approached for donation.

There are a number of reasons why living donors may be more likely to be women. Giving an organ to save or improve the life of a loved-one may seen as an extension of the care-giving role, which is traditionally seen as the domain of women. Clinicians involved with living donation report that in families where living donation is an option, a female family member is more likely to be seen as a potential donor by both providers and other family members than is a male family member. Living donors face possible disability, poor health, long recovery times, and loss of income following donation. Regardless of realities, both providers and families may perceive women as more able to deal with the aftermath of living donation and less essential to the financial well-being of the family unit, even when they are heads of households or part of a dual income family (Bloembergen et al., 1996).

CONCLUSION

In this chapter we have explored some of the perceived and real deficiencies of the U.S. healthcare system in providing healthcare for women and minorities. We viewed organ transplantation as an example of how medical, social, cultural, and economic forces converge to produce an unsettling, but dynamic picture of our healthcare system today. And we discussed the diversity of beliefs related to organ transplantation that enrich this picture in ways that, ultimately, enlarge our understanding of the meanings of organ transplantation. Throughout, we have underscored the important role that beliefs and biases of patients and providers play in the transplantation process.

Clearly, education is needed to increase awareness and understanding in minority communities about transplantation as a treatment option and about the realities of organ donation. A number of such initiatives have been launched, and their impact is under evaluation (Callender et al., 1995, 1996, 1997). However, these education initiatives must be developed with attention to language and comprehension issues, as well as relevant cultural and religious beliefs. Educators must be attentive to how their efforts to "target" minority communities to increase rates of organ donation are perceived and interpreted by members of those communities. In sum, communities and health care systems need to join forces to address broader issues such as access to care and patient rights, and to develop strategies to improve health and health care choices so that the need for transplantation is minimized.

For providers, more attention needs to be paid to recognizing and understanding biases in medicine based on gender and ethnicity. The studies reviewed in this chapter provide evidence that social and racial biases against members of minority groups can undermine the processes involved in transplantation, resulting in narrower treatment choices for these patients, particularly as the severity of disease increases. Stereotyped views of patients who are women or members of ethnic or religious minorities can result in harm for patients, providers, and the larger health care system, and should not be tolerated.

We end this chapter with some thoughts and questions about survival following transplantation as it relates to women and minorities. The aftermath of transplant involves increased intensity of medical surveillance, the presence of both expected and unexpected medical sequelae, and ultimately, a body's acceptance or rejection of the organ. For those who survive transplantation to discharge, ability and willingness to comply with the medical régime can be complicated by all of the factors we have identified in this chapter.

Survival as a straight medical outcome does not represent a true assessment of the success or failure of transplantation. The quality of life experienced by post-transplant patients and their families varies greatly and is the more meaningful outcome; however, it is rarely the subject of study. It is well known that caring for family members has traditionally fallen on women. Who provides post-transplant care to female transplant recipients? How do transplant patients with limited economic resources obtain medications or even get transportation to attend important follow-up appointments? How do non-English speaking or patients for whom English is a second language become informed about what to expect from post-transplant medications, many of which can have serious or disturbing side effects, or what they must do to promote healthy functioning of the new organ? How do cultural and religious beliefs about the consequences of removal of body parts affect patients and families as they deal with life post transplant? And finally, for those patients who do not survive, how is their death understood by their families – as a failure or as a blessing? The values, beliefs, and prejudices that make up the fabric of our society are an undeniable presence in organ transplantation. Addressing that reality through education and standards for quality of care that take into account the needs of patients, families, and communities will go a long way toward improving equity in the health care system for all.

ACKNOWLEDGMENTS

We would like to thank Umi Chong, M. B. E., and Diana Harris, M. B. E., for their research assistance. We are also grateful to Janet Theophano, Ph. D., for her critical review of the chapter and her insightful comments.

REFERENCES

Alexander, G. C., & Sehgal, A. R. (1998). Barriers to cadaveric renal transplantation among blacks, women, and the poor. *JAMA*, *280*, 1148–1152.

Andrulis, D. P. (1998). Access to care is the centerpiece in the elimination of socioeconomic disparities in health. *Ann Intern Med.*, *129*, 412–416.

Angell, M. (1993). Caring for women's health – what's the problem? *N Engl J Med.*, *329*, 271–272.

Annual report of the U.S. scientific registry for transplant recipients and the organ procurement and transplantation network: transplant data: 1988–1997. Rockville, MD, UNOS Richmond, VA; 1998. U.S. Department of Health and Human Services, Health Resources and Services Administration, Office of Special Programs, Division of Transplantation.

Apple, R. D. (1990.) *Women, Health, and Medicine in America: A Historical Handbook*. New York: Garland Publishing, Inc.

Arnold, R. M., & Youngner, S. J. (1993a). The dead donor Rule – should we stretch it, bend it, or abandon it? *Kennedy Inst Ethics J.*, *3*, 263–278.

Arnold, R. M., & Youngner, S. J. (1993b). Ethical, Psychosocial, and Public Policy Implications of Procuring Organs from Non-Heart-Beating Cadavers. *Kennedy Inst Ethics J.*, *3*, 103–277.

Ayanian et al. (1999). The effect of patients' preferences on racial differences in access to renal transplantation. *N Engl J Med.*, *341*, 1661–1669.

Baird, K. L. (1999). The new NIH and FDA medical research policies: targeting gender, promoting justice. *Journal of Health Polit Policy Law*, *24*, 531–565.

Bennett, J. C. (1993). Inclusion of women in clinical trials – policies for population subgroups. *N Engl J Med.*, *329*, 288–292.

Blendon et al. (1989). Access to medical care for black and white Americans; a matter of continuing concern. *JAMA*, *261*, 278–281.

Bliatout, B. T. (1982). *Hmong Unexpected Noctural Death Syndrome: A Cultural Study*. Portland, OR: Sparkling Publishing Enterprises.

Bloembergen et al. (1996). Gender discrepancies in living related renal transplant donors and recipients. *J Am Soc Nephrol.*, *7*, 1139–1144.

Burstin et al. (1992). Socioeconomic status and risk for substandard medical care. *JAMA*, *268*, 2383–2387.

Callender et al. (1995). A national minority organ/tissue transplant education program: the first step in the evolution of a national minority strategy and minority transplant equity in the U.S.A. *Transplant Proc.*, *27*, 1441–1443.

Callender et al. (1996). An assessment of the impact of the national minority organ tissue transplant education program. *Transplant Proc.*, *28*, 394–397.

Callender et al. (1997). A national minority transplant program for increasing donation rates. *Transplantation Proceedings*, *29*, 1482–1483.

Cantor et al. (1998). Effect of an intensive educational program for minority college students and recent graduates on the probability of acceptance to medical school. *JAMA*, *280*, 772–776.

Carlisle et al. (1995). Racial and ethnic differences in the use of invasive cardiac procedures among cardiac patients in Los Angeles County, 1986 through 1988. *Am J Public Health*, *85*, 352–356.

Carrese, J. A., & Rhodes, L. A. (1995). Western bioethics on the Navajo reservation. benefit or harm? *JAMA*, *274*, 826–829.

Cheung et al. (1998). Cultural attitudes of Asian-Americans toward death adversely impact organ donation. *Transplant Proc.*, *30*, 3609–3610.

Chindarsi, N. (1976). *The Religion of the Hmong Njua*. Bangkok, Thailand: Siam Society.

Collins et al. (1998). *Health concerns across a woman's lifespan. The Commonwealth Fund 1998 Survey of Women's Health.*

Commonwealth Fund. (1995). *National Comparative Survey of Minority Health Care*. New York.

Corbie-Smith et al. (1999). Attitudes and beliefs of African Americans toward participation in medical research. *J Gen Intern Med*, *14*, 537–546.

Council on Ethical and Judicial Affairs: American Medical Association. (1991). Gender disparities in clinical decision making. *JAMA*, *266*, 559–562.

Creecy et al. (1992). Discriminators of willingness to consider cadaveric kidney donation among Black Americans. *Soc Work Health Care*, *18*, 93–105.

Daniels et al. (1998). Organ and tissue donation: are minorities willing to donate? *Ann Transplant*, *3*, 22–24.

Delano et al. (1997). Gender and racial disparity in peritoneal dialysis patients undergoing kidney transplantation. *ASAIO J.*, *43*, M 861–864.

Doniger, W. (1996). Transplanting myths of organ transplants. In: S. J. Youngner, R. C. Fox & L. J. O'Connell (Eds), *Organ transplantation: meanings and realities* (pp. 194–220). Madison: University of Wisconsin Press.

Dorff, E. N. (1996). Choosing life: Aspects of Judaism Affecting Organ Transplantation. In: S. J. Younger, R. C. Fox & L. J. O'Connell (Eds), *Organ transplantation: meanings and realities* (pp. 168–193). Madison: University of Wisconsin Press.

Eckhoff et al. (1998). Race: A critical factor in organ donation, patient referral and selection, and orthotropic liver transplantation? *Liver Transpl Surg.*, *4*, 499–505.

Eggers, P. W. (1995). Racial differences in access to kidney transplantation. *Health Care Financ Rev.*, *17*, 89–103.

Ferguson et al. (1998). Racial disparity in cardiac decision making: results from patient focus groups. *Arch Intern Med.*, *158*, 1450–1453.

Gamble, V. N. & Blustein, B. E. (1994). Racial differentials in medical care. In: A. C. Mastroianni, R. Faden & D. Federman, (Eds), *Women and health research: ethical and legal issues of including women in clinical studies*. Vol. 2. Washington, D.C.: National Academy Press.

Gaston et al. (1993). Racial equity in renal transplantation. *JAMA*, 270, 1352–1356.

Griffin, L. W. & Bratton, L. B. (1995). Fewer black kidney donors: what's the problem? *Soc Work Health Care*, *22*, 19–42.

Guadagnoli et al. (1999). The influence of race on approaching families for organ donation and their decision to donate. *Am J Public Health*, *89*, 244–247.

Hartwig et al. (1993). Effect of organ donor race on health team procurement efforts. *Arch Surg.*, *128*, 1331–1335.

Irish et al. (Eds) (1993). *Ethnic variations in dying, death, and grief: diversity in universality.* Washington DC: Taylor and Francis.

Jones, J. (1992). The Tuskegee legacy, AIDS, and the Black community. *Hastings Center Report*, *22*, 38–40.

Jones, J. (1993). *Bad blood: The Tuskegee syphilis experiment: A tragedy of race and medicine*, (expanded edition). NY; The Free Press.

Joun et al. (1997). Attitudes of Korean-Americans in and around New York City toward organ transplantation. *Transplant Proc.*, *29*, 3751–3752.

Kahn et al. (1994). Healthcare for black and poor hospitalized Medicare patients. *JAMA*, *271*, 1169–1174.

Kasiske, B. L. (1998). The evaluation of prospective renal transplant recipients and living donors. *Surg Clin North Am.*, *78*, 27–39.

Kasiske et al. (1991). The effect of race on access and outcome in transplantation. *N Engl J Med.*, *324*, 302–307.

Kasiske et al. (1998). Race and socioeconomic factors influencing early placement on the kidney transplant waiting list. *J Am Soc Nephrol.*, *9*, 2142–2147.

Kjellstrand, C. M. (1988). Age, sex, and race inequality in renal transplantation. *Arch Intern Medicine*, *148*, 1305–1309.

Klassen et al. (1998). Factors influencing waiting time and successful receipt of cadaveric liver transplant in the United States, 1990–1992. *Med Care*, *36*, 281–294.

Lee et al. (1997). Medicare treatment differences for blacks and whites. *Med Care*, *35*, 1173–1189.

McCabe, M. (1994). Patient Self-Determination Act: a Native American (Navajo) perspective. *Camb Q Healthc Ethics*, *3*, 419–421.

Merkatz et al. (1993). Women in clinical trials of new drugs. A change in food and drug administration policy. The working group on women in clinical trials. *N Engl J Med.*, *329*, 292–296.

Narva et al. (1996). Access of Native Americans to renal transplantation in Arizona and New Mexico. *Blood Purif.*, *14*, 293–304.

O'Connor, B. B. (1995). Hmong cultural values, biomedicine, and chronic liver disease. In: *Health Traditions: Alternative Medicine and the Health Professions*. Philadelphia: University of Pennsylvania Press.

Palepu et al. (1998). Minority faculty and academic rank in medicine. *JAMA*, *280*, 767–771.

Pappas et al. (1993). The increasing disparity in mortality between socioeconomic groups in the U.S., 1960 and 1986. *N Engl J Med.*, *329*, 103–109.

Pappas et al. (1997). Potentially avoidable hospitalizations: inequalities in rates between U.S. socioeconomic groups. *Am J Public Health*, *87*, 811–816.

Phipps, E., & True, G. *Inconsistencies in Values and Treatment Preferences around End-of Life: A Qualitative Study of Five Culturally Diverse Communities*. Presentation at the annual meeting of the American Society for Bioethics and Humanities, Philadelphia, PA, October 1999.

Randall, V. R. (1996). *Slavery, segregation, and racism: trusting the health care system ain't always easy! An African American perspective on bioethics*. St Louis: University Publishers.

Rodin, J., & Ickovics, J. R. (1990). Women's health. Review and research agenda as we approach the 21st century. *Am Psychol., 45*, 1018–1034.

Rosser, S. V. (1994.) *Women's Health: Missing from U.S. Medicine*. Bloomington, IN: Indiana University Press.

Schulman et al. (1999). The effect of race and sex on physicians' recommendations for cardiac catheterization. *N Engl J Med., 340*, 618–626.

Schwartz et al. (1990). Black/white comparisons of deaths preventable by medical intervention; United States and the District of Columbia 1980–1986. *Int J Epidemiol. 19*, 591–598.

Siminoff et al. (1995). Public policy governing organ and tissue procurement in the United States. Results from the national organ and tissue procurement study. *Ann Intern Med., 123*, 10–17.

Siminoff, L. A. (1997). African American perspectives on organ donation. Presented at the Fourth International Society for Organ Donation Congress. Washington, D.C.

Soucie et al. (1992). Race and sex differences in the identification of candidates for renal transplantation. *Am J Kidney Dis., 19*, 414–419.

Thao, X. (1986). Hmong perceptions of illness and traditional ways of healing. In: G. L. Hendricks, B. T. Downing, & A. Deinard, (Eds), *The Hmong in Transition*. New York: Center for Migration Studies.

Thomas, S., & Quinn, S. (1991). The Tuskegee syphilis study: implications for HIV education and AIDS risk education programs in the black community. *Am J Public Health, 81*, 1498–1505.

Wenger et al. (1993). Cardiovascular health and disease in women. *N Engl J Med., 329*, 247–256.

Wenneker, M. B., & Epstein, A. M. (1989). Racial inequalities in the use of procedures for patients with ischemic heart disease in Massachusetts. *JAMA, 261*, 253–257.

Whittle et al. (1993). Racial differences in the use of invasive cardiovascular procedures in the Department of Veterans Affairs medical system. *N Engl J Med., 329*, 621–627.

Yergan et al. (1987). Relationship between patient race and intensity of hospital services. *Med Care, 26*, 1111–1114.

Youngner, S. J. (1996). Some must die. In: S. J. Youngner, R. C. Fox & L. J. O'Connell (Eds). *Organ transplantation: meanings and realities* (pp. 32–55). Madison: University of Wisconsin Press.

14. ORGAN TRANSPLANTATION ISSUES IN MINORS

Marilyn A. Fisher

INTRODUCTION

Just as adults may experience vital organ failure, so, too, may children become impaired by failure of their major organs. The death of a child due to organ failure is even more tragic than the death of an adult from the same etiology, when one considers the number of years of potential life lost.

Without organ transplantation, even if a child does not die, but is able to accomplish marginal survival with severe chronic organ failure, the psychological/social/developmental effects of his illness pervade every aspect of his life. While there is no guarantee that receipt of a donor organ will suddenly cure the child's illness, the chance exists that organ transplantation may improve his quality of life.

Considerable attention has been focused on the ethics of procurement of vital organs from minors. At first glance, it would seem to be unethical to remove vital organs (heart, lungs, etc.) from a living individual. However, in certain scenarios, exactly that has been done. The development of a definition of brain death has given society the ability to declare an individual dead, even though his heart may be beating. Debate has occurred regarding whether an infant born without the cerebral cortex might be brain dead. If he is incapable of experiencing any thought processes, emotions, or relationships with other individuals, is not such an infant brain dead? His existence seems to confer no benefit to himself or to society, and only consumes society's resources. So, would it not be best if he were to be considered brain dead, and allowed to

The Ethics of Organ Transplantation, Volume 7, pages 339–366.

ISBN: 0-7623-0764-1

donate vital organs to a child who has a chance of survival if he receives a donated organ?

Vital organs for transplantation may also be harvested from fetuses. Fetuses have been deliberately conceived in order to remove their organs or tissues for donation, usually to a needy family member. Generally, removal of organs or tissues from a fetal donor results in death of the fetus. If a fetus' existence is brought about solely to serve such a purpose (that is, the fetus is regarded as worthless otherwise), is it wrong to use its organs for donation? Even if there is an urgent need for fetal organs by a deserving family member, is it ethical to regard the fetus as an organ farm?

Such individuals cannot protect themselves or stand up for their rights and are, therefore, among the most vulnerable members of society. At times they may be chosen by society, and by their surrogate decision makers, to be donors of vital organs. In this chapter, we will discuss the ethically charged issues regarding organ procurement from the infant born without a cerebral cortex and from the fetus.

ORGAN PROCUREMENT AND THE ANENCEPHALIC INFANT

If debate exists in other areas of pediatric organ donation, the issue of anencephalic patients donating organs is a virtual Pandora's box of hotly argued controversy. Anencephaly occurs in approximately 1 of 1000 to 2000 live births in the United States (Medical Task Force on Anencephaly, 1990). Its incidence is decreasing with improved prenatal testing technology, as some prospective parents opt for elective termination of these pregnancies. In anencephaly, the cerebral hemispheres of the brain are completely, or nearly completely, absent and, therefore, the patient is permanently unconscious. Acrania, absence of the bones of the cranial vault of the skull, exists, along with an extensive open defect of the spine. The cranial vault is open, with the remains of brain tissue appearing from the outside as a spongy vascular mass consisting mostly of hindbrain structures (a rudimentary brain stem: medulla, pons, cerebellum; and usually midbrain). The eyes are usually present, but the face is severely malformed, as the forehead and cranial vault of the skull are absent. Death usually occurs from either overwhelming central nervous system infection, since the central nervous system from the level of the rudimentary brain tissue down the length of the spinal cord is completely exposed to the environment, or from apnea (cessation of spontaneous breathing) due to lack of brain tissue. Other causes of death include endocrine dysfunction, low blood pressure, aspiration pneumonia, and hypothermia. Statistically, less than 10%

of these neonates survive to 1 week of age. Without heroic, and probably inappropriate, intervention, all anencephalics die in the newborn period. Any type of intervention which prolongs an anencephalic's life will also prolong his death, is futile, and is, therefore, believed by most to be unethical. The American Academy of Pediatrics has set forth guidelines for the care of anencephalic infants stating, "Customary medical care for anencephalic infants includes (provision of) warmth and feeding but no major medical interventions" (American Academy of Pediatrics, 1992).

Because anencephalic patients have a completely hopeless prognosis, and, aside from the abnormal central nervous system, generally have no organ anomalies, organs derived from these patients would seem to be perfect donor organs. Legally, vital organs from any patient, including an anencephalic, may be procured for organ donation only once death has occurred. Death may be declared by virtue of brain death or via cardiac death. With the onset of cardiac arrest, the organs experience lack of adequate blood flow and oxygenation. For this reason, donation of tissues/organs from a non-heart-beating donor is frequently restricted to use only of the heart valves and, rarely, skin and corneas, whereas, use of organs from heart-beating neonates, such as anencephalics, could reduce the shortage of vital organs donated to small children. For these reasons, there has been significant motivation to find ways to limit the hypoxic-ischemic damage to the potential donor anencephalic's organs and tissues.

In order to procure more useful donor organs, many have advocated that donation of the organs from the anencephalic neonate should occur *before* the heart has stopped beating. In fact, legislation has been proposed (then withdrawn) to modify the standards for determining human death as set forth in the Uniform Determination of Death Act (UDDA) so that they will include anencephalic infants with beating hearts. Another piece of legislation (New Jersey Assembly Bill No. 3367) permits parents of an anencephalic neonate to donate its organs before the patient actually meets death requirements as set forth in the Uniform Anatomical Gift Act (UAGA). Reasons cited to justify this practice are multiple.

(1) The demand for neonatal organs exceeds supply (Purvis, 1987).
(2) An anencephalic infant is, scientifically, an ideal organ donor because, while he is still breathing and has a heartbeat, there has not been irreversible hypoxemic damage to his tissues/organs.
(3) Anencephalics have been called "brain absent" (Harrison, 1986, 1986). The absence of cerebral cortex causes the anencephalic to be permanently unconscious without any shred of hope of gaining any neurologic function.

The fact that such an infant has always been unconscious, including *in utero*, and will always be unconscious, makes it impossible for him to ever have his own interests to protect.

(4) The anencephalic neonate carries a completely hopeless prognosis and, by virtue of his diagnosis, from the moment of birth, is clearly and definitely dying. Anencephaly is distinct diagnosis; most physicians believe that no misdiagnosis of this condition is possible. No amount of medical technology can cure or save such an infant. If placed on artificial mechanical ventilation due to apneas, the amount of time that his heart is beating may be prolonged, but he will continue to be unconscious or, in the absence of any neurological function, brain-dead. The ultimate outcome is that the patient will certainly die, whether or not he donates his organs.

(5) The parents of an anencephalic infant may derive some emotional benefit in donating multiple organs from their infant, realizing that some good can come of a tragic situation.

(6) Donation of multiple organs from an anencephalic is perceived to be an altruistic act, being beneficial to society in terms of saving lives, and in term of decreasing society's long-term financial and emotional costs of patients struggling to survive with chronic organ failure.

The Definition of Death

A key issue in the debate about procurement of organs from an anencephalic patient is whether the anencephalic patient must be dead before his organs are donated. Related issues include the definition of brain death and whether the definition of brain death should be altered in order to allow organ procurement from these patients while their hearts are still beating.

For time immemorial, death has been determined to occur when all bodily functions, especially heart beat and respiratory efforts, have ceased. Since the advent of life-sustaining medical technology in the past half century, circulation, respiration, and nourishment may be artificially continued, even if a patient has no spontaneous respiratory effort, nor ability to take in nutrition on his own. In the late 1960s, medical studies showed that complete absence of brain function provided an alternate means of establishing death. Beginning in 1970, various states gave recognition to *two* means of assessing death: the long-standing assessment of irreversible cessation of circulatory and respiratory function, and the new assessment of *irreversible cessation of all functions of the entire brain*. In 1982, the Uniform Determination of Death Act (UDDA), recognizing both these means of assessing death, arose from efforts of the National Conference of Commissioners on Uniform State Laws, the American

Medical Association, the American Bar Association, and the President's Commission. Since that time, the UDDA has been adopted in the majority of states of the United States, either explicitly or implicitly (Capron, 1987).

Some may argue that the term "brain death" is misleading because it suggests that organs, rather than organisms, die. In a patient declared brain dead, the heart continues to beat, the various organs continue to function, and the person is even able to reproduce. For these reasons, physiologists may not agree that complete absence of neurologic function is tantamount to death.

Currently, only those patients with total cessation of intracranial function can be declared brain dead. An anencephalic infant is not generally brain dead at birth. He usually has some initial respiratory efforts at birth and, therefore, does not initially have total cessation of brainstem function. This prevents him from being given an initial diagnosis of brain death.

The anencephalic neonate has no cerebral cortex and has, indeed, been called "brain-absent" (Harrison, 1986, 1986). His present, past, and future consist of permanent unconsciousness. He has not, has never had, and never will have, a potential to establish human relationships. He will never develop any cognitive function and will remain in a persistent vegetative state until he dies. By virtue of his diagnosis, he is dying. Neural tube defects, including anencephaly, lie on a continuum of developmental defects of the central nervous system. Some of the affected infants will have absolutely no cerebral tissue, while others will have rudimentary cerebral tissue. Regardless of the degree of affliction, the anencephalic will die of his malformation. He has severe structural brain damage, but is not completely brain-absent.

Since an anencephalic infant initially has both a heartbeat and respiratory effort, he satisfies neither the circulatory/respiratory nor the brain death criteria for death. Yet, because he has no potential for human relationship, an argument has been made (Paris et al., 1983) that such an infant should not have life artificially sustained. This does not mean, however, that vital organs should be removed from the patient while he is, by definition, still alive.

Certain maneuvers have been performed in attempts to have enough laboratory evidence to determine brain death in a heart beating anencephalic infant, so that his vital organs may be donated. Radionuclide cerebral angiography has been utilized to demonstrate unequivocal arrest of carotid circulation to the brain. Absence of intracranial arterial circulation is a valid diagnostic test for brain death in the neonate. If such a test can demonstrate complete lack of blood flow to the entire brain, including the brain stem which is responsible for respiratory efforts and reflexes, brain death can be inferred. However, in the case of neonates with anencephaly, two factors cause the radionuclide cerebral angiography to be inadequate to diagnose brain death.

First, such infants usually still have arterial blood flow to the hindbrain. Therefore, the study does not infer brain death. Second, clinical correlation is always needed with such testing. An anencephalic infant with respiratory effort is not clinically brain dead, regardless of the results of the radionuclide cerebral angiography!

If a breathing, heart-beating anencephalic neonate's organs are considered fair game for organ donation because of his state of permanent unconsciousness, his lack of personal interest in the past, present, and future, and his progression toward inevitable death, it must be expected that the next logical step will be the evaluation of other classifications of brain-damaged individuals for their acceptability for organ donation. Thus begins the so-called "slippery slope" argument. Should unconscious, breathing, heart-beating individuals with severe congenital brain malformations, who apparently contribute nothing to society, be considered brain-damaged enough to donate organs, even though they do not technically meet the criteria for brain death?

Hydranencephaly is a congenital structural deformity of the brain in which, like anencephaly, the cerebral cortex is absent at birth, but the brainstem remains intact. Like the anencephalic patient, the hydranencephalic patient remains in a state of permanent unconsciousness, but may retain brainstem reflexes, including breathing, sucking and swallowing, for months. Unlike anencephaly, hydranencephaly is associated with no external deformity; the cranial vault is present and appears grossly normal. Fluid fills the intracranial space which should have been occupied by brain tissue. Patients with hydranencephaly tend to survive longer than do anencephalics because their central nervous systems are not open to the environment and are not subject to overwhelming central nervous system infection. Hydranencephalic patients generally succumb to apnea or aspiration pneumonia within the first several years of life. In terms of type, function, and amount of brain tissue present, anencephaly and hydranencephaly are equal. However, the mechanisms by which these structural deformities develop are different. Anencephaly occurs because of failure of the cranial end of the neural tube to close during the fourth week of embryonic life. Hydranencephaly occurs after previously normal fetal development of the cerebral hemispheres. Sometime during fetal life, an obstruction of blood flow to the arteries of the brain occurs, leading to necrosis and reabsorption of the cerebral cortex. So, like the anencephalic patient, the hydranencephalic patient is in a state of permanent unconsciousness. However, unlike the anencephalic patient, the hydranencephalic at one time during fetal life did possess a cerebral cortex, may have experienced sensations, and so may have had some interest in life, although never an opportunity to express his interests to anyone. In comparing anencephaly vs. hydranencephaly, it might be argued that a brain which had never developed any personal interest nor self-awareness, should be treated differently than a brain which had previously developed normally, but then experienced damage, albeit in utero. Therefore, should the hydranencephalic neonate's vital organs be considered less seriously for donation than should those of the anencephalic? Similarly, might it be more easily justified to take vital organs from a living, previously neurologically competent, but now incompetent, patient who had decided to donate his organs if his prognosis became hopeless, than to take organs from a vulnerable anencephalic patient who never had an opportunity to realize or express his own personal interest? Should unconscious, breathing, heart-beating individuals with other acquired brain abnormalities such as porencephalic cysts, cerebral infarction and necrosis, hydrocephalus, progressive neurologic dysfunction, Alzheimer's disease, and sequelae of head trauma be considered brain-damaged enough to donate vital organs, even though they do not technically meet the criteria for brain or cardiac death? Because these lesions are acquired, some of these patients may have had an opportunity to let their personal interests be known before onset of their neurologic dysfunction. Once they have become brain-damaged, are their previously stated personal interests valid any longer? Consideration must also be given to whether the brain damage is reversible or irreversible. If the brain damage is potentially reversible (for instance, following head trauma), even though certain patients may have never voiced their own personal interests previously, someday they might, theoretically, be neurologically competent enough to make their interests known.

Societal Issues in Anencephaly

The controversial practice of removing vital organs from heart beating, non-brain dead anencephalics could potentially be legally sanctioned in several ways.

(1) The definition of brain death could be legally changed. If brain death is redefined to require only non-function of the cerebral cortex, then any patient in a persistently vegetative state with regular respiratory efforts could be legally deemed brain dead. He would, therefore, be eligible to donate his vital organs. Along these utilitarian lines of thought, the Harvard Committee Report on the Definition of Death (Ad Hoc Committee of the Harvard Medical School to Examine the Definition of Brain Death, 1968) sought to declare "irreversible coma as a new criterion for death because obsolete criteria for the definition of death can lead to controversy in obtaining organs for transplantation." Should death be defined in

whichever way maximizes the benefit to society, or is the definition of death independent of societal factors? If the definition of death can be changed with the times in order to maximize the good to society, then certain individuals, such as anencephalics, could be legally eliminated if their existence does not serve the purposes of society.

(2) Rather than redefining death, the law could be changed to permit removal of vital organs from heart beating non-brain dead anencephalics. These patients would be regarded as a unique group of people with regards to vital organ donation. Therefore, it would be legal to take vital organs solely from this particular group of living patients. Like the previous proposal, this proposal may also be considered excessively utilitarian. In an attempt to ethically justify this proposal, it could be argued that anencephalics have no self-interest in the past, present, or future, so that no personal interest of theirs is violated by removal of their vital organs. However, once the law is relaxed to allow certain living individuals to be killed by removal of their vital organs, other individuals in society may gradually be considered to be fair game for vital organ removal. It is likely that tight legal restrictions would have to be enacted in order to prevent abuse of such vulnerable patients.

(3) In order to justify removal of his vital organs, it could be argued that an anencephalic is not a human being. He may be a collection of human chromosomes, tissues, and organs which, scientifically, appear to function, but there is no self-interest, no capacity for any human relationships, no personality, no desire, and no thought process. He is an inanimate object. Thus, he may be proclaimed to be never alive, or neither alive nor dead (Veatch, 1992, 1993).

If anencephalics are eventually regarded as legitimate organ donors, to what lengths will society go in order to acquire organs from anencephalics? Anencephaly is often diagnosed prenatally. At that point, the mothers are offered a therapeutic abortion, or the option to deliver the moribund infant at term. Will women carrying anencephalic infants eventually be pressured to carry these defective fetuses to term and to deliver by cesarean section in order to maximize the chances that the fetus/future organ donor survives the delivery process? This would optimize the health and usefulness of the vital organs earmarked for donation. However, the mother would be subject to excessive risks: the risk of carrying a pregnancy to term, the risk of cesarean section, the emotional risks of carrying a moribund fetus for a prolonged time. Even if the mother subjects herself to such excessive risk in order to salvage her anencephalic infant's organs, there is no guarantee that the organs will be able to be used.

Relaxation of the brain death standard so that vital organs may be retrieved from non-brain dead anencephalic patients will have impact on more than just the areas of organ donation and anencephaly; it will affect the debate on euthanasia. It has been argued that sustaining medical therapies, including nutrition and hydration, can legally be withheld from anencephalics (Ashwal et al., 1992) because they are dying, will never recover, and have no interest in living. If they have no interest in living, it has been argued, how can actively causing their deaths by removal of their vital organs be more injurious to them than passive killing by withholding treatment? It has been argued that a difference must be recognized between allowing an anencephalic to die by removing, or not increasing the level of, life-support *versus* actively killing the patient by removing his vital organs. This difference exists, perhaps, not in the final outcome, which is inevitable death, but in the means by which that final outcome is achieved. All living beings, including anencephalics, no matter how ill, should be afforded a certain level of dignity and respect. If active killing of a certain group of patients were legalized, this would symbolize a weakening of society's commitment to respect and protect life. If taking vital organs from living anencephalics leads to unjustifiable organ removal from other incompetent patients, this would establish an unhealthy precedent, and should either not be done, or rigid safeguards to protect against abuse should be delineated. Once a patient lacks his own interests, it must be determined which is most important: the benefit to society of having more organs available for transplantation, or respect for society's prohibition against killing. It may be that this symbolic loss of respect for human life could cause the degeneration of the ethical, social, and moral nature of the community (Ascher, 1987).

As an addendum to the influence such a policy could have on society, and irrelevant to the moral issue of organ donation, our voluntary system of organ procurement depends on public confidence that organ donation does not harm the interests of donors. Public concern may arise over a changing definition of brain death. When physicians pronounce a patient brain-dead, the public may wonder whether the patient is really dead, or if the prognosis is just so dismal that it might be more utilitarian to take out the patient's organs for donation, and bring about death so that the severly-damaged patient does not usurp hospital resources. If organs are taken from neurologically incompetent, living donors, such practice may discourage the idealistic, altruistic public from committing to organ donation.

Yet another controversial issue that has been brought up involves the utilization of resources to achieve organ donation from anencephalic patients.

Medical technology, health care professionals, and space in a neonatal intensive care unit are expensive and limited in terms of their availability. Some believe that it may be unethical to transfer such resources from the care of standard critically ill infants to an unproven, experimental project such as the maintenance of infants with anencephaly, not for their own good, but solely for the purpose of organ donation (Bioethics Committee, Canadian Paediatric Society, 1990).

Even if agreement is established that anencephalics should not be killed by removal of vital organs, another debate exists as to whether non-vital organs/ tissues, such as bone marrow, blood, or one of two functioning kidneys may be harvested from an anencephalic donor. Removal of such organs/tissues would not directly cause the death of such a patient, although the surgical procedure itself might provide additional physical stressors which could, theoretically, hasten death by increasing the risk of infection, apnea, blood loss, and fluid/ electrolyte abnormalities. It has been suggested that non-vital organs may be taken from children and other incompetent patients if such patients derive a net benefit from the donation and are not harmed. In order to proceed with this manner of reasoning, the terms "benefit" and "harm" must be defined. Both have been defined in terms of their physical, emotional, psychosocial, and religious aspects. It is unlikely that a patient can have any physical benefit, and may, indeed, be subject to significant physical harm to his own body by donating non-vital organs/tissues.

The benefit realized by donation of non-vital organs by children to family members is sometimes measured in terms of its emotional/psychosocial effect. That is, if a child successfully donates blood, bone marrow, or one of two functioning kidneys to his parent or sibling, this may result in the saving of the life of that family member. The net emotional/psychosocial benefit to the donor child in not having to face the death of a family member may outweigh the physical risk to the donor child. In the case of a donor with anencephaly, however, there is neither physical benefit from the donation of non-vital organs nor emotional or psychosocial benefit. Emotional/religious/psychosocial benefit cannot be realized by the anencephalic patient himself, since he possesses no awareness of the life or death of any family member, nor awareness of any good effects which he may be imparting to a family member or a member of his community by virtue of the donation of his non-vital organs/tissues. Any emotional benefit to an anencephalic infant of providing heroic organ donation would rest in the improbability that the diagnosis of anencephaly, and thus the lethal prognosis, is incorrect, and that the patient may not die and may someday be cognizant of the survival of a family or community member. The "benefit" derived by an anencephalic upon donation of his (non-vital) organs may be a societal one, one appreciated by his family and by the organ recipient and the recipient's family, but not by the anencephalic patient himself.

Similarly, the definition of "harm" must also be clarified. Does removal of non-vital organs/tissues from an anencephalic cause "harm"? Risk to the body is likely in the event that an unnecessary surgical procedure is performed on an anencephalic. Does this risk constitute harm? Risks of surgery include risk of infection, risk of blood loss, risk of anesthesia/mechanical ventilation, and risk of poor wound healing. Or, does "harm" mean interfering with the patient's desire to proceed toward certain goals? Since the anencephalic has neither conscious desires nor interests of his own, is harm to him even possible? Should the desires and interests that his family projects onto him be considered valid? Or, are the interests of the anencephalic patient distinct from those of his parents? If so, who is qualified to determine what his interests are? It has been argued that an anencephalic should not be referred to as a prospective organ donor, since "donor" refers to one who voluntarily chooses to give a gift. As permanently unconscious individuals who have no interest in themselves or in others, anencephalics are incapable of making such a choice. Removal of non-vital organs from an anencephalic may not directly lead to his death, and, therefore, may not legally be considered homicide, but may be best defined as assault.

There seems to be a willingness of society to use such incompetent patients as a means to an end (i.e. helping others). Is this ethically correct? To help others at the possible expense of the interests of the anencephalic may be a violation of the respect and dignity that is due all humans, regardless of their health or intellectual capacity.

Mechanisms of Procuring Organs

The Use of Anesthesia in Anencephaly

If harvesting non-vital organs from anencephalic infants is acceptable, the mechanism by which such organs might be procured must be considered. Does an anencephalic being prepared for organ donation require anesthesia in the operating room? The absence of the cerebral cortex makes it impossible for the anencephalic to consciously perceive pain or pleasure, but the presence of an, albeit, poorly functioning brainstem, makes it possible for primitive spinal reflexes to occur in response to painful stimuli.

If anesthesia is necessary, another concern becomes the actual mechanism of providing anesthesia to the anencephalic infant in the operating room. Should such a patient be stabilized on mechanical ventilation during the operative procedure (while he is under the influence of general anesthesia) in order to keep the donor tissues well oxygenated? Once the effects of general anesthesia have worn off, and the patient is no longer apneic (having breath-holding spells) as a result of the general anesthesia, the patient should be removed from the mechanical ventilator. If the patient then develops apneas apparently associated with anencephaly rather than with the general anesthesia, is it ethical to withhold placing him back on mechanical ventilation, even though this decision may well result in cardiorespiratory death? Some would argue that an apneic anencephalic (not under the influence of general anesthesia) is brain-dead by virtue of his apneas. That is, even his rudimentary brain stem has ceased to function. It may be ethical to withhold mechanical ventilation from an apneic anencephalic, even if he is not brain-dead, if the apnea is related to his primary diagnosis, and not to an effect of the anesthesia. But how does the medical practitioner determine the exact etiology of the apneas? There is no test to differentiate one etiology from the other.

Anticipation of Death

Since it is morally, ethically, and, currently, legally homicide to remove vital organs from the permanently unconscious, including anencephalics, several proposals have been drawn up to permit retrieval of fairly well-oxygenated vital organs from dead anencephalics. In one scenario, the anencephalic infant is allowed to suffer a respiratory arrest due to apneas associated with his neurologic dysfunction. With lack of breathing and inadequate oxygenation, the heart eventually stops beating. The infant is then pronounced dead. His body is then resuscitated with cardiopulmonary resuscitation, medications to improve cardiac output and blood pressure, and even with mechanical ventilation in hopes of re-establishing adequate organ perfusion and oxygenation. The living organs are then surgically removed from the newly pronounced dead infant, even though the heart rate may have returned during the resuscitation of the "dead" infant's body. If the heart resumes beating after resuscitation, the organs will be healthier and more likely to be harvested successfully than if the heart fails to resume beating. If after resuscitation, hearts beat and, perhaps, even respiratory effort return, was the patient really dead? In retrospect, in this scenario, the cessation of heart rate and, perhaps, respiratory effort was reversible. The definition of death, as established by the Task Force on Brain Death in Children (Task Force on Brain Death in Children, 1987) states that, in order for death to be determined, an individual must have sustained: (1) *irreversible* cessation of circulatory and respiratory functions, or (2) *irreversible* cessation of all functions of the entire brain, including the brainstem. For what amount of time must an anencephalic be without heartbeat, respiratory effort, or neurologic function in order to ensure irreversibility of his death? How much time may an anencephalic be without heartbeat, respiratory effort, or neurologic function before his organs/tissues are no longer suitable for donation? Is there overlap between these two periods of time, or are they distinct from each other? Also, of note, resuscitation is not generally done for patients with anencephaly, because it will simply prolong the dying process. Unlike other organ donors, when anencephalics are placed on mechanical ventilation, it is never for their own benefit, but rather for the benefit of prospective organ recipients, or the emotional benefit of their families, or for the benefit of society. From the point of view of the helpless anencephalic, is it ethical to prolong his dying in this way? Since he is incapable of perceiving discomfort, is his suffering being prolonged?

Another method to legally procure organs from anencephalics is to monitor such infants for apnea, which is then interpreted as an indication of whole brain death. When a terminal apnea occurs, brain death can be declared, even in the presence of a weakly beating heart, and the organs can then be harvested. A problem with this proposal is that such an infant may have many apneas from which he spontaneously recovers before encountering his final, terminal apnea. There are no markers to determine which breath is the last breath, which apnea is the final apnea. Minutes after cessation of the heart and respiratory efforts, resuscitative efforts or spontaneous endogenous factors occasionally cause return of heart rate and respiratory efforts. Therefore, as in the previous proposal, irreversibility of death cannot be ensured.

A third proposal investigated in Canada and in one U.S. institution (Peabody et al., 1989) involves resuscitation and mechanical ventilation of anencephalic infants at birth, maintaining organ viability in this way until brain death occurs. Once brain death occurs, as manifested by loss of respiratory effort, the infants are pronounced dead and their organs harvested. It may take days or weeks, or longer, for an anencephalic infant to manifest brain death, especially if the mechanical ventilator breaths mask his apneas. The usurping of hospital resources for a prolonged period of time awaiting brain death of an anencephalic patient may not be appropriate.

A final proposal set forth to legally attempt to accomplish organ donation from anencephalics involves deliberately cooling the patient. When the patient becomes apneic, the apnea is interpreted as whole brain death. In addition, cardiac arrest may occur with the onset of hypothermia-induced apnea. Removal of the vital organs is then carried out (Fletcher et al., 1986). The hypothermia is believed to help preserve organ function in the presence of poor organ blood flow and hypoxia. Proponents of this proposal argue that the terminal apnea may not be induced by the hypothermia, but may be secondary to the patient's neurologic dysfunction. That may or may not be true, but if the terminal apnea occurs during deliberately induced hypothermia, and the patient has not previously experienced a terminal apnea during normothermia, the induction of hypothermia appears, at least, to be responsible for the terminal apnea. Again, there are no markers to determine whether such an apnea is due to hypothermia or to the patient's primary neurologic diagnosis. In addition, in the practice of medicine, a hypothermic individual (for instance, someone pulled from an icy lake) should not be pronounced dead from a cardiac nor neurologic standpoint until he has been rewarmed to a normal body temperature. This is because a hypothermic individual who has no heart beat nor respiratory effort may exist in a state akin to suspended animation (due to hypothermia-induced lowering of basal metabolic rate) and, upon rewarming, may have return of neurologic and organ function. If a hypothermic anencephalic has a cardiorespiratory arrest or a terminal apnea, it may likely be reversible if the hypothermia is corrected. So, if hypothermia has the ability to reversibly halt cardiac, respiratory, and neurologic function, it is probably unethical to declare any hypothermic individual, including the anencephalic, dead unless he remains lifeless upon rewarming.

If no consensus can be reached on how to procure organs from heart-beating anencephalic patients, then organ donation from these patients should be forbidden.

It must be determined why some argue that organs can be removed from anencephalic patients. Is it because the anencephalics are brain-dead? What exactly is brain-death? Is it because they are brain-damaged enough that they have no personal interests? Is homicide ethically permissible if the individual to be killed is going to die anyway? This goes a step beyond euthanasia, which is currently illegal. Is homicide permissible if the killing of one person could save the life of one or several people? Who has the qualifications to determine whose life is more valuable?

Summary

In summary, the donation of organs is a much-needed act, accomplishing a desirable end. Parents who have chosen to offer their infant's organs have made a difficult and noble decision. However, extreme caution must be exercised in the *mechanism* by which this is justified and accomplished. The definition of death should not be relaxed in order to accomplish this deed, as this may have far-reaching negative implications on the moral and ethical foundation of society. For the same reason, bending and distorting the law in order to justify the killing of anencephalics by removal of vital organs or by administration of hypothermia should be forbidden. In order to protect society's high moral and ethical structure, potential donor organs from anencephalics may, unfortunately, have to be forfeited. The medical professional must remember, "Above all, do no harm".

ORGAN TRANSPLANTATION AND THE FETUS

The Fetus as a Patient

In this modern era, invasive and transplacental therapy, including transplantation with donor cells or tissues, is increasingly able to treat a variety of pathological fetal conditions. There are several situations in which a fetus may be treated with transfused or transplanted donor tissue. A severely anemic fetus may require a red blood cell transfusion in utero in order to survive. Donated bone marrow and liver cells have been used to treat fetuses with immunodeficiency states, hematologic disorders, and inborn errors of metabolism. The fetus is uniquely suited early in gestation to have immunotolerance induced by receipt of donor cell suspensions. Therefore, when an eventual need for organ transplantation is recognized early in gestation, it may be possible to induce donor-specific tolerance by transfusing, in utero, the future organ recipient with blood from the future organ donor (Crombleholme, 1991).

Ethical Decisions in Treating a Fetus

Is it morally correct to risk the mother's health in an attempt to treat her ailing fetus? The ability of a pregnant woman to make an autonomous medical decision is composed of the following elements. First, there must be disclosure by the physician to the patient of pertinent information relating to the patient's condition and its management. Second, there must be understanding of such information by the patient. Finally, there must be a voluntary decision by the patient to authorize or refuse such management. In the discussion of treatment of a fetus, issues of surrogacy further complicate the ethical decision-making process. That is, the mother of the fetus may or may not be an appropriate individual to authorize treatment of the fetus. However, any treatment of the fetus that is carried out will, of necessity, affect the mother, in whose womb the fetus dwells. Therefore, it is expected, but not guaranteed, that the mother of the fetus will exercise her responsibilities to protect the well being of her fetus as part of her beneficence-based obligations to her fetus. Autonomy-based self-protection should also play a role in the mother's decision-making process as to whether to treat her fetus.

In medical literature and, especially, in the practice of maternal-fetal medicine, the fetus is often referred to as a patient in its own right. That the fetus is considered in this way is a result of technological advances in maternal-fetal medicine, rather than due to careful ethical consideration of the concept of the fetus as a patient and the associated clinical implications. Whether a fetus should be regarded as a patient in its own right, and should receive treatment as such, may be dependent on the independent moral status of the fetal patient. However, there has been no authoritative determination as to how to assess the independent moral status of a fetus. Independent moral status may begin at the moment of conception or implantation (Bopp, 1985), may be acquired in steps as fetal development progresses, or may occur only when the infant can survive ex utero.

Conversely, it may be that a patient does not need to possess independent moral status in order to be regarded as a patient. An individual may be considered to be a patient when he is presented to a physician with the expectation that diagnosis and treatment may be carried out if such diagnosis and treatment modalities are expected to result in greater good than harm to the future of that individual. When the fetus is a considered to be a patient, both the physician and the mother have beneficence-based obligations to it; they are both expected to act, within reason, to protect and promote the interests of the fetus (Chervenak & McCullough, 1996). A viable fetus will eventually become a child with independent moral status as long as biological (and technical factors, if necessary) support it up until that point. For instance, a fetus at 24 weeks gestation (16 weeks short of its due date) is generally considered to be viable. It may mature within the uterus until its due date with the cooperation of favorable maternal biological factors, or, if born prematurely, may mature in an intensive care setting with maximal technical support. In each of these scenarios, its independent moral status, distinct from its mother, is recognized.

On the other hand, the only way that a *previable* fetus can become a child with independent moral status is through the pregnant woman's autonomy as she decides whether or not to carry the pregnancy to viability. If favorable biological factors are withdrawn by the mother, as in an elective termination of pregnancy, the fetus will die. Likewise, if the fetus is spontaneously born prematurely at a period of previability, no amount of technical support is capable of making the fetus survive to become a child with independent moral status. An extreme form of previability is the fertilized ova or *in vitro* embryo in a test tube, which is available for implantation into a woman's reproductive tract. Like the previable fetus, the fertilized ova or *in vitro* embryo may be regarded as a patient only when the woman who is to carry the fetus confers that status upon it. Eventual independent moral status of the previable fetus, fertilized ova, or *in vitro* embryo rests solely on the exercise of the woman's (not the sperm donor's) autonomy as she makes the decision to carry the pregnancy. A pregnant woman is under no ethical obligation to confer the status of being a patient onto her previable fetus (or fertilized ova or embryo) simply because there exists a fetal therapy that can be done for the previable fetus to eventually make it an independent individual.

A viable fetus may be considered a patient in its own right, since its survival does not depend completely on maternal autonomy. Beneficence-based obligations of the mother and the physician toward the fetus must be tempered, however, with beneficence-based obligations of the physician toward the mother and autonomy-based obligations of the mother to herself. This is because, since the viable fetal patient dwells within the mother's womb, therapy of the fetus necessarily involves physical, mental, and financial risks to the mother. The mother is ethically obligated to accept only reasonable risks to herself in order to attempt to benefit her fetus. This ethical obligation to treat the viable fetus exists when all of the following are true: (1) invasive therapy of the viable fetus is expected to have a very high probability of being life saving or of preventing serious and irreversible disease, injury, or handicap for the fetus and for the child the fetus can become, (2) when such therapy is expected to involve low mortality risk and low risk of serious disease, injury, or handicap to the viable fetus and the child it can become, and (3) when the mortality risk to the pregnant woman is judged to be very low, and the risk of disease, injury, or handicap to the pregnant woman is judged to be low or manageable. A physician should not recommend fetal therapy unless all of the above factors are true. If, after receiving all pertinent information, a woman declines fetal therapy for her viable fetus when all three of the above facts are true, then the mother has made an unethical decision to forego fetal intervention, and the physician may have to resort to respectful persuasion, or even to an ethics committee mediation (Chervenak & McCullough, 1996).

If the three above factors are not met, the mother's autonomy may be enhanced by offering her experimental fetal therapies which may expand the range of treatment options for her viable fetus, and may enhance the accumulation of knowledge which may benefit future patients with similar problems. A physician may offer, but not recommend, such experimental therapies; consultation with an institutional review board for human experimentation is suggested. In contrast to the case of a viable fetus, neither a pregnant woman nor the physician has any moral obligation to regard a previable fetus as a patient, unless, while exercising her autonomy, a pregnant woman confers the status of being a patient upon her previable fetus. Therefore, a pregnant woman may ethically withhold or withdraw treatments from her previable fetus, and is under no moral obligation to consent to experimental therapies, regardless of lack of risk of therapy to herself.

The Fetus as an Organ Donor

The Brave New World of Technological Possibilities

While there has been some controversy as to whether fetuses should have therapeutic tissue/organ transplantation, there has been intense debate as to whether donation of tissue from a fetus is morally permissible. In order to clarify the nomenclature used in the following discussion, it must be noted that the term "fetus", technically, to the medical community, refers to an *in utero* being which has developed in maturity to a point beyond that of an embryo. An "abortus" is a fetus born before it is of sufficient maturity to be viable. In this discussion, however, the term "fetus" is used both correctly to describe an *in utero* being, as well in the vernacular to describe an *ex utero* abortus, which is a fetal-like previable infant who has no chance for survival outside of the uterus. Therefore, such a "fetus" must be dying.

The question of the morality of fetal tissue donation came about recently because it has only recently become technically possible to transplant fetal tissue into other living beings. Transplantation of fetal tissue offers certain advantages compared to transplantation of tissue that is more mature. Fetal tissue, especially that procured relatively early in gestation, in general, has a lower expression of histocompatibility antigens than does tissue procured from more mature donors, so the risk of organ rejection by the recipient is lessened. Early gestation fetal cells are superior in their abilities to grow, proliferate, and differentiate *in vivo*. They have the ability to produce trophic substances that not only increase their own ability to survive and proliferate but also promote regeneration of adjacent damaged tissue. Fetal tissues produce angiogenic factors, which promote blood vessel formation, which increases perfusion and, thus, survival of the fetal tissue. Fetal neural tissue secretes nerve growth factors that assist in neural tissue regeneration (Consultants to the Advisory Committee to the Director, 1988). Success has been demonstrated in the donation of fetal tissues and organs to treat recipient kidney, liver, thymus, heart, pancreas, hematologic, muscle, neurologic, and reproductive tissue disease.

It is technically possible to transplant fetal ovarian tissue into another living female, where the transplanted ovarian tissue releases ova (eggs). Using this technique, a female fetus who has never survived outside of the womb could become the genetic mother of another individual. There are certain issues to be addressed regarding the transplantation of fetal ovaries. For the sake of this discussion, we will set aside debate on the mechanism by which the ovarian tissue is obtained, as this topic will be discussed in a subsequent section. First of all, it may be preferable to use donor fetal ova as compared to ova of an older female, because the fetal ova have probably not had exposure to environmental toxins and radiation, both of which are known to cause chromosomal abnormalities. Also favoring the use of fetal cells is the fact that ova from elderly mothers have a clear association with genetic defects of the ova. These defects may arise both as a result of the age of the mother, and the resultant length of time that the ova have existed unfertilized within her body, as well as the fact that, the older the mother, the greater the amount of time that the ova may have been exposed to environmental toxins.

Some have argued against the use of fetal ova on scientific grounds. Reasons that are cited include the fact that the ova being fertilized are most likely the ones that would not have ordinarily been fertilized by natural means. By the fifth month of gestation, the ovaries of the average female fetus will have approximately 7 million ova, only 400,000 of which will remain at puberty, with less than 500 of these being ovulated during her reproductive years with the potential to create a human being (Sadler, 1990). If some of these ova which would have ordinarily not been fertilized become fertilized via technology such as fetal ovarian tissue transplantation, then ova which have not been subject to natural selection pressures are being allowed to develop into individuals. This may result in defective genes being propagated, in the production of defective individuals, and may work against the theory of "survival of the fittest". This argument assumes that some ova are superior to others, and it is this superiority of certain ova that leads to their being ovulated and to their opportunity to be fertilized (Berkowitz, 1995).

Similarly, cells from primordial male reproductive organs from male rat fetuses and neonates have been transplanted (Jiang, 1995) into the lumen of seminiferous tubules of recipient adult male rats, where they produce sperm. By its transplanted testicular tissue producing sperm in this manner, a male fetus who has never survived outside of the womb could become the genetic father of another individual. Monumental religious, psychosocial, and ethical arguments against fetal ovarian and testicular tissue transplantation also exist.

The research that has been done thus far in the field of fetal organ, tissue, and cell transplantation has been performed on fetal animals which have been surgically removed from the wombs of their mothers, or which have had surgery performed while the fetuses were still *in utero*. In humans, due to ethical and legal reasons, if fetal organs, tissues, or cells are considered for use in transplantation, they are most likely to be acquired from fetuses that have experienced spontaneous expulsion from the uterus. Spontaneous pregnancy losses yield minimal usable tissue for human transplantation because of a lack of adequate quantity of embryonic or fetal tissues, delayed collection of tissue which is no longer viable, decomposition, bacterial or viral contamination, or genetic abnormality of such tissue. Spontaneously aborted fetuses have a higher risk of chromosomal abnormalities than do fetuses from elective termination of pregnancy and fetuses from ectopic pregnancies. In one study (Hainline et al., 1995), 13.8% of mothers with spontaneous abortion or ectopic (Fallopian tubal) pregnancy at 5–30 weeks gestation gave consent for their products of conception to be evaluated for possible organ, tissue, cell donation. 18.4% of tissues yielded samples of good to excellent quality for potential organ/tissue transplantation and 66% grew pathogenic bacteria. Two percent of fetuses in the study originated from mothers who were positive for hepatitis C. Seventy-seven percent of fetuses originated from mothers infected with cytomegalovirus. None of the mothers tested in this particular study was infected with the human immunodeficiency virus, the human t-lymphotrophic virus, syphilis, nor hepatitis B virus. Only 4% of fetal brain samples were potential candidates for human tissue transplantation. Negligible numbers of viable fetal hepatocytes were identified. With such little usable tissue able to be utilized from products of spontaneous abortions and ectopic pregnancies, and with the development of early abortifacient medications (the "morning-after pill"), there is predicted to be a shortage of tissue able to be obtained from both spontaneously aborted and electively aborted fetuses.

Ethics of Fetal Organ Procurement

What prerequisites must be satisfied in order to make fetal tissue transplantation morally acceptable? First, consent from the woman donating the tissues of the abortus would seem to be necessary. Even this, however, is debatable because some would hold that, once she gives consent for an abortion, or for an *in utero* procedure that would jeopardize the life of her fetus, she is no longer seeking the best interest of the fetus and should lose her rights of surrogate decision maker for that fetus. Second, other modes of therapy (for the ailing individual in need of donor organs/tissue) must not be available. Some, however, would argue that, even if fetal tissue transplantation were the only mode of therapy known, transplantation of fetal tissue is still not ethical because the woman's decision to have an abortion and her decision to donate the fetal tissue are too closely interrelated. The third criterion that may need to be met in order to make fetal tissue transplantation morally acceptable is that the good expected to come of the procedure must outweigh the harm/risk of the procedure. Risk-benefit ratios are difficult to determine since each individual will use a different measuring unit by which to judge risk and benefit. Finally, pain and suffering of the fetus must be avoided. Fetal pain and suffering is difficult to detect, however, because the fetus cannot express its discomfort. Moreover, some may argue that fetuses in the early stages of gestation cannot experience pain because the neural pathways responsible for transmitting painful impulses are not developed. Others may argue that, in order to ensure that a fetus experiences no pain related to donating tissue, health care professionals should wait until it is clearly dead (i.e., exhibits cessation of the heartbeat) before harvesting its tissues.

In 1977, the National Commission for the Protection of Human Subjects of Biomedical and Behavioral Research (Destro, 1977) stated that moral concern should extend to all who share human genetic heritage, and that the fetus, regardless of its life prospects, should be treated respectfully and with dignity. The Commission, at that time, imposed boundaries restricting freedom of scientific inquiry out of respect for the fetus. It stated that, with regards to the field of fetal tissue transplantation (non-therapeutic for the fetus), only minimal risk could be accepted as permissible for such non-consenting subjects. The Commission regarded research being performed on dying fetuses less risky than research being performed on non-dying fetuses because it believed that a dying fetus could not be harmed, except to increase its suffering during the dying process. The Commission did see as unethical, however, any procedure which would alter the length of the dying process of such fetuses. The removal of vital organs from these fetuses, therefore, would be deemed unethical by the Commission. Some may argue, however, that the removal of vital organs, thus shortening the life (and, therefore, length of suffering) of a dying fetus, may be the most humane procedure for such a fetus. The process of terminating the life of a dying individual, including a fetus, is termed euthanasia, however, and is currently illegal and possibly unethical.

There may exist a double standard here. Why should research be permitted on non-consenting dying fetuses when it is prohibited on non-consenting dying adults? A possible explanation for this paradox is that a fetus never possessed self-interest or the ability to express itself, so its family may consent to research on its tissues, whereas, a dying adult has (or, at least, had) self-interest and may have let his wishes regarding research be known either via a legal document or via past conversations with his family and friends.

If it is ethically permissible to use fetal tissue for donation, which fetuses are eligible to have their tissues harvested? Fetuses who seem to be candidates for tissue donation include those delivered at a previable gestational age due to spontaneous abortion as well as those delivered at a previable age as a result of an elective termination of pregnancy. Women who simply do not desire to bring children into the world may seek abortion for some fetuses. Women who have an ulterior motive beyond simply the termination of the pregnancy may seek abortion for other fetuses. Such a fetus may have been deliberately conceived in order to use its tissues or organs for transplantation to another needy individual. Is it acceptable to obtain fetal tissue from an abortus who was conceived solely for the use of his tissues? Is it acceptable to eat cattle raised on a cattle farm solely for their meat products? Some would say that an abortus, having no consciousness, has no self-interest, and therefore no right to life, whereas a cow does. However, it is uncertain as to when a fetus develops consciousness and self-interest. On the contrary, others would state that a human fetus, unlike a cow, should have a right to be protected by mankind because it contains the genetic pool of a human being, and has the *potential* to become a conscious, reasoning human being.

Because fetal tissue may be useful in treatment of certain diseases, but the process of obtaining fetal tissue may cause death or damage to the fetus, there exist ethical dilemmas in how procurement of human fetal tissue should be accomplished. The literature documents the plan of a woman to provide her husband with kidneys donated from a fetus conceived and electively aborted at 5 to 6 months gestation solely for the purpose of kidney donation (Warren, et al., 1978). Another woman whose father suffered from Alzheimer's disease requested to be artificially inseminated with her father's sperm. She then intended to provide her father with fetal neural tissue for transplantation, although she knew that the procedure to harvest the fetal tissue would result in the death of the fetus (Lewin, 1987). The sale of fetal tissue for financial gain has also been reported.

In Europe, these ethical conflicts have been addressed by the 13 medical centers participating in the Network of European CNS (Central Nervous System) Transplantation and Restoration (NECTAR) (Brotchi, 1995). NECTAR has proposed the following ethical guidelines pertaining to the procurement of human embryonic and fetal tissue:

(1) Tissue for transplantation or research may be obtained only from dead embryos or fetuses, their death resulting from ***legally induced*** or spontaneous abortion. Death of an intact embryo or fetus is defined as absence of respiration and heartbeats. Brain death of a fetus or embryo has not been defined.
(2) Keeping intact embryos or fetuses alive artificially, for the purpose of removing usable material, is not allowed as per NECTAR guidelines. Interestingly, it is ***legally*** permissible for neonates, children, and adults, as well as fetuses, to be pronounced dead based on brain death or cardiorespiratory criteria, then to have efforts made to restart or maintain the functions of the organs with the intention of salvaging those organs for donation. NECTAR does not define how embryos and fetuses could be kept alive artificially against its guidelines. Theoretically, embryos could

have been created *in vitro* in the laboratory and could be kept alive for a short period of time for the theoretical purpose of tissue donation. Practically speaking, the quantity of tissue obtainable from such a small embryo is so small, however, that it would not be of any use in tissue donation. Fetuses, on the other hand, could theoretically be kept alive *ex utero* in order to eventually donate their tissues/organs. However, if such fetuses can be kept alive on mechanical ventilation and other types of highly specialized technology, they may actually be viable living infants. Therefore, removal of their organs/tissues would be unethical.

(3) The decision to terminate pregnancy must, under no circumstances, be influenced by the possible or desired subsequent use of the embryo or fetus, and must therefore precede any introduction of the possible use of the embryonic or fetal tissue. There should be no link between the donor and the recipient, nor designation of the recipient by the donor or the donor's surrogate decision maker. This particular guideline is careful to declare that the termination of pregnancy must not be influenced by intent to donate tissue from the fetus, and that the donation of fetal tissue should not be directed by the mother to any particular recipient. Otherwise, the act might be interpreted as murder (or sacrifice, if you will) of a living being of little worth in order to help a person of greater inherent worth. Certainly, those opposed to abortion would find these statements unappealing. Also, many may believe that a fetus is just as worthy of life as an individual who is already born. If a fetus, unable to defend itself, is representative of those humans which are helpless, and, if it is ethically correct to take organs from the fetus without its consent, which results in the death of the fetus, is it also ethical to take organs from other helpless people such as newborns, the brain-damaged, and the mentally ill?

(4) The procedure of abortion, or of its timing, must not be influenced by the requirements of the transplantation activity when this would be in conflict with the woman's interests, or would increase embryonic or fetal distress. In the event that a woman requests an elective abortion for reasons unrelated to organ and tissue transplantation, but has incidentally agreed to donation of her fetus' organs/tissues, is it ethical to ask her to prolong the pregnancy so that there will be a greater chance for successful transplantation of her fetus' organs/tissues? Prolongation of the pregnancy may expose the woman to a longer duration of the risks of pregnancy, and may require that a different, less safe, means of performing the abortion is carried out. NECTAR guidelines suggest, therefore, that it would be unethical to request that the woman delay

performance of an abortion simply so that the fetal organs are more favorable for donation. In a sense, in this scenario *in utero* prolongation of such a pregnancy could be considered unethical and, ironically, artificial by NECTAR.

(5) No fetal material may be used without informed consent of the woman involved. This informed consent should, whenever possible, be obtained prior to abortion.
(6) Screening of the woman for transmissible diseases requires informed consent.
(7) Nervous tissue may be used for transplantation only as suspended cell preparations or tissue fragments.
(8) All members of the hospital or research staff directly involved in any of the procedures must be fully informed.
(9) The procurement of embryos, fetuses or their tissue must not involve profit or remuneration.
(10) The local ethics committee must approve every transplantation or research project involving the use of embryonic or fetal tissue.

These guidelines, believed to be ethical by the members of NECTAR, are not law. Members of NECTAR, and others, may choose to follow these guidelines if local law allows, but are not legally bound to follow them.

It has been debated whether the procurement of tissue from an already aborted pre-viable fetus is unethical, or whether it is the abortion/termination of fetal life that is the unethical issue. It is possible that transplantation of tissue from an already aborted pre-viable fetus is ethically acceptable, as long as the transplantation process is distinct and separate from the decision to proceed with abortion. However, if the two processes are linked, as in the previously mentioned cases, then there may have been unethical decisions made to abort each fetus in order to bring about the tissue transplantation.

Who Shall Decide?

Anatomic gifts of fetal tissue must always be authorized by a surrogate decision-maker, rather than by the fetus itself, since the fetus has never had the capacity to make such a decision. There are certain ethical issues regarding who may serve as surrogate decision-maker in the procurement of fetal tissue. Regarding tissue donation, when a pregnancy ends in spontaneous abortion (miscarriage), the role of the mother of the dead fetus is analogous to the role of any close relative of a deceased individual. However, when the mother of the fetus deliberately brings about the death of her fetus by consenting to an abortion, and then chooses to donate the organs of the fetus, it may be that the purpose of the abortion was primarily to donate tissue to another living being. It may also be argued that a woman choosing to have an elective abortion is not concerned about the best interests of the fetus and, therefore, she should lose her capacity as the abortus' surrogate decision maker to decide what should be the disposition of the abortus' organs and tissues.

The National Commission for the Protection of Human Subjects of Biomedical and Behavioral Research (National Commission for the Protection of Subjects of Biomedical and Behavioral Research, 1975) has stated that research on living but non-viable fetuses is acceptable because the consent obtained is based on the "principle of proximity". Under this principle, knowledge obtained from such research would be used on the type of beings "close to" the fetus, such as other fetuses, neonates, and pregnant women.[35] Ironically, if the fetus "wants" to help others of his class and community, it must be in a completely altruistic manner since the donation of his tissues to another individual usually causes death of the fetus, thereby excluding him from continuing his membership within that very community which he is striving to assist (Mahowald et al., 1987).

Do tissues/organs belong to the donor individual and his family? If so, then they may be available for donation to others out of an act of kindness and altruism. Some would argue that the owner of such personal belongings should be allowed to sell such possessions for financial gain. Or, do such tissues/organs belong to the community? If so, then they may be routinely salvaged from the body of the dead individual.

When a fetus is aborted, and his tissues/organs donated to another individual, these tissues are deemed an anatomical "gift". Yet, the mother of the fetus chose to have the fetus aborted because it was worthless to her. Can a "gift" be worthless? A potential organ/tissue recipient would view these tissues as priceless. It has been noted that something cannot be simultaneously "worthless" and "priceless" (Nolan, 1988). Since a pregnant woman desiring an abortion obviously assigns different value to her living fetus than does a person in need of donor tissue/organs from that same fetus, one can only conclude that one person's trash is truly another person's treasure.

Legal Issues

Federal regulations do not govern the acquisition and disposal of fetal remains. Federal regulations do state that activities involving the dead fetus and its tissues be conducted in accordance with any applicable state or local laws. Transplantation of fetal tissue is permitted under the Uniform Anatomical Gift

Act (UAGA), originally drafted in 1968, and passed by all fifty states. *Roe v. Wade* was passed in 1973, stating that the fetus possesses no constitutional rights (including the right to life) until after its birth. *Roe v. Wade* gave the pregnant woman the legal right to terminate a pregnancy within its first two trimesters. Furthermore, the unborn child does not qualify as a dependent in the eyes of the law, and is not eligible for benefits under the Social Security Act. (However, virtually every American jurisdiction permits financial recovery in the tort system for prenatal injuries which a child might have incurred as a fetus; and an unborn fetus has been allowed to become a beneficiary of property under a bequest [Louisell, 1969]). In 1987, a group of lawyers, ethicists, and neuroscientists revised the UAGA, concluding that retrieval and transplantation of fetal tissue "is analagous to the transplantation of organs or tissue obtained from adult human cadavers." The 1987 revisions to the UAGA did not specifically address the passage of *Roe v. Wade*. Legally, under the UAGA, either parent of a fetus (in the absence of objection from the other) can authorize the donation of fetal tissue, and he/she may designate the recipient. Generally, in the event that the parents of the fetus are unmarried, only the mother's authorization is required to donate her fetus' tissue. Thus, the UAGA would permit a woman to deliberately conceive and abort a fetus in order to treat a family member in need of fetal tissue. The states of Massachusetts and Michigan have laws that prohibit abortion if it depends on the use of fetal tissue. In order to avoid abortions being performed in order to use the fetal tissue to attempt to save a loved one's life, Arizona, Indiana, Ohio, and Oklahoma have laws restricting use of fetal remains for any type of medical experimentation if the tissue comes from a fetus of an induced abortion. Many states, including New York, have laws prohibiting carrying out an abortion at or after the 24th week gestation. An incidental effect of these laws is that larger fetal organs are, therefore, not available for transplantation. Financial remuneration for fetal tissue donations is prohibited by the 1987 UAGA revisions. Hospital personnel or the organ procurement officers are required by the UAGA to request that families consider the donation of any dead fetus's tissues.

Although not required by law, consent forms for the release of fetal tissue for research purposes are already a feature of abortion consent forms in some academic centers; modification of such forms to include therapeutic use of such tissue would authorize transplantation of fetal tissue.

Experimentation on an aborted fetus determined to be viable is legally prohibited. "Viability" is defined as the ability to survive after induced or spontaneous delivery, even if utilizing a high level of medical technology.

Currently, in the year 2000, viability generally refers to infants of at least 23–24 weeks gestation. These infants are, in fact, extremely premature infants, not fetuses. If a fetus is non-viable (only transiently alive, but not viable), non-therapeutic research is permitted only if: (1) vital functions are not artificially maintained, and (2) procedures performed on the fetus that would terminate its heartbeat or respiratory effort are not used, and (3) the purpose of the research is to obtain scientific information not otherwise obtainable.

Summary

Currently, medical ethics may place tighter restrictions on the procedures involved in fetal organ and tissue transplantation than does the legal system. Although it may be legal to do certain procedures, and, recently, technically possible to do certain procedures, careful attention must be devoted to ethical considerations in the field of fetal organ/tissue transplantation. Simply because there are no legal or technical barriers to doing some of these procedures does not necessarily mean that performance of these procedures is morally correct.

REFERENCES

Ad Hoc Committee of the Harvard Medical School to Examine the Definition of Brain Death (1968). A Definition of Irreversible Coma. *Journal of the American Medical Association, 205*, 337–340.

American Academy of Pediatrics (1992). Policy Statement. Infants with anencephaly as organ sources: ethical considerations (RE9253). Policy Reference Guide 1993:354. *Pediatrics, 89*(6), 1116–1119.

Ascher, N. (1987). Pediatric transplantation needs and potential donors. In: H. H. Kaufman (Ed.), *Pediatric brain death and organ/tissue retrieval: medical, ethical, and legal aspects*, Chapter 24 (pp. 233–235). New York: Plenum Medical Book Co.

Ashwal et al. (1992). When too much is not enough. *Pediatric Annals, 21*(5), 311–317.

Berkowitz, J. M. (1995). Mummy was a fetus: motherhood and fetal ovarian transplantation. *Journal of Medical Ethics, 21*, 298–304.

Bioethics Committee, Canadian Paediatric Society (1990). Transplantation of organs from newborns with anencephaly. *Canadian Medical Association Journal, 142*(7), 715–717.

Bopp, J. Jr. (1985). Protection of disabled newborns: are there constitutional limitations? *Issues in Law and Medicine, 1*(3), 173–200.

Brotchi, J. (1995). Use of Fetal Tissue for Grafting. In: Y. Englert (Ed.), *Organ and Tissue Transplantation in the European Union: management of difficulties and health risks linked to donors*, Chapter 19 (pp. 147–148). Norwell, Massachusetts: M. Nijhoff/Kluwer Academic Publishers.

Capron, A. M. (1987). Anencephalic donors: separate the dead from the dying. *Hastings Center Report, 17*, 5–9.

Chervenak, F. A., McCulloughm, L. B. (1996). The fetus as a patient: an essential ethical concept of maternal-fetal medicine. *Journal of Maternal-Fetal Medicine, 5*(3), 115–119.

Consultants to the Advisory Committee to the Director (1988). Report of the Human Fetal Tissue Transplantation Research Panel. Bethesda, MD: National Institutes of Health; D28-D31;2.

Crombleholme et al. (1991). Transplantation of fetal cells. *American Journal of Obstetrics and Gynecology, 164*, 218–230.

Destro, R. A. (1977). A Symposium on the Report and Recommendations of the National Commission for the Protection of Human Subjects of Biomedical and Behavioral Research: Research on the Fetus. *Villanova Law Review, 22*, 297–417.

Fletcher et al. (1986). Primates and anencephalics as sources for organ transplants. *Fetal Ther., 1*, 154–160.

Hainline et al. (1995). Fetal tissue derived from spontaneous pregnancy losses is insufficient for human transplantation. *Obstetrics and Gynecology, 85*(4), 619–624.

Harrison, M. R. (1986). Organ procurement for children: the anencephalic fetus as donor. *Lancet, 2*(8520), 1383–1385.

Harrison, M. R. (1986). The anencephalic newborn as organ donor. Commentary. *Hastings Center Report, 16*(2), 21–23.

Jiang, F.X, & Short, R. V. (1995). Male germ cell transplantation in rats: apparent synchronization of spermatogenesis between host and donor seminiferous epithelia. *International Journal of Andrology, 18*(6), 326–330.

Lewin, T. (1987). Medical Use of Fetal Tissue Spurs New Abortion Debate. *The New York Times, 1*, August 16.

Louisell, D. W. (1969). Abortion, the Practice of Medicine and the Due Process of Law. *UCLAL Rev., 16*, 233–254.

Mahowald et al. (1987). The Ethical Options in Transplanting Fetal Tissue. *Hastings Center Report, 17*(1), 9–15.

Medical Task Force on Anencephaly (1990). The infant with anencephaly. *N. Engl. J. Med., 322*, 699-674.

The National Commission for the Protection of Subjects of Biomedical and Behavioral Research (1975). Research on the Fetus: Report and Recommendations. DHEW Publication No. (OS), 76–127, p. 87, Washington.

Nolan, K. (1988). Genug ist Genug: A Fetus is Not a Kidney. *Hastings Center Report, 18*(6), 13–19.

Paris, J. J., & McCormick, R. A. (1983). Saving defective infants: options for life or death. *America, 143*, 313–317.

Peabody et al. (1989). Experience with anencephalic infants as prospective organ donors. *N. Engl. J. Med., 321*, 344–350.

Purvis, J. F. (1987). Organ transplantation and neurosurgeons. *Neurosurgery, 20*, 650–651.

Sadler, T. X. (1990). *Langman's medical embryology* (pp. 10–11). London: Williams and Wilkins.

Task Force on Brain Death in Children. (1987). Guidelines for the Determination of Brain Death in Children. *Pediatrics, 80*, 298–300.

Veatch, R. M. (1992). Brain death and slippery slopes. *Journal of Clinical Ethics, 3*(3), 181–187.

Veatch, R. M. (1993). The impending collapse of the whole-brain definition of death. *Hastings Center Report, 23*(4), 18–23.

Warren et al. (1978). Can the Fetus be an Organ Farm? *Hastings Center Report, 8*(5), 23–25.